Angiotensin and the Heart

H. Grobecker, G. Heusch,
B. E. Strauer (Eds.)

Angiotensin and the Heart

Steinkopff Verlag Darmstadt
Springer-Verlag New York

The Editors:
Prof. Dr. med. H. Grobecker
Institut für Pharmakologie
der Universität Regensburg
Universitätsstraße 31
8400 Regensburg

Prof. Dr. med. B. E. Strauer
Med. Klinik und Poliklinik B
der Heinrich-Heine-Universität
Abt. für Kardiologie, Pneumologie
Moorenstraße 5
4000 Düsseldorf 1

Prof. Dr. med. Gerd Heusch
Abt. Pathophysiologie
Zentrum Innere Medizin
Universitätsklinikum Essen
Hufelandstraße 55
4300 Essen

Die Deutsche Bibliothek — CIP-Einheitsaufnahme

Angiotensin and the heart / H. Grobecker ... (ed.).
Darmstadt: Steinkopff; New York: Springer, 1993
(Supplement to Basic research in cardiology; Vol. 88,1)
ISBN-13: 978-3-7985-0936-8 e-ISBN-13: 978-3-642-72497-8
DOI: 10.1007/978-3-642-72497-8
NE: Grobecker, Horst [Hrsg.]; Basic research in cardiology / Supplement

Basic Res. Cardiol, ISSN 0300-8428
Indexed in Current Contents.

Softcover reprint of the hardcover 1st edition 1993

Medical Editor: Sabine Müller—English Editor: James C. Willis—Production: Heinz J. Schäfer

Typesetting: Graphische Textverarbeitung Hans Vilhard

Printed on acid-free paper

Foreword

In the last decade, ACE inhibitors have become a cornerstone of cardiovascular drug therapy. Beneficial effects in patients with hypertension, heart failure, and post myocardial infarction have been established in large clinical trials. In parallel, experimental research has shifted the interest from the immediate homeostatic function of the circulating renin-angiotensin-system to the multiple paracrine functions of local tissue renin-angiotensin-systems, including hypertrophy, hyperplasia, athergoenesis, and vasomotion.

It was the aim or a symposium held in Hamburg, October 22—24, 1992, to bring together an international panel of experimental and clinical scientists and to discuss the most recent findings on the role of angiotensin and associated mediators in cardiovascular adaptation and disease, with a particular emphasis on the treatment of such disease by ACE inhibitors.

The meeting and this publication were generously supported by Astra Chemicals.

H. Grobecker
G. Heusch
B. E. Strauer

Contents

Foreword ... V

Introduction

Local expression and pathophysiological role of renin-angiotensin in the blood vessels and heart
Dzau, V. J. ... 1

Myocardial Perfusion

Angiotensin, ACE-inhibitors and endothelial control of vasomotor tone
Lüscher, T. F. ... 15

Local and neurohumoral control of coronary blood flow
Krajcar, M., G. Heusch ... 25

ACE-inhibitors in coronary artery disease?
Vogt, M., W. Motz, B. E. Strauer ... 43

Myocardial Hypertrophy

Molecular mechanisms of cardiac gene expression
Nadal-Ginard, B., V. Mahdavi ... 65

Myocardial perfusion dependent and independent mechanisms of regional myocardial dysfunction in hypertrophy
Vatner, S. F., L. Hittinger ... 81

ACE-inhibitors and coronary microcirculation
Strauer, B. E., M. Vogt, W. Motz ... 97

Ventricular Remodelling

Myocardial fibrosis: role of angiotensin II and aldosterone
Weber, K. T., C. G. Brilla, S. E. Campbell, E. Guarda, G. Zhou, K. Sriram ... 107

Ventricular remodeling after myocardial infarction. Experimental and clinical studies
Ertl, G., P. Gaudron, K. Hu ... 125

Infarct Size, Reperfusion, Restenosis

"Cardioprotection" by ACE-inhibitors in acute myocardial ischemia and infarction?
Przyklenk, K., R. A. Kloner 139

Effect of angiotensin-converting enzyme inhibitors on myocardial ischemia/reperfusion injury: an overview
Zaghaib, M. E., J.-Z. Sun, R. Bolli 155

Angiotensin-converting enzyme inhibitor in a human model of restenosis
Heyndrickx, G. R. 169

Heart failure

Pathophysiology of heart failure and the renin-angiotensin-system
Holtz, J. 183

Angiotensin-converting enzyme inhibitors in the treatment of clinical heart failure
Pouleur, H. 203

Summary and Perspectives

A. Basic aspects
Grobecker, H. 211

B. Clinical aspects
Strauer, B. E. 219

Subject Index 223

Local expression and pathophysiological role of renin-angiotensin in the blood vessels and heart

V. J. Dzau

Division of Cardiovascular Medicine, Falk Cardiovascular Research Center, Stanford University School of Medicine, Stanford, California, USA

Summary: While the circulating renin-angiotensin system (RAS) plays an important role in short-term maintenance of cardiovascular homeostasis, recent studies point to a role in long-term cardiovascular regulation for endogenous RAS in target tissues. This article focuses on the multiple effects of tissue angiotensin enzyme (ACE) and angiotensin II (Ang II), its active peptide product. Ang II has been shown to be a potent growth factor in vascular smooth muscle cells. Depending on the local conditions, the vascular response may be either hypertrophy or hyperplasia. The molecular mechanisms involved in the interactions of Ang II with endothelium- and smooth muscle-derived cell products may play important roles in the modulation of vascular structure in hypertension and vascular injury. Evidence also points to a role for Ang II in the development of left ventricular hypertrophy in hypertension. In addition, cardiac RAS may contribute to the pathophysiology of heart failure. Experimental and clinical studies with ACE inhibitors point to a role for tissue ACE activity in the development of atherosclerosis, as well as cardiac hypertrophy and remodeling.

Key words: Angiotensin converting enzyme; angiotensin II; growth factors; inhibitors; myocardial infarction; vascular hypertrophy

Traditionally, it has been thought that the renin-angiotensin system (RAS) is an endocrine system whose effects are exerted entirely through the peptide hormone angiotensin II (Ang II) in the circulation. Ang II results from two proteolytic steps in the processing of the precursor angiotensinogen. The action of renin produces the decapeptide Angiotensin I (Ang I). The subsequent cleavage of Ang I by angiotensin converting enzyme (ACE) produces the active octapeptide Ang II.

Circulating Ang II binds to receptors at multiple end organs and plays a role in short-term cardiac homeostasis. The activated receptors mediate systemic vasoconstriction, adrenal aldosterone release, hypophyseal vasopressin secretion, and renal sodium reabsorption. These activities affect cardiac function as well as preload and afterload. As an endocrine system, circulating RAS is subject to feedback inhibition. It is activated under conditions of reduced blood pressure, sympathetic stress, or volume contraction and is inactivated when these conditions are normalized.

In the last 10 years, many laboratories have reported evidence for tissue RAS in addition to the endocrine system. The synthesis of endogenous angiotensinogen, renin, and angiotensin converting enzyme has been reported within blood vessels, the heart, kidneys, and adrenal glands. The extrarenal expression of RAS messenger RNAs (mRNA) and their protein products has been demonstrated through Northern blot techniques, in situ hybridization, and biochemical techniques (8, 17, 19, 23, 28, 36, 40, 68).

- **Expression of angiotensinogen, renin, ACE mRNAs**
    - **Heart**
    - **Kidney**
    - **Vasculature**
- **Ang I → Ang II conversion in tissue ex vivo**
- **Ang I → Ang II conversion in isolated, perfused vascular beds**

Fig. 1. Functional tissue RAS: supporting evidence.

Further evidence for endogenous synthesis of tissue RAS components comes from the demonstration of Ang I to Ang II conversion in isolated perfused hearts (49). Similarly, local synthesis of Ang II was demonstrated in isolated rat limb artery (36, 57). In vivo support for vascular tissue Ang II production was demonstrated by kinetic analysis of arterial-venous Ang I and Ang II differences in sheep and humans (2, 7).

Characteristics and distribution of the angiotensin converting enzyme

Angiotensin converting enzyme (ACE) is a key enzyme in the RAS that converts Ang I to the active peptide hormone, Ang II. ACE has been cloned, allowing a detailed study of its molecular structure (3, 4). Structural analysis has shown ACE to be primarily a membrane-bound protein with both intracellular and extracellular domains. The active site is thought to be included in the extracellular domain. ACE has been localized to the endothelial cells (22) lining all vascular tissue. Circulating Ang I is thus exposed to the active site of the membrane-bound ACE and is subsequently converted to Ang II. The local production of Ang II exerts both autocrine and paracrine effects on vascular cells and adjacent tissues.

In studies using site-directed mutagenesis, evidence supports the existence of two functionally active sites in the ACE molecule (3, 4). The substrate selectivity for these sites has not been determined, however, a differential preference for various substrates may be possible. Several ACE substrates are known. For example, ACE degrades bradykinin and other peptides in addition to converting Ang I to Ang II (71). Thus, the activity of ACE will lead to an increased level of Ang II and decreased bradykinin levels (9). Bradykinin can exert effects on the endothelium by activating arachidonic acid conversion to prostacyclin as well as stimulating the release of endothelium-derived relaxing factor (EDRF) or nitric oxide (5).

ACE is characterized by a ubiquitous distribution and is found in many parenchymal tissues as well as in blood vessels. An autoradiographic study of radiolabeled ACE inhibitor binding in sectioned rat tissues (42, 69) shows a wide distribution. High levels were detected in testes, adrenal medulla and cortex, and in the kidney, particularly in the cortico-medullary junction in the proximal tubule brush border. ACE is present in the heart and its vessels. High densities of ACE can be detected in the myocardium, especially in the microvasculature, the endocardium and the valves, the ascending aorta, pulmonary artery, and pulmonary vein, etc. (79). The ubiquitous distribution of ACE has been confirmed in human tissues. Human kidney and endomyocardial biopsies, adrenal heart and aortic samples obtained from surgery show ACE mRNA expression as reported in a recent study using polymerase chain reaction technology to amplify ACE mRNA isolated from these tissues (59).

Direct RAS effects

The direct effects of Ang II binding to target receptors include the activation of phospholipase C, which results in increased hydrolysis of phosphatidylinositol biphosphate to diacyl glycerol and inositol triphosphate (34). These metabolites modulate calcium-sensitive protein kinase and cytoplasmic calcium concentrations. Calcium mobilization will then alter the contractility of smooth muscle while increasing secretion of aldosterone (52). Ang II also has a direct inotropic effect on cardiac muscle, independent of adrenergic potentiation (45, 46). In addition to these short-term effects, Ang II can exert long-term effects on the structures of the cardiovascular system.

Angiotension effects in vascular smooth muscle cells

Current evidence points to long-term effects of Ang II on cells by activating gene expression. Of particular interest is the potential role of Ang II as a growth promoter. A measurement of uridine and leucine incorporation in cultured smooth muscle cells exposed to Ang II, shows a dose-dependent increase in RNA and protein synthesis (30, 41). Thus, Ang II may exert a hypertrophic effect on vascular smooth muscle cells.

Several mechanisms appear to be involved in the growth-promoting effects of Ang II. First, the expected activation of protein kinase C will result in a series of events which lead to cell growth. Second, Ang II may promote growth by stimulating the expression of the proto-oncogenes c-fos, c-myc, c-jun, and others (47, 53, 54, 73). The cells exposed to proto-oncogenes will enter an S-phase in the cell cycle and become responsive to growth factors. Ang II is also known to stimulate the subsequent expressions of platelet-derived growth factor (PDGF), basic fibroblast growth factor (FGF), and transforming growth factor beta-1 (TGF β-1) by vascular smooth muscle (32, 33, 53).

The sequential activation of proto-oncogenes and growth factor may explain, in part, the hypertrophic effect of Ang II on vascular smooth muscle. More recent data (32, 33) shows that the growth response to Ang II is dependent on the interactions of PDGF, FGF, and TGF β-1. The data suggest that if TGF β-1 activation is inhibited or minimized, the principal effect of angiotensin is mitogenesis or hyperplasia resulting from the activation of FGF and PDGF. The simultaneous activation of TGF β-1 results in an inhibition of cell proliferation and leads to hypertrophy.

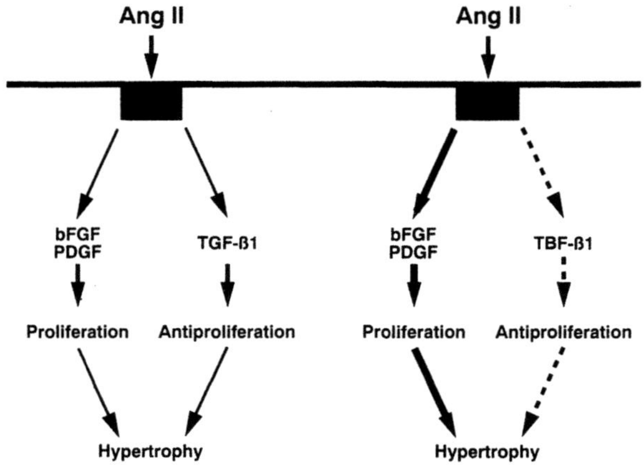

Fig. 2. Effect of angiotensin on vascular smooth muscle cell growth.

Angiotensin effects in the myocardium

In the myocardium, in addition to exerting a contractile effect, Ang II exerts a hypertrophic effect. The primary site of intramyocardial production of Ang II is the microvascular capillary. Due to the extensive capillary network in the myocardium and the presence of ACE in these capillaries, Ang I will be readily converted to Ang II. Subsequent transport or infusion to the interstitium will lead to Ang II binding in the myocyte receptors. The activation of receptors will result in increased contraction and a stimulation of myocyte hypertrophy (44, 51, 74). These effects are amplified by angiotensin's ability to stimulate norepinephrine release by sympathetic nerve endings, leading to positive inotropic and hypertrophic effects (80). Recent evidence (75) suggests the existence of a second myocardial enzyme, A1 convertase, which can convert Ang I to Ang II. This enzyme was found to be abundant and confirms the ability of the myocardium to produce Ang II in vitro, independent of that delivered by the circulation. However, its in vivo relevance is still unclear at this time.

RAS may also contribute to myocardial fibrosis through aldosterone stimulation in hypertension. Increased aldosterone levels have been linked to cardiac fibroblast growth and fibrillar collagen accumulation in the myocardium (78). In addition, Ang II infusion into rats has been shown to stimulate fibronectin mRNA expression in cardiac fibroblasts in vivo (12).

Tissue ACE in cardiovascular diseases

Vascular ACE in hypertension and vascular injury

Several studies have demonstrated the existence of endogenous RAS in blood vessels (20, 68). Evidence for the activation of ACE in the vasculature comes from an earlier study of experimental hypertension (56). Animals made hypertensive by a one-kidney, one-clip procedure show normal endocrine renin and ACE levels. However, aortic and vascular ACE is significantly increased over time with the development of hypertension. It appears that under an increase in pressure and concomitant wall tension, the vasculature activates ACE mRNA transcription and subsequently increases ACE production (21). The structural changes caused by Ang II stimulation of vascular hypertrophy may amplify vasoconstriction and perpetuate hypertension (27).

There is also evidence for the induction of ACE expression following vascular injury (64). After vessel wall injury and the removal of the endothelium, activated platelets release a variety of biologically active mediators, including PDGF (67). Injured endothelial cells also release FGF (76). These growth factors will initiate the process of smooth muscle activation, replication, migration, and proliferation leading to intimal hyperplasia. In addition, there is evidence for increased Ang II formation as a result of increased ACE expression within the neointima following vascular injury. Our in vitro studies show that angiotensin exerts a synergistic effect on these growth factors leading to further proliferation of the intima (31). Indeed, in vivo Ang II infusion after vascular injury results in marked enhancement of vascular smooth cell proliferation (14).

Previous studies have shown that ACE inhibitors can reduce neointimal formation (63). More recent studies in our laboratory (65) show a significant linear relationship ($r = .881$) between vascular ACE and intimal lesion size. Rat carotid arteries were subjected to balloon injury and the animals were treated with different doses of ACE inhibitor. We observed that a complete suppression of lesions was only seen in those animals treated with high doses. It is hypothesized that higher doses of ACE inhibitor are required to suppress tissue ACE activity and local Ang II concentration which may play a determinant role in lesion development. These observations may have clinical implications since the recent MERCATOR study of cilazapril (ACE inhibitor) on human restenosis (35) failed to demonstrate an effect of the drug. This trial employed a low dose (1/10 the effective dose in animal study) that was initiated after angioplasty (while animal studies administered drug prior to and after angioplasty). Thus, it may be speculated that the negative outcome of MERCATOR is due to ineffective suppression of tissue ACE due to low dose of cilazapril. However, one cannot exclude the possibility that ACE inhibitor effect on restenosis is species specific.

In addition to the inhibition of angiotensin formation, ACE inhibitors may further limit neointima formation by enhancing bradykinin and nitric oxide levels. Recent data (26) show that while the angiotensin receptor antagonist DuP 753 is able to suppress the lesion, a greater inhibition is seen with ACE inhibitor. In addition, part of the lesion attenuating activity of ACE inhibitor is blocked by the kinin antagonist, Hoechst 140, indicating a link between the ACE inhibitor's ability to increase kinin concentration and its ability to block lesion formation. Indeed, kinin has been shown to increase nitric oxide production, which is known to inhibit smooth muscle proliferation and migration.

Vascular ACE and atherosclerosis

Studies in Watanabe heritable hyperlipidemic rabbits treated with ACE inhibitor show a marked reduction in atherosclerosis of the descending thoracic aorta, when

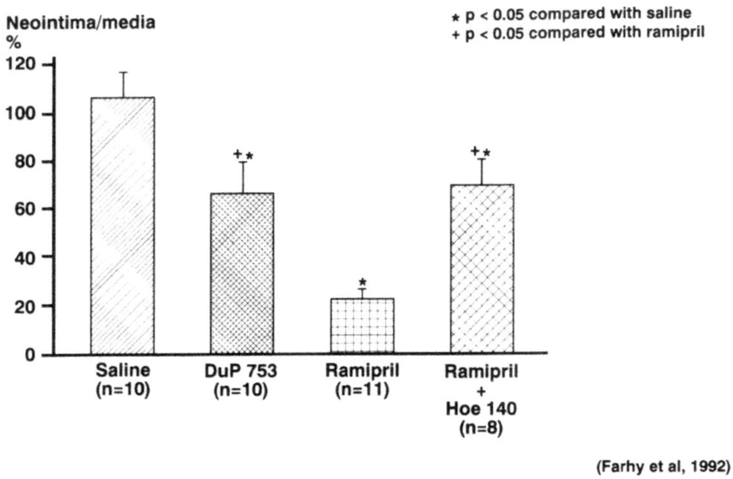

Fig. 3. Changes in neointima formation.

compared to controls (11, 12). In addition, the atherosclerotic plaques were thinner and less cellular in the treated group. Since cholesterol levels are not affected by ACE inhibitors, it is hypothesized that their effect is through a decreased cellularity, and decreased cell proliferation and migration. Similar results were reported in cynomolgus monkeys fed with cholesterol. Treatment with ACE inhibitors significantly reduced the development of atherosclerotic lesions, particularly in the coronary arteries (1). In cholesterol-fed rabbits, evidence exists for nitric oxide involvement in addition to Ang II inhibition in preventing atherosclerosis. After 4 months of cholesterol feeding, rabbits showed impaired production of nitric oxide and endothelium-dependent relaxation in aortic rings. Impairment of endothelium-mediated relaxation in response to acetylcholine is an early marker of endothelial dysfunction and atherosclerosis in rabbits (43, 66). The administration of ACE inhibitor restored endothelial relaxation (5). These observations have recently been confirmed by other researchers (77).

Recent genetic evidence (6) identifies a deletion polymorphism in the ACE gene as a potent risk factor for myocardial infarction in men. In a multi-site study looking for genetic markers as predictors of myocardial infarction, it was found that the ACE deletion polymorphism was significantly more frequent in patients with heart attacks than in controls. In patients with normal LDL cholesterol, body mass index (low-risk patients), the presence of homozygote deletion polymorphism of the ACE gene is associated with a threefold increase in risk for myocardial infarction. It is interesting to note that a previous study reported that patients homozygous for the deletion polymorphism are also associated with an increased plasma level of ACE, thus further suggesting a link between ACE activity and factors leading to the development of coronary heart disease.

Cardiac ACE and left ventricular hypertrophy

In experiments with pressure overload left ventricular hypertrophy, ACE activity in the ventricle was increased under conditions of increased pressure loading (70).

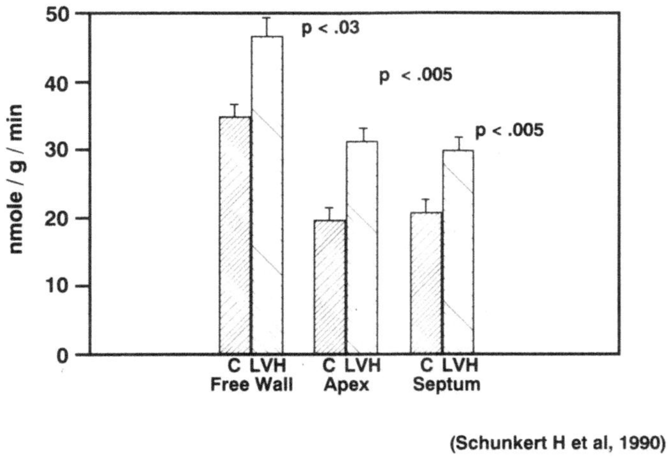

Fig. 4. Cardiac ACE activity in experimental LVH.

The expression of ACE mRNA was increased threefold in hearts with ventricular hypertrophy when compared to controls. Ang I conversion to Ang II was also increased in perfused beating hearts from experimental animals. This evidence suggests that, under pressure, there is an increased expression of ACE mRNA and subsequent increases in ACE and Ang II. The myocardial Ang II may in turn play a role in adaptive hypertrophy through its growth promoter effect.

Several in vivo studies now suggest a direct effect of angiotensin on cardiac hypertrophy. In a rat model of hypertension and cardiac hypertrophy induced by constriction of the abdominal aorta, hypertension was reduced by three different agents, ramipril, nifedipine, and dihydralazine. While all of the antihypertensive agents reduced blood pressure, only the ACE inhibitor was able to regress cardiac hypertrophy as well. Regression of cardiac hypertrophy was also seen in animals treated with the ACE inhibitor ramipril at doses which were not antihypertensive (50). This evidence suggests a direct role for Ang II in cardiac hypertrophy which is separate from its hemodynamic effect. In humans, several experimental and clinical studies (24, 29, 55, 58) point to the efficacy of ACE inhibitors in the regression of LVH. In recent meta-analysis of 109 studies by Dahlöf (15), ACE inhibitors were found to be superior to other hypertensive agents in reducing left ventricular mass in humans.

Cardiac ACE and myocardial infarction

In myocardial infarction (MI) the unaffected segments of the ventricle compensate for the infarcted segment. They are subjected to greater working load and uneven distribution of wall tension. In rat models (61) with moderate to large infarcts, left ventricle (LV) weight increased acutely and then progressively decreased to normal values as inflammation and edema developed. During resolution of the inflammatory response, LV dilatation was observed in relation to infarct size. In the early phase, chamber stiffness remained within normal range, but decreased significantly during

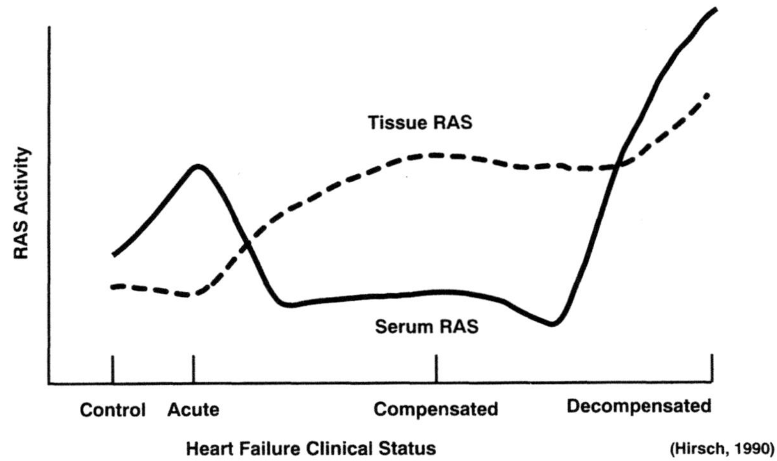

Fig. 5. Renin-angiotensin systems in heart failure.

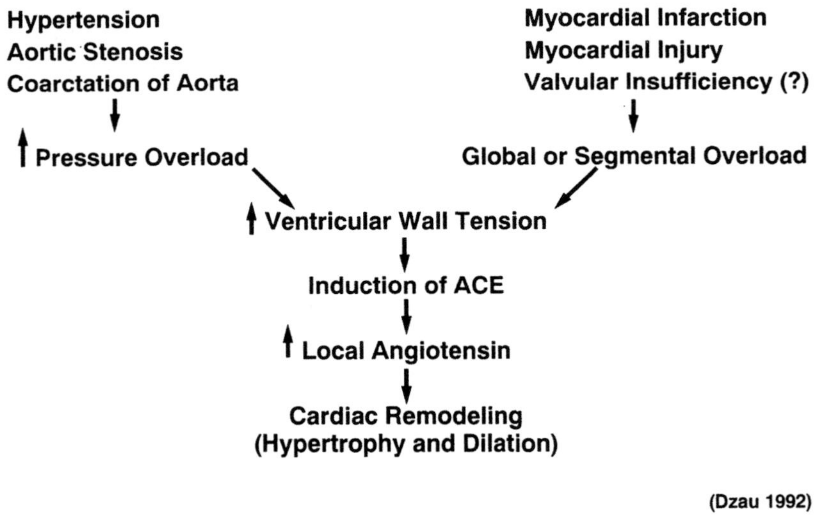

Fig. 6. Cardiac angiotensin and remodeling.

the late phase. In the late post-infarction phase, marked changes were observed in volume-to-mass ratio, where volume increased and mass decreased and then increased in rats with moderate to large infarcts. Treatment with ACE inhibitors following MI significantly attenuated the characteristic cardiac remodeling observed in this animal model (60).

Overload following MI may also lead to the induction of ACE and the local generation of Ang II (38). In a study of relative contributions of plasma and tissue RAS during the course of congestive heart failure, it was found that plasma levels are elevated during acute myocardial infarction and cardiac decompensation. In compensated heart failure, tissue RAS is activated while the circulating RAS activity returns to normal (18). The plasma RAS is elevated again in end-stage or decompensated states and tissue RAS is further activated (37). It is hypothesized that in patients with compensated cardiac function and asymptomatic left ventricular dysfunction, that cardiac tissue RAS continues to be activated locally, while the circulating RAS is normal (18, 48). The continuing presence of Ang II may lead to cardiac remodeling through the local mechanism discussed previously.

Studies in rat MI models support this hypothesis (16, 25). In rats undergoing cardiac remodeling, hypertrophy, and dilatation, the circulating RAS levels remain normal. When the ACE levels are measured in the lung, vasculature, kidney, and heart, only local cardiac ACE activation is observed. The degree of cardiac RAS activity is positively correlated to MI size (38). More specifically, when the left ventricle is infarcted, an increase in ACE activity is observed in the right ventricle and the septum. The increased pressure observed in these areas and myocardial neurosympathetic activity may be responsible for the local ACE activation. The increased local Ang II production may participate in cardiac remodeling (hypertrophy and dilatation) after myocardial infarction. The efficacy of ACE inhibition in preventing experimental cardiac remodeling may be due to local inhibition of cardiac ACE.

In two major clinical trials, ACE inhibitors were found to be useful in patients with asymptomatic left ventricular dysfunction. In the SOLVD study (72) most of the patients with asymptomatic left ventricular dysfunction (LVD) and ejection fractions of 0.35 or less received either ACE inhibitor or placebo on an average approximately 1 year after MI. ACE inhibitor was shown to significantly reduce (36%) hospitalizations due to heart failure. Although not statistically significant, a trend to reduced mortality was also found among the ACE inhibitor-treated group. In the SAVE study (62), patients with left ventricular dysfunction were treated with an ACE inhibitor 3 to 16 days after MI. Mortality from all causes was significantly reduced (19%) in the ACE inhibitor-treated group. In addition, a significant reduction in morbidity was observed with a reduction in both fatal and nonfatal cardiovascular events. The development of severe heart failure was reduced by 37% with ACE treatment. These benefits were observed both in the presence or absence of additional therapeutics including thrombolytic therapy, aspirin, or beta-blockers. These results indicate an incremental improvement in outcome for patients receiving ACE inhibitors following MI.

Conclusions and discussion

The activation of RAS results in both short-term and long-term effects. The short-term effects exerted by the circulating RAS include sodium and water retention through aldosterone secretion, vasoconstriction, and positive inotropic and arrhythmogenic effects in the heart. The tissue RAS exerts long-term effects such as intraglomerular hypertension, and vascular and myocardial hypertrophy. Thus, the sequential effects of ACE inhibitors include both functional and structural changes in the cardiovascular system.

In order to address the long-term tissue effects, ACE inhibitors must be designed to optimize ACE-binding as well as tissue permeability and bioavailability. Some

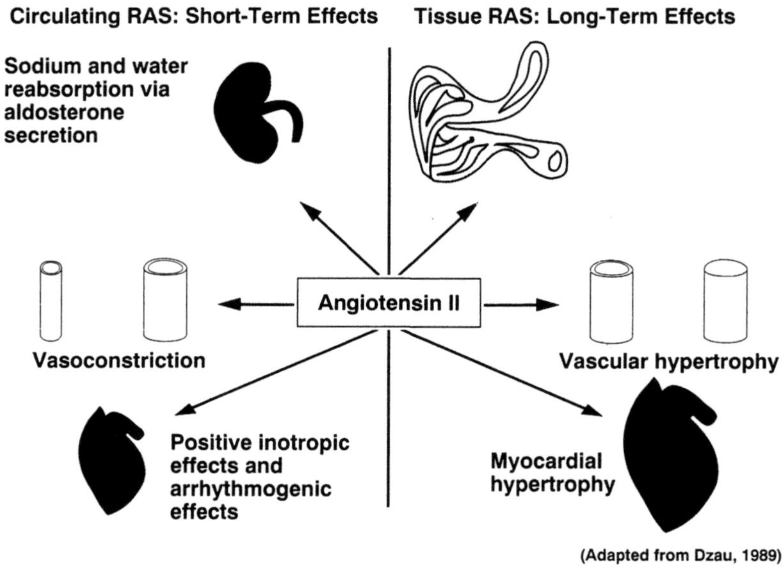

Fig. 7. RAS: short-term and long-term effects.

experimental evidence already exists for differential tissue RAS activity among ACE inhibitors (10, 39). Future studies along these lines may further elucidate differences among ACE inhibitors in their ability to block specific tissue ACE effects and prevent subsequent cardiovascular disease in humans.

References

1. Aberg G, Ferrer P (1990) Effects of captopril on atherosclerosis in cynomolgus monkeys. J Cardiovasc Pharmacol 15 (suppl 5):S65—S72
2. Admiraal PJJ, Derkx FHM, Jan Danser AH, Pieterman H, Schalenkamp MADH (1990) Metabolism and production of angiotensin I in different vascular beds in subjects with hypertension. Hypertension 15:44—55
3. Alhenc-Gelas F, Soubrier F, Hubert C, Allegrini J, Corvol P (1989) The peculiar characteristics of the amino acid sequence of angiotensin I-converting enzyme, as determined by cDNA cloning of the human endothelial enzyme. J Cardiovasc Pharmacol 14 (suppl 4):S6—S9
4. Alhenc-Gelas F, Soubrier F, Hubert C, Allegrini J, Lattion AL, Corvol P (1990) The angiotensin I-converting enzyme (kininase II): progress in molecular and genetic structure. J Cardiovasc Pharmacol 15 (suppl 6):S25—S29
5. Becker RHA, Weimer G, Linz W (1991) Preservation of endothelial function by ramipril in rabbits on a long-term atherogenic diet. J Cardiovasc Pharmacol 18 (suppl 2): S110—S115
6. Cambien F, Poirier O, Lecerf L, Evans A, Cambou JP, Arveller D, Luc G, Bard JM, Bara L, Ricard S, Tiret L, Amouyel P, Alhenc-Gelas F, Soubrier F (1992) Deletion polymorphism in the gene for angiotensin-converting enzyme is a potent risk factor for myocardial infarction. Nature 359:641:644
7. Campbell DJ (1985) The site of angiotensin production. J Hypertension 3:730:737

8. Campbell DJ (1987) Circulating and tissue angiotensin systems. J Clin Invest 79:1—6
9. Carretero OA, Miyazaki S, Scicli AG (1981) Role of kinins in the acute antihypertensive effect of the converting enzyme inhibitor, captopril. Hypertension 3:18—22
10. Chevillard C, Brown NL, Jouquey S, Mathiou M-N, Laliberte F, Gamon G (1989) Cardiovascular actions and tissue-converting enzyme inhibitory effects of chronic enalapril and trandolapril treatment of spontaneously hypertensive rats. J Cardiovasc Pharmacol 14:297—301
11. Chobanian AV (1990) The effects of ACE inhibitors and other antihypertensive drugs on cardiovascular risk factors and atherogenesis. Clin Cardiol 13:VII—43—VII—48
12. Chobanian AV, Haudenschild CC, Nickerson C, Drago R (1990) Antiatherogenic effect of captopril in the Watanabe heritable hyperlipidemic rabbit. Hypertension 15:327—331
13. Crawford DC, Chobanian AV, Brecher P (1992) Angiotensin II increases fibronectin expression in rat cardiac fibroblasts in vivo (Abstr). Circulation 86 (suppl I):I—89
14. Daemen MJAP, Lombardi DM, Bosman FT, Schwartz SM (1991) Angiotensin II induces smooth muscle cell proliferation in the normal and injured rat arterial wall. Circ Res 68:450—456
15. Dahlöf B, Pennert K, Hansson L (1992) Reversal of left ventricular hypertrophy in hypertensive patients. A metaanalysis of 109 treatment studies. Am J Hypertension 5:95—110
16. Drexler H, Lindpaintner K, Lu W, Schieffer B, Ganten D (1989) Transient increase in the expression of cardiac angiotensinogen in a rat model of myocardial infarction and failure (Abstr). Circulation 80:(suppl II):II—459
17. Dzau V (1987) Vascular angiotensin pathways: new therapeutic target. J Cardiovasc Pharmacol 10 (suppl 7):S9—S16
18. Dzau VJ, Colucci WS, Hollenberg NK, Williams GH (1981) Relation of the renin-angiotensin-aldosterone system to clinical state in congestive heart failure. Circulation 63:645—651
19. Dzau VJ, Ellison KE, Brody T, Ingelfinger J, Pratt RE (1987) A comparative study of the distributions of renin and angiotensinogen messenger ribonucleic acids in rat and mouse tissues. Endocrinology 120:2334—2338
20. Dzau VJ, Gibbons GH (1987) Autocrine-paracrine mechanisms of vascular myocytes in hypertension. Am J Cardiol 60:991—1031
21. Dzau VJ, Gibbons GH, Pratt RE (1991) Molecular mechanisms of vascular renin-angiotensin system in myointimal hyperplasia. Hypertension 18 (suppl II):II—100—II—105
22. Dzau VJ, Pratt RE (1986) Renin-angiotensin system: biology, physiology and pharmacology. In: Haber E, Morgan H, Katz A, Fozzard H (eds) Handbook of experimental cardiology; Raven Press, New York, pp 1631—1661
23. Dzau VJ, Re RN (1987) Evidence for the existence of renin in the heart. Circulation 73 (suppl I):1134—1136
24. Eichstaedt H, Danne O, Langer M, Cordes M, Schubert C, Felix R, Schmutzler H (1989) Regression of left ventricular hypertrophy under ramipril treatment investigated by nuclear magnetic resonance imaging. J Cardiovasc Pharmacol 13 (suppl 3):S75—S80
25. Fabris B, Jackson B, Kohzuki M, Perich R, Johnston CI (1990) Increased cardiac angiotensin-converting enzyme in rats with chronic heart failure. Clin Exp Pharmacol Physiol 17:309—314
26. Farhy RD, Ho KL, Carretero OA, Scicli AG (1992) Kinins mediate the antiproliferative effect of ramipril in rat carotid artery. Biochem & Biophys Res Comm 182:283—288
27. Folkow B (1990) "Structural factor" in primary and secondary hypertension. Hypertension 16:89—101
28. Ganten D, Hutchinson JS, Haebara H, Schelling P, Fischer H, Ganten U (1976) Tissue iso-renins. Clin Sci Mol Med 51:117S—120S
29. Garavaglia GE, Messerli FH, Nunez BD, Schmieder RE, Frohlich ED (1988) Immediate and short-term cardiovascular effects of a new converting enzyme inhibitor (lisinopril) in essential hypertension. Am J Cardiol 62:912—916

30. Geisterfer AAT, Peach MJ, Owens GK (1988) Angiotensin II induces hypertrophy, not hyperplasia, of cultured rat aortic smooth muscle cells. Circ Res 62: 749—756
31. Gibbons GH, Pratt RE, Dzau VJ (1989) Angiotensin is a bifunctional modulator of vascular smooth muscle cell growth: Interaction with basic fibroblast growth factor (abstract). Hypertension 14:358
32. Gibbons GH, Pratt RE, Dzau VJ (1992) Vascular smooth muscle cell hypertrophy vs. hyperplasia: autocrine transforming growth factor-β1 expression determines growth response to angiotensin II. J Clin Invest 90:456—461
33. Gibbons GH, Pratt RE, Dzau VJ (1992) Role of autocrine transforming growth factor-β1 expression and activation in determining vascular myocyte growth response to angiotensin II versus basic fibroblast growth (Abstr). Clin Res 39:287A
34. Griendling KK, Berk BC, Ganz P, Gimbrone MA, Alexander RW (1987) Angiotensin II stimulation of vascular smooth muscle phosphoinositide metabolism: state of the art lecture. Hypertension 9 (suppl 3):III—181—III—185
35. Hermans WR, Rensing BJ, Foley DP, Deckers JW, Rutsch W, Enamuelsson H, Danchin N, Wijns W, Chappuis F, Serruys PW (1992) Therapeutic dissection after successful coronary balloon angioplasty: No influence on restenosis or on clinical outcome in 693 patients. J Am Coll Cardiol 20:767—780
36. Hilgers KF, Kuczera M, Wilhem MJ, Wiecek A, Ritz E, Ganten D, Mann JFE (1989) Angiotensin formation in the isolated rat hindlimb. J Hypertension 7:789—798
37. Hirsch AT, Dzau VJ (1990) Tissue renin-angiotensin systems in the pathophysiology of heart failure. In: Brachmann J, Dietz R, Kubler W (eds) Heart failure and arrhythmias; Springer-Verlag, Heidelberg
38. Hirsch AT, Talsness CE, Schunkert H, Paul M, Dzau VJ (1991) Tissue-specific activation of cardiac angiotensin-converting enzyme in experimental heart failure. Circ Res 69:475—482
39. Hirsch AT, Talsness CE, Smith AD, Schunkert H, Ingelfinger JR, Dzau VJ (1992) Differential effects of captopril and enalapril on tissue renin-angiotensin systems in experimental heart failure. Circulation 86:1566—1574
40. Ichikawa I, Brenner BM (1984) Glomerular actions of angiotensin II. Am J Med 76:43—49
41. Itoh H, Pratt RE, Dzau VJ (1990) Atrial natriuretic factor inhibits hypertrophy of vascular smooth muscle cells. J Clin Invest 86:1690—1697
42. Jackson B, Mendelsohn FA, Johnston CI (1991) Angiotensin-converting enzyme inhibition: prospects for the future. J Cardiovasc Pharmacol 18 (suppl 7):S4—S8
43. Jayakody L, Kappagoda T, Senaratne MPJ, Thomson ABR (1988) Impairment of endothelium-dependent relaxation: an early marker for atherosclerosis in the rabbit. Br J Pharmacol 94:335—346
44. Katoh Y, Komuro I, Shibasaki Y, Yamaguchi H, Yazaki Y (1989) Angiotensin II induces hypertrophy and oncogene expression in cultured rat heart myocytes (Abstr). Circulation 80 (suppl II):II—450
45. Koch-Weser J (1964) Myocardial actions of angiotensin II. Circ Res 14:337—344
46. Koch-Weser J (1965) Nature of the inotropic action of angiotensin on ventricular myocardium. Circ Res 16:230—237
47. Komuro I, Kurabayashi M, Takaku F, Yazaki Y (1988) Expression of cellular oncogenes in the myocardium during the developmental state and pressure-overloaded hypertrophy of the rat heart. Circ Res 62:1075—1079
48. Kubo SH, Clark M, Laragh JH, Borer JH, Cody RJ (1987) Identification of normal neurohormonal activity in mild congestive heart failure and stimulating effect of upright posture and diuretics. Am J Cardiol 60:1322—1328
49. Lindpaintner K, Jin M, Wilhelm MJ, Suzuki F, Linz W, Schoelkens BA, Ganten D (1988) Intracardiac generation of angiotensin and its physiologic role. Circulation 77 (suppl 1):1—18

50. Linz W, Scholkens BA, Ganten D (1989) Converting enzyme inhibition specifically prevents the development and induces regression of cardiac hypertrophy in rats. Clin Exper Hypertens A11(7):1325—1350
51. Michel JB, Cattion AL, Salzmann JL, de Lourdes Cerol M, Phillipe M, Camilleri JP, Coruol P (1988) Hormonal and cardiac effects of converting enzyme inhibition in rat myocardial infarction. Circ Res 62:641—650
52. Muller J, Lund EG, Hofstetter L, Brunner DB, Haldy P (1982) Stimulation of aldosterone biosynthesis by sodium sequestration: role of angiotensin II. Am J Physiol 243:E450—E457
53. Naftilan AJ, Pratt RE, Dzau VJ (1989) Induction of platelet-derived growth factor A-chain and c-myc gene expressions by angiotensin II in cultured rat vascular smooth muscle cells. J Clin Invest 83:1419—1424
54. Naftilan AJ, Pratt RE, Eldridge CS, Lin HL, Dzau VJ (1989) Angiotensin II c-fos expression in smooth muscle via transcriptional control. Hypertension 13:706—711
55. Nakashima Y, Fouad FM, Tarazi RC (1984) Regression of left ventricular hypertrophy from systemic hypertension by enalapril. Am J Cardiol 53:1044—1049
56. Okamura T, Myazcki M, Inagemi T, Toda N (1986) Vascular renin-angiotensin system in two-kidney, one-clip hypertensive rats. Hypertension 8:560—565
57. Oliver JA, Sciacca RR (1984) Local generation of angiotensin II as a mechanism of regulation of peripheral vascular tone in the rat. J Clin Invest 74:1247—1251
58. Oren S, Messerli FH, Grossman E, Garavaglia GE, Frolich ED (1991) Immediate and short-term effects of fosinopril, a new angiotensin converting enzyme inhibitor, in patients with essential hypertension. J Am Coll Cardiol 17:1183—1187
59. Paul M, Schunkert H, Allen P, Dzau VJ (1990) Widespread distribution of angiotensin converting enzyme mRNA in human tissues. J Hypertens 8 (suppl 3):S36
60. Pfeffer JM, Pfeffer MA (1988) Angiotensin converting enzyme inhibition and ventricular remodeling in heart failure. Am J Med 84:37—44
61. Pfeffer JM, Pfeffer MA, Fletcher PJ, Braunwald E (1991) Progressive ventricular remodeling in rat with myocardial infarction. Am J Physiol 260(Pt. 2):H1406—1414
62. Pfeffer et al, The SAVE Investigators (1992) Effect of captopril on mortality and morbidity in patients with left ventricular dysfunction after myocardial infarction. N Engl J Med 327:669—677
63. Powell JS, Clozel JP, Muller RKM, Kuhn H, Hefti F, Hosang M, Baumgartner HR (1989) Inhibitors of angiotensin-converting enzyme prevent myointimal proliferation after vascular injury. Science 245:186—188
64. Rakugi H, Jacob HJ, Ingelfinger JR, Krieger JE, Dzau VJ, Pratt RE (1990) Angiotensinogen gene expression in the myointima after vascular injury (abstract). Hypertension 16:345
65. Rakugi H, Krieger J, Wang DS, Dzau VJ, Pratt RE (1991) Induction of angiotensin converting enzyme in neointima after balloon injury. Circulation 84 (suppl II):II—113
66. Ragazzi E, Froldi G, Pandolfo L et al. (1989) Segmental impairment of endothelium-mediated relaxation in thoracic aortas from atherosclerotic rabbits. Comparison to cholesterol infiltration and energy metabolism. Artery 16:327—345
67. Reidy MA, Fingerle J, Au YP, Majesky MW (1989) Correlation of mRNA expression of cellular mitogens and smooth muscle cell proliferation in arteries denuded of endothelium (Abstr). J Cell Biochem 13E (suppl 13):194
68. Rosenthal JH, Pfieffer B, Mecheilor ML, Pschorr J, Jacob ICM, Dahlheim H (1984) Investigations of components of the renin-angiotensin system in rat vascular tissue. Hypertension 6:383—390
69. Sakaguchi K, Chai SY, Jackson B, Johnston CI, Mendelsohn FA (1988) Inhibition of tissue angiotensin converting enzyme. Quantitation by autoradiography. Hypertension 11:230—238
70. Schunkert H, Dzau VJ, Tang SS, Hirsch AT, Apstein CS, Lorell BH (1990) Increased rat cardiac angiotensin converting enzyme activity and mRNA expression in pressure overload left ventricular hypertrophy: effects on coronary resistance, contractility, and relaxation. C Clin Invest 86:1913—1920

71. Skidgel RA, Defendini R, Erdos EG (1988) Angiotensin I converting enzyme and its role in neuropeptide metabolism. In: Turner AJ (ed) Neuropeptides and their peptidases; Ellis Horwood-VCH, pp 165—188
72. The SOLVD Investigators (1992) Effect of enalapril on mortality and the development of heart failure in asymptomatic patients with reduced left ventricular ejection fractions. N Engl J Med 327:685—691
73. Taubman MB, Berk BC, Izumo S, Tsuda T, Alexander RW, Nadal-Ginard B (1989) Angiotensin II induces c-fos mRNA in aortic smooth muscle. Role of Ca^{++} mobilization and protein kinase C activation. J Biol Chem 264:526—530
74. Urata H, Healey B, Stewart RW, Bumpus FM, Husain A (1989) Angiotensin II receptors in normal and failing human hearts. J Clin Endocrinol Metab 69:54—66
75. Urata H, Healey B, Stewart RW, Bumpus FM, Husain A (1990) Angiotensin II-forming pathways in normal and failing human hearts. Circ Res 66:883—890
76. Vlodavsky I, Folkman J, Sullivan R, Fridman R, Ishai-Michaeli R, Sasse J, Klagsbrun M (1987) Endothelial cell-derived basic fibroblast growth factor: Synthesis and deposition into subendothelial extracellular matrix. Proc Natl Acad Sci USA 84:2292—2296
77. Webb RC, Finta KM, Fisher M, Lee L, Pitt B (1992) Ramipril reverses impaired endothelium-dependent relaxation in arteries from rabbits fed an atherogenic diet. The FASEB Journal 6(No. 5:Part I):Abstract 3022
78. Weber KT, Brilla CG, Janicki JS, Reddy HK (1991) Myocardial fibrosis: role of ventricular systolic pressure, arterial hypertension, and circulation hormones. Basic Res Cardiol 86 (suppl 3):25—31
79. Yamada H, Fabris B, Allen AM, Jackson B, Johnson CI, Mendelsohn FAO (1991) Localisation of angiotensin converting enzyme in the rat heart. Circ Res 68:141—149
80. Xiang J, Linz W, Becker H, Ganten D, Lang RE, Schoelkens B, Unger T (1984) Effects of converting enzyme inhibitors: ramipril and enalapril on peptide action and sympathetic neurotransmission in the isolated rat heart. Eur J Pharmacol 113:215—223

Author's address:
Victor J. Dzau, M.D.
Professor of Medicine
Stanford University School of Medicine
Chief, Division of Cardiovascular Medicine
Falk Cardiovascular Research Center
300 Pasteur Dr., Rm. 269
Stanford, CA 94305-5246
USA

Angiotensin, ACE-inhibitors and endothelial control of vasomotor tone

T. F. Lüscher

Department of Medicine, Division of Clinical Pharmacology,
University Hospital Basel, Basel, Switzerland

Summary: The renin angiotensin system and endothelium-derived vasoactive substances are both important regulators of vascular tone. Recent evidence suggests that the two systems may be tightly interconnected and drugs interfering with one system may also affect the other. Beside the circulating renin angiotensin system, a vascular wall renin angiotensin system has been postulated and various components of it have been demonstrated in endothelial and vascular smooth muscle cells. Of particular importance is the angiotensin converting enzyme (ACE) which is identical to kininase II, which breaks down bradykinin into inactive components. Bradykinin is a potent activator of the L-arginine nitric oxide system (endothelium-derived relaxing factor). Hence, ACE-inhibitors not only deactivate the pressor system, but increase the local concentrations of bradykinin and thereby stimulate a potent endothelium-derived vasodilator system. Angiotensin II not only can activate vascular smooth muscle cells (where it causes contraction and proliferation), but also endothelial cells. In certain blood vessels, angiotensin II can stimulate prostacyclin production; in addition, angiotensin II activates endothelin messenger RNA in endothelial cells. This activation of the endothelin vasopressor system increases vascular tone and enhances the local vasoconstrictor responses (due to the amplifying effects of endothelin on noradrenaline- and serotonin-induced contractions).

Although the acute effects of ACE-inhibitors in isolated blood vessels are restricted to inhibition of angiotensin I-induced contractions and augmentation of bradykinin-induced endothelium-dependent relaxations, chronic therapy with the drugs appears to enhance endothelium-dependent responses to several agonists, particularly in hypertensive animals. Hence, this mechanism of action of ACE-inhibitors may account for an important vascular protective effect of the drugs.

Thus, in summary, the renin angiotensin system and endothelium-derived vasoactive substances are tightly interconnected. This may be important under physiological and pathophysiological conditions, and is of importance for the action of currently available cardiovascular drugs, in particular, ACE-inhibitors.

Key words: L-arginine; nitric oxide; endothelin; prostaglandins; bradykinin

Introduction

The renin angiotensin system is an important regulator of the cardiovascular system (20, 28). Both a circulating and local vascular renin angiotensin system have been proposed (13, 14). While the physiology and pathophysiology of the circulating renin angiotensin system has been well characterized, less is known about the local functional importance of angiotensin II produced within the blood vessel wall. Several structures of the blood vessel wall have been shown to express parts or the entire renin angiotensin system. In particular, endothelial cells express the angiotensin converting enzyme (6) which activates angiotensin I to the more powerful vasoconstrictor angiotensin II (Fig. 1) (6). In addition, other parts of the renin angiotensin

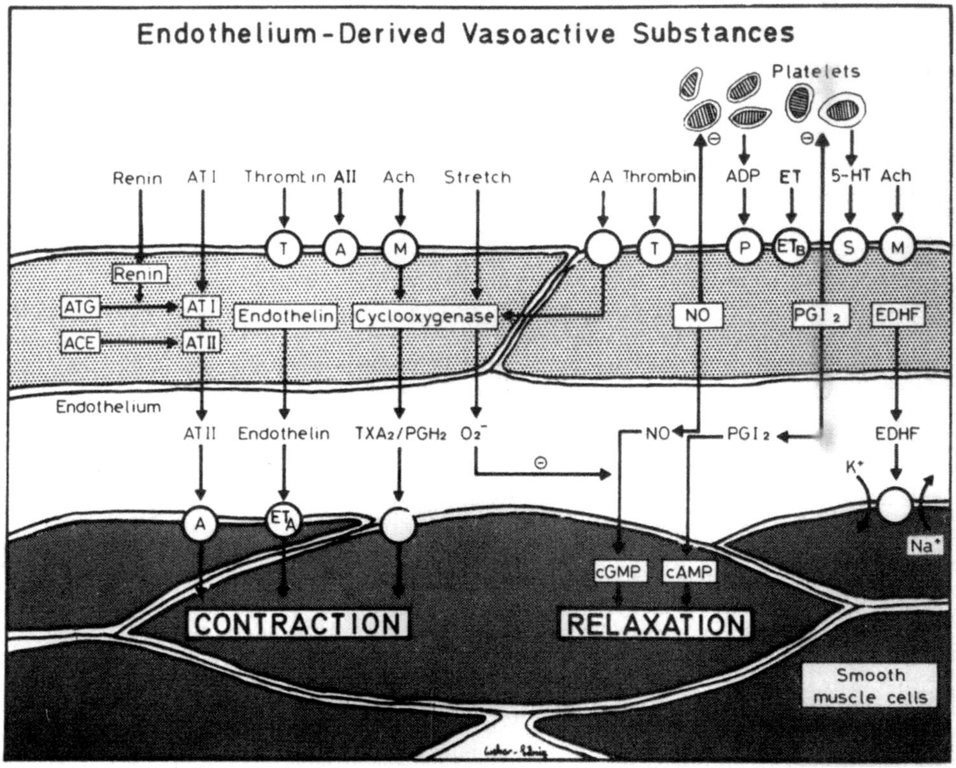

Fig. 1. Endothelium-derived vasoactive substances: The endothelium releases relaxing factors (right part) and contracting factors (left part). The relaxing factors include nitric oxide (NO), prostacyclin (PGI_2) and endothelium-derived hyperpolarizing factor (EDHF). NO and PGI_2 not only cause relaxation but also inhibition (⊖) of platelet function. The contracting factors include the local vascular renin angiotensin (AT) system, endothelin (ET) and cyclooxygenase-derived contracting factor such as thromboxane A_2 (TXA_2) and prostaglandin H_2 (PGH_2). In addition, the cyclooxygenase pathway is a source of oxygenderived free radicals (O_2^-). A = angiotensin receptor, AA = arachidonic acid, ADP = adenosin diphosphate, ATG = angiotensinogen, ACE = angiotensin converting enzyme, Ach = acetylcholine, cAMP = cyclic adenosinmonophosphate, cGMP = cyclic guanosinmonophosphate (from (20) by permission).

system have been shown to be expressed in endothelial cells, although the physiological importance of these findings has not been established yet. Similarly, vascular smooth muscle cells do express components of the renin angiotensin system (13).

The renin angiotensin system can also interact with substances involved in endothelium-dependent regulation of vascular tone (Fig. 1; 20). This review summarizes the local vascular effects of angiotensin, ACE-inhibitors, with particular emphasis on their relation to endothelium-dependent regulation of vascular tone.

Angiotensin and endothelium-derived prostaglandins

In the renal and femoral artery of the dog, angiotensin II stimulates prostaglandin production, indicating that angiotensin receptors are present in endothelial cells and are linked to the activation of phospholipase A_2 and cyclooxygenase (27). Prostaglandins may act as modulators of the contractile response to angiotensin II which is related to activation of AT_1-receptors on vascular smooth muscle.

Angiotensin and endothelium-derived relaxing factor

It is conceivable that the activity of the local vascular renin angiotensin system may counteract the formation or action of endothelium-derived relaxing factors such as nitric oxide (17, 24, 30, 33) and endothelium-derived hyperpolarizing factor (20, 26, 30, 33) and that activation or inhibition, respectively, of either system may effect physiological responses of isolated blood vessels. However, under most circumstances, pretreatment of isolated blood vessels with either an ACE-inhibitor or an AT_1-angiotensin receptor antagonist such as DuP 753 does not affect endothelium-dependent relaxations to acetylcholine (the classical activator of the L-arginine nitric oxide pathway) (Fig. 2) (10). This indicates that under in vitro conditions there seems to be no tonic activity of the vascular renin angiotensin system, at least not in the sense that it would inhibit the effects of the L-arginine nitric oxide pathway.

However, the response to bradykinin, another endothelium-dependent vasodilator which activates the L-arginine nitric oxide pathway, is profoundly affected by ACE-inhibitors (15, 16, 23, 34). Indeed, in the human saphenous vein, pretreatment of the blood vessel with enalapril markedly increases the sensitivity to bradykinin, indicating that the endothelial ACE continuously inactivates part of the bradykinin

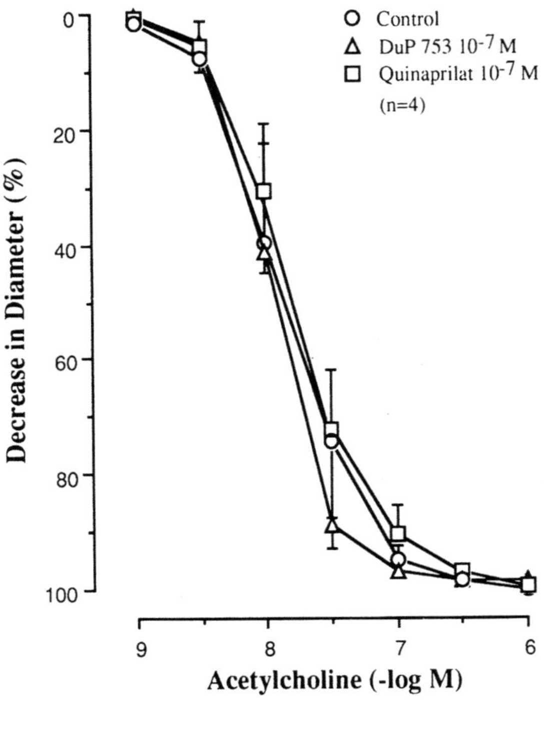

Fig. 2. Effects of the ACE-inhibitor quinaprilat and the angiotensin receptor antagonist DuP 753 on endothelium-dependent relaxations to acetylcholine in rat mesenteric resistance arteries: Neither drug effects endothelium-dependent relaxations to acetylcholine, indicating that, in normal resistance arteries, the local vascular renin angiotensin system is not interacting with the endothelial L-arginine nitric oxide pathway (from (10) by permission).

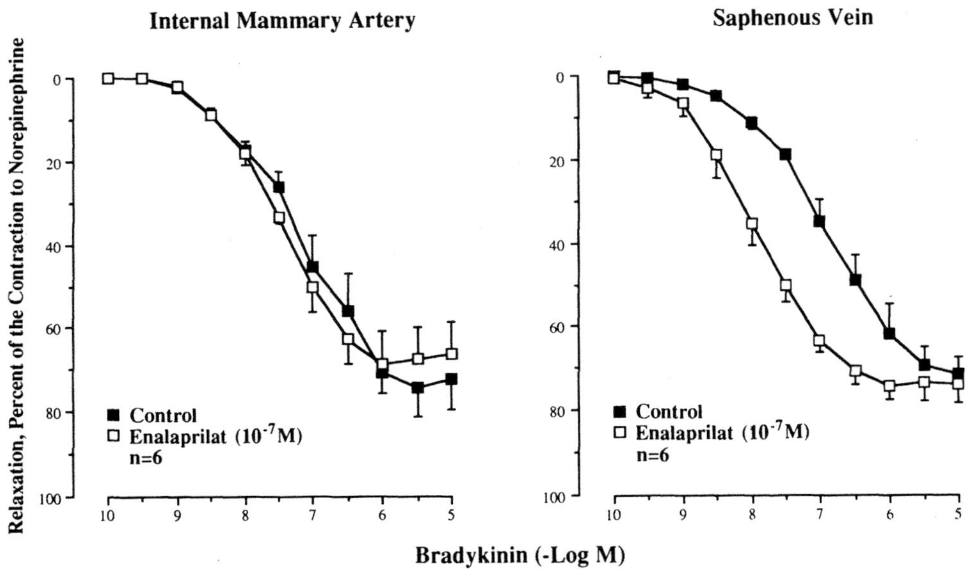

Fig. 3. Endothelium-dependent relaxations to bradykinin in the human internal mammary artery (left panel) and saphenous vein (right panel). Pretreatment with enalaprilat significantly increase the sensitivity to bradykinin in the saphenous vein but not mammary artery, indicating that, in the vein, angiotensin converting enzyme continuously breaks down bradykinin and thereby partially inhibits the response to this endothelium-dependent vasodilator (from (34) by permission).

added to the blood vessel (Fig. 3; 34). In contrast, in the human internal mammary artery, ACE activity does not seem to be as pronounced. However, in the human coronary artery, ACE-inhibitors also increase endothelium-dependent relaxations to bradykinin. Indeed, in the presence of low concentrations of bradykinin, ACE-inhibitors cause endothelium-dependent relaxations (Fig. 4; 1). These differences indicate a heterogeneity of the activity of the ACE (or kinase II) in different human blood vessels.

It is of interest that endothelial cells can produce and release bradykinin locally, particularly in response to flow (most likely due to the shear forces exerted by the circulating blood; 2, 5, 31). Locally released bradykinin may then bind to bradykinin receptors on endothelial cells and activate the endothelial L-arginine nitric oxide pathway (as well as other endothelium-derived relaxing factors such as the putative hyperpolarizing factor; 30). It is uncertain, however, to what degree this mechanism is important under resting conditions, as in the human forearm circulation, infusion of captopril does not increase local blood flow. However, the response may be important with increased flow rates, for instance, during exercise, and it may participate in flow-induced vasodilator responses (see (22)).

Angiotensin and endothelin

Angiotensin II has been shown to express to endothelin messenger RNA in endothelial cells in culture (Fig. 5) (11, 22, 35). In addition, angiotensin II appears to

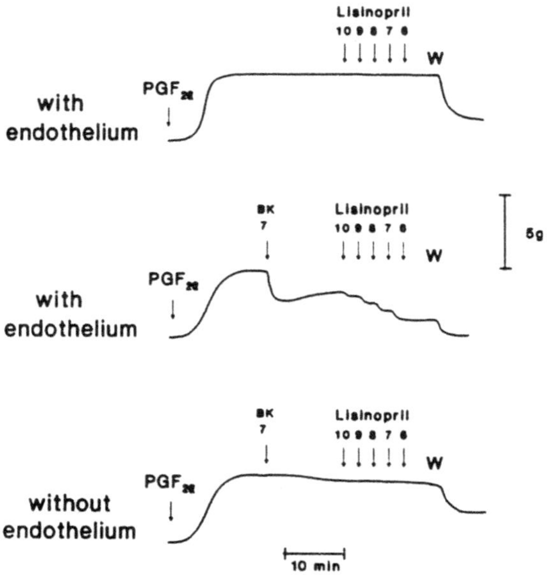

Fig. 4. Original registration of the response to lisinopril (10^{-10}—10^{-6} M) in human coronary artery contracted with $PGF_{2\alpha}$ (10^{-6} M). Top: ring with endothelium not stimulated with bradykinin. Middle: ring with endothelium in the presence of bradykinin (BK; 10^{-7} M). Bottom: ring without endothelium in the presence of bradykinin (BK; 10^{-7} M) (from (1) by permission).

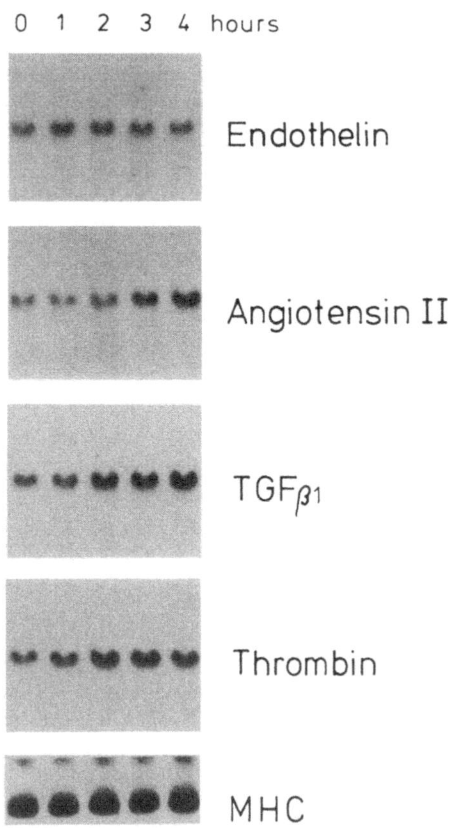

Fig. 5. Northern blot analysis of endothelin gene expression using a cDNA probe for endothelin in cultured porcine aortic endothelial cells: Zero to 4 h after stimulation with either endothelin, angiotensin II, transforming growth factor$_{\beta 1}$ ($TGF_{\beta 1}$) or thrombin, endothelin messenger RNA is expressed with the three latter agonists, but not by endothelin itself. MHC = control experiments using major histocompatability complex (From (11), by permission of the American Heart Association).

exert similar effects in endothelial cells obtained from the rat mesenteric microcirculation (11). Expression of endothelin in response to angiotensin II may contribute to the vasoconstrictor effects of angiotensin. Indeed, in perfused mesenteric resistance arteries of the spontaneously hypertensive rat (SHR), perfusion with

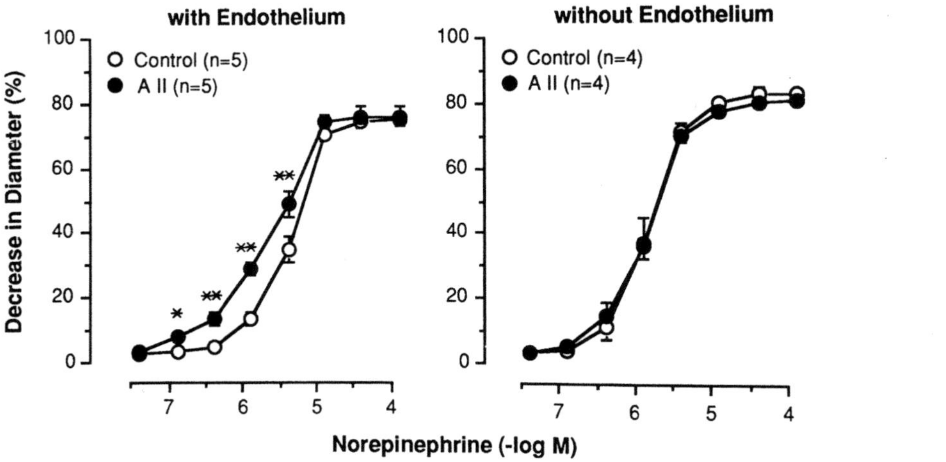

Fig. 6. Line graphs show concentration-response curves to norepinephrine obtained before (○) and after (●) stimulation with angiotensin II (A II) (10^{-7} M for 5 h) in mesenteric resistance arteries with (left panel) and without (right panel) endothelium of spontaneously hypertensive rats. Note that the contractions induced by low and moderate concentrations of norepinephrine were potentiated after the stimulation with angiotensin II in arteries with, but not in those without endothelium. * $p < 0.01$, ** $p < 0.005$ as compared with control (from (11) by permission of the American Heart Association).

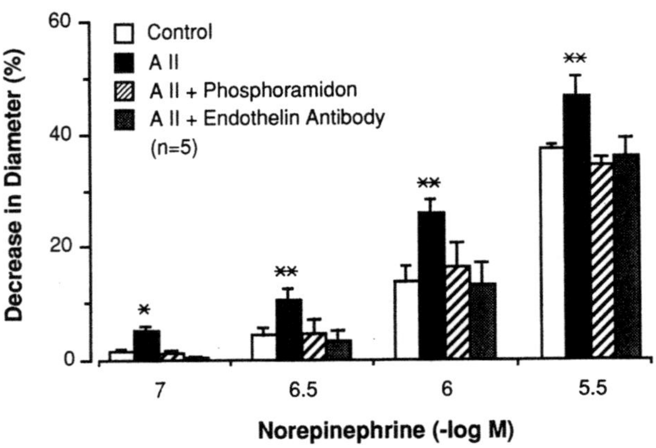

Fig. 7. Histogram shows effects of phosphoramidon (10^{-5} M) and endothelin antibody on the potentiation of contraction to norepinephrine by angiotensin II (A II) (10^{-7} M) in mesenteric resistance arteries with endothelium obtained from spontaneously hypertensive rats. Note that the potentiation was prevented both by the inhibitor of the endothelin converting enzyme, phosphoramidon, and an endothelin antibody. * $p < 0.01$, ** $p < 0.005$ as compared with control (from (11) by permission of the American Heart Association).

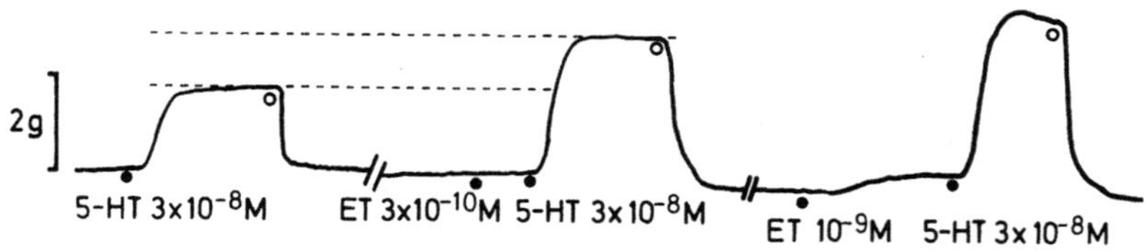

Fig. 8. Potentiating effects of endothelin 1 in the human coronary artery: Low and threshold concentrations of endothelin, which by themselves do not cause significant contraction, considerably augment contractile responses to serotonin. o washout (from (32) by permission of the American Heart Association).

angiotensin II causes a transient contraction, but after again reaching basal tone, the concentration response curve to norepinephrine is significantly shifted to the left (Fig. 6) (11). This effect of angiotensin II is endothelium-dependent, requires — as does the in vitro production of endothelin (4) — 4 h to be expressed, and can be inhibited by endothelin antagonists and inhibitors of the endothelin converting enzymes such as phosphoramidone (Fig. 7) (11). Hence, it appears that angiotensin II stimulates the local vascular production of endothelin and thereby enhances vasoconstrictor responses to noradrenaline.

Similarly, potentiating effects to exogenous endothelin-1 have been demonstrated in the human coronary artery suggesting that it might play a role as well in the human (Fig. 8) (32). As the circulating levels of endothelin under most circumstances are rather low, these indirect potentiating effects of endothelin-1 may have great physiological and pathophysiological importance (22).

ACE-Inhibitors and endothelium-dependent relaxations

Acute effects

As mentioned above, ACE-inhibitors have limited acute effects on vascular tone. Indeed, in vitro the addition of ACE-inhibitors such as enalapril or benazepril does not change local vascular tone of mesenteric and coronary arteries of the rat or the human mammary artery or saphenous vein (10, 29, 34). Also, endothelium-dependent relaxations are not affected by the drugs (Fig. 2) (29, 34) except if bradykinin and substance P are used (which are both inactivated by kininase II or ACE in the blood vessel wall; (7, 13).

Chronic effects

Chronic therapy with ACE-inhibitors, besides lowering blood pressure and reducing the local and circulating levels of angiotensin II (which is a vasoconstrictor and possibly also proliferative agent; 13) provides the possibility to chronically increase the bradykinin-induced stimulation of the L-arginine nitric oxide pathway and possibly also that of endothelium-derived hyperpolarizing factor. This may keep the blood vessel wall in a continuous state of vasodilation, thereby improving blood flow and lowering peripheral vascular resistance and blood pressure and may also be important for the antithrombotic properties of the endothelium (as nitric oxide is a potent inhibitor of platelet-function; 25). Furthermore, this may also be important for the regulation of vascular growth (18). Indeed, nitric oxide has also been implicated as a antiproliferative agent in the blood vessel wall. Hence, chronic therapy with ACE-inhibitors may be vascular protective in various parts of the circulation and possibly also in the coronary circulation.

In experimental animals, chronic therapy with ACE-inhibitors augments endothelium-dependent relaxations, not only to bradykinin, but also to other agonists such as acetylcholine. This effect can be demonstrated in the aorta of normotensive rats (3) as well as in the aorta and mesenteric resistance arteries of spontaneously hypertensive rats (8, 12). Most likely, this is an effect seen with all forms of ACE-inhibitors.

The effects of chronic therapy with ACE-inhibitors on endothelium-dependent vasodilation in normotensive man has not been investigated yet, but two studies have reported on the effects of captopril, enalapril (9) and cilazapril (19) on endothelium-dependent vasodilation induced by acetylcholine in the forearm circulation of hypertensive patients. In contrast to the experimental data in the rat (12), ACE-inhibitors were unable to improve or even normalize the impaired endothelium-dependent vasodilation in hypertensive patients. The lack of effect, which contrasts with experimental data, may be related to the duration of therapy, the time when therapy was started and/or to ineffectiveness of this approach in the human. In clinical practice, most patients with hypertension are already at the more advanced stage of the disease once they are seen by a clinician and effectively treated. In contrast, experimental animals are usually treated early in life when hypertension develops. Furthermore, 8 weeks of treatment in the rat may be sufficient, while a similar treatment duration may be inefficient in humans, particularly with fully established hypertension. Hence, studies with more prolonged and early treatment with ACE-inhibitors are required to reach a final conclusion on these effects of the drugs.

ACE-Inhibitors and endothelin

Acute effects

The activation of endothelin by angiotensin II in perfused mesenteric resistance arteries of the SHR can also be obtained with angiotensin I (11). This indicates that even in these small vessels, enough ACE is expressed to transform angiotensin I locally into the more active component angiotensin II. Hence, ACE-inhibitors not only would augment endothelium-dependent relaxations to certain agonists, but also inhibit the activation of endothelin gene by local or systemic angiotensin I.

Chronic effects

Not much is known about the effects of chronic treatment with ACE-inhibitors on endothelin production. However, in SHR antihypertensive therapy with benazepril partially restores the paradoxically decreased sensitivity of mesenteric resistance arteries to endothelin (11).

Conclusion

The close interaction between the circulating and local vascular renin angiotensin system and endothelium-derived vasoactive substances provides new insights in the regulation of vascular tone under physiological and pathophysiological conditions. In addition, it provides new mechanisms of action of currently used cardiovascular drugs as well as of those in development.

Acknowledgment. The authors wish to acknowledge the assistance of Amanda N. de Sola Pinto and Bernadette Weber-Libsig. Own research reported in this manuscript was supported by grants from the Swiss National Research Foundation (No. 32-32541.91), the Helmut Horten Foundation, Merck Sharp & Dohme, Glattbrugg/Switzerland and Gödecke Parke-Davis, Freiburg, Germany.

References

1. Auch-Schwelk W, Bossaller C, Claus M, Graf K, Gräfe M, Fleck E (1992) Endothelium-dependent relaxations to angiotensin-converting enzyme inhibitors in isolated coronary arteries stimulated with bradykinin. J Cardiovasc Pharmacol 20 (in press)
2. Boglie RG, Coade SB, Moncada S, Pearson JD, Mann GE (1991) Bradykinin and ATP stimulate L-arginine uptake and nitric oxide release in vascular endothelial cells. Biochem Biophys Res Commun 180:926—932
3. Bossaller C, Auch-Schwelk W, Weber F, Götze S, Gräfe M, Graf K, Fleck E (1992) Endothelium-dependent relaxations are augmented in rats chronically treated with the angiotensin-converting enzyme inhibitor enalapril. J Cardiovasc Pharmacol 20 (in press)
4. Boulanger CM, Lüscher TF (1990) Endothelin is released from the porcine aorta: Inhibition by endothelium-derived nitric oxide (rapid publication). J Clin Invest 85:587—590
5. Busse R, Lamontagne D (1991) Endothelium-derived bradykinin is responsible for the increase in calcium produced by angiotensin-converting enzyme inhibitors in human endothelial cells. Naunyn Schmiedebergs Arch Pharmacol 344:126—129
6. Caldwell PRB, Seegal BC, Hsu KC, Das M, Sooffer RL (1976) Angiotensin converting enzyme: vascular endothelial cell location. Science 191:1050—1051
7. Cascieri MA, Bull HG, Mumford RA, Patchett AA, Thornberry NA, Liang T (1983) Carboxyl-terminal tripeptidyl hydrolysis of substance P by purified rabbit lung angiotensin-converting enzyme and the potentiation of substance P activity in vivo by captopril and MK-422. Molec Pharmacol 25:287—293
8. Clozel M (1991) Mechanism of action of angiotensin converting enzyme inhibitors on endothelial function in hypertension. Hypertension 18 (Suppl II) II37—II42
9. Creager MA, Roddy M-A, Coleman SM, Dzau VJ (1992) The effect of ACE inhibition on endothelium-dependent vasodilation in hypertension. J Vasc Res 29:97
10. Dohi Z, Hahn AWA, Boulanger CM, Lüscher TF (1991) Vascular renin angiotensin system and endothelial function: Effect of ACE-inhibitors. In: Current Advance in ACE-Inhibition II, pp. 226—229. MacGregor EA, Safar PS, Caldwell D, Hollenberg NK, eds., Churchill Livingstone, Edinburgh, London, Melbourne, New York and Tokyo
11. Dohi Y, Hahn AWA, Boulanger CM, Bühler FR, Lüscher TF (1992) Endothelin stimulated by angiotensin II augments contractility of spontaneously hypertensive rat resistance arteries. Hypertension 19:131—137
12. Dohi Y, Criscione L, Pfeiffer K, Lüscher TF (1992) Angiotensin blockade or calcium antagonists improve endothelial dysfunction in hypertension: Studies in perfused mesenteric resistance arteries (submitted)
13. Dzau VJ (1986) Significance of the vascular renin-angiotensin pathway. Hypertension 8:553—559
14. Dzau VJ (1989) Short- and long-term determinants of cardiovascular function and therapy: Contributions of circulating and tissue renin-angiotensin systems. J Cardiovasc Pharmacol 14 (Suppl 4):S1—S5
15. Félétou M, Germain M, Teisseire B (1990) Converting-enzyme inhibitors potentiate bradykinin-induced relaxation in vitro. Am J Physiol 262:H839—H845
16. Félétou M, Teisseire B (1990) Converting enzyme inhibition in isolated porcine resistance artery potentiates bradykinin relaxation. Eur J Pharmacol 190:159—166

17. Furchgott RF, Zawadzki JV (1980) The obligatory role of endothelial cells in the relaxation of arterial smooth muscle by acetylcholine. Nature 299:373—376
18. Garg UC, Hassid A (1989) Nitric oxide-generating vasodilators and 8-bromo-cyclic guanosine monophosphate inhibit mitogenesis and proliferation of cultured rat vascular smooth muscle cells. J Clin Invest 83:1774—1777
19. Kiowski W, Linder L (1992) personal communication
20. Lüscher TF, Vanhoutte PM (1990) The endothelium modulators of cardiovascular function. Boca Raton, Florida, USA, pp 1—115
21. Lüscher TF, Diederich D, Siebenmann R, Lehmann K, Stulz P, von Segesser L, Yang Z, Turina M, Grädel E, Weber E, Bühler FR (1988) Difference between endothelium-dependent relaxations in arterial and in venous coronary bypass grafts. N Engl J Med 319:462—467
22. Lüscher TF, Boulanger CM, Dohi Y, Yang Z (1992) Endothelium-derived contracting factors. Hypertension 19:117—130
23. Mombouli J-V, Nephtali M, Vanhoutte PM (1991) Effects of the converting enzyme inhibitor cilazaprilat on endothelium-dependent responses. Hypertension 18 (Suppl II):II22—II29
24. Palmer RMJ, Ferrige AG, Moncada S (1987) Nitric oxide release accounts for the biological activity of endothelium-derived relaxing factor. Nature 327:524—526
25. Radomski MW, Palmer RMJ, Moncada S (1987) The anti-aggregating properties of vascular endothelium: interactions between prostacyclin and nitric oxide. Br J Pharmacol 92:639—646
26. Richard V, Tanner FC, Tschudi M, Lüscher TF (1990) Different activation of L-arginine pathway by bradykinin, serotonin, and clonidine in coronary arteries. Am J Physiol 259:H1433—H1439
27. Satoh H, Hosono M, Satoh S (1984) Distinctive effect of angiotensin II on prostaglandin production in dog renal and femoral arteries. Prostaglandins 27:807—820
28. Sealey JE, Laragh JH (1990) The renin angiotensin aldosterone system for normal regulation of blood pressure and sodium and potassium homeostasis. In: Laragh JH, Brenner BM, eds. Hypertension, Pathophysiology, Diagnosis, and Management. New York: Raven Press, pp 1287—1317
29. Tschudi M, Criscione L, Lüscher TF (1991) Effect of aging and hypertension on endothelial function of rat coronary arteries. J Hypertension 9 (Suppl 6):164—165
30. Vanhoutte PM (1987) The end of the quest. Nature 327:459—460
31. Wiemer G, Scholkens BA, Becker RH, Busse R (1991) Ramiprilat enhances endothelial autocoid formation by inhibiting breakdown of endothelial derived bradykinin. Hypertension 18:558—563
32. Yang Z, Richard V, von Segesser L, Bauer E, Stulz P, Turina M, Lüscher TF (1990) Threshold concentrations of endothelin-1 potentiate contractions to norepinephrine and serotonin in human arteries: A new mechanism of vasospasm? Circulation 82:188—195
33. Yang Z, von Segesser L, Bauer E, Stulz P, Turina M, Lüscher TF (1991) Different activation of endothelial L-arginine and cyclooxygenase pathway in human internal mammary artery and saphenous vein. Circ Res 68:52—60
34. Yang Z, Arnet U, von Segesser L, Siebenmann R, Turina M, Lüscher TF (1993) Different effects of angiotensin-converting enzyme inhibition in human arteries and veins. J Cardiovasc Pharmacol (in press)
35. Yanagisawa M, Kurihara H, Kimura S, Mitsui Y, Kobayashi M, Watanabe TX, Masaki T (1988) A novel potent vasoconstrictor peptide produced by vascular endothelial cells. Nature 332:411—415

Author's address:
Thomas F. Lüscher, M.D., F.A.C.C.
Department of Medicine
Division of Clinical Pharmacology
University Hospital
4031 Basel, Switzerland

Local and neurohumoral control of coronary blood flow

M. Krajcar, G. Heusch

Abteilung für Pathophysiologie, Zentrum für Innere Medizin
Universitätsklinikum Essen

Summary: The powerful local metabolic regulation adjusting coronary blood flow to myocardial oxygen consumption under normal conditions is beyond doubt. However, despite substantial experimental efforts the responsible mediators are still largely unknown. Adenosine, a purported mediator of local metabolic control of coronary blood flow, is probably only involved in transient flow adaptations, but not in steady-state coronary autoregulation. Even below the autoregulatory range a substantial vasodilator reserve persists. Recruitment of such vasodilator reserve results in improved regional myocardial blood flow and attenuated regional ischemic dysfunction.

β-adrenergic coronary dilation is of minor functional importance. α-adrenergic coronary constriction acts to attenuate increases in coronary blood flow during sympathetic activation under normal conditions, such that myocardial oxygen extraction increases to match the increased oxygen consumption. α-adrenergic coronary constriction remains operative in ischemic myocardium, thus precipitating or contributing to acute myocardial ischemia during sympathetic activation and exercise in experimental animals as well as in patients with stable angina. The vagal transmitter acetylcholine — upon exogenous intracoronary infusion — induces critical constriction of epicardial coronary arteries with endothelial dysfunction and atherosclerosis. However, a vagal initiation of coronary spasm or myocardial ischemia has not been documented so far. Similarly, peptide hormones/transmitters such as NPY, vasopressin, and angiotensin can induce myocardial ischemia upon exogenous administration. Their pathophysiological role in myocardial ischemia and reperfusion, however, remains to be established.

Key words: Coronary vasomotor tone; myocardial ischemia; coronary reserve; α-adrenoceptors; angiotensin; ACE-inhibitors

The control of coronary blood flow has been extensively reviewed elsewhere (5, 35). The current article will focus on only three selected aspects of coronary pathophysiology, i.e., 1) the persistence of coronary dilator reserve in ischemic myocardium, 2) the role of α-adrenergic coronary constriction in stress-induced myocardial ischemia, and 3) the role of the renin-angiotensin system in myocardial ischemia and reperfusion.

Persistence of coronary dilator reserve in ischemic myocardium

Traditionally, myocardial ischemia has been viewed as the most potent coronary dilator stimulus causing maximal dilation of the ischemic coronary resistance vessels (9, 57). However, in the last decade a number of experimental studies unanimously demonstrated the persistence of some coronary vasomotor tone in ischemic myocardium which could be removed by pharmacological dilation (3, 14, 41, 44, 53, 80). At a coronary perfusion pressure as low as 35 mm Hg (3, 80) or 30 mm Hg (23, 44) and in the presence of a significant reduction in regional myocardial blood flow (3, 14, 23, 44, 80), ischemic contractile dysfunction (3, 23, 80) and net lactate production (53, 80), intracoronary infusion of adenosine, nevertheless, significantly increased regional myocardial blood flow. Subepicardial vasodilator reserve persisted even to a perfusion pressure as low as 25 mm Hg (14). The resulting effects of such pharmacological recruitment of coronary dilator reserve on the ischemic myocardium remain controversial. In one study in anesthetized dogs a significant adenosine-induced increase in regional myocardial blood flow was associated with a moderate, yet significant increase in regional contractile function (3), whereas the recruitment of coronary dilator reserve by intracoronary adenosine in two other studies using anesthetized dogs (23) or pigs (80) neither attenuated regional dysfunction nor lactate production. The recruitment of coronary dilator reserve by intravenous nifedipine during exercise-induced myocardial ischemia in conscious dogs was once more associated with an attenuation of ischemic contractile dysfunction (53). In conscious resting and closed-chest, anesthetized dogs no dilator reserve can be pharmacologically recruited in ischemic myocardium (15), suggesting that recruitable dilator reserve is related to increased vasoconstrictor tone, in particular, α-adrenergic vasoconstrictor tone, which becomes apparent under open-chest conditions (51) or during exercise (53).

Two pioneering studies from Hoffman's laboratory (2, 23) recently pointed out that the distribution of both resting blood flow and coronary reserve is extremely heterogeneous and that small patchy areas with and without persistent coronary dilator reserve may coexist in ischemic myocardium (23). On the one hand, these studies may reestablish the view of maximal coronary dilation during myocardial ischemia on a microregional level. On the other hand, the impact of recruiting coronary dilator reserve on regional contractile function may depend on the extent of dilator reserve in each microregion and the number of such microregions involved. More detailed analyses comparing regional blood flow distribution and regional contractile function with similar spatial resolution are required.

α-Adrenergic coronary constriction in stress-induced myocardial ischemia

Experimental myocardial ischemia

Bassenge et al. (4) in 1967 first observed a shift from metabolic coronary dilation to coronary constriction during intracoronary norepinephrine infusion when coronary perfusion pressure in anesthetized dogs was progressively reduced (Fig. 1). This important dependence of norepinephrine-induced coronary vasomotion on the preexisting coronary vasomotor tone was not further pursued until Buffington and Feigl (12) in 1981 demonstrated the persistence of α-adrenergic coronary vasoconstriction distal to a moderate stenosis during intracoronary norepinephrine infusion. This poststenotic α-adrenergic coronary vasoconstriction was powerful enough to limit oxygen supply up to the point of cardiac failure. However, net lactate production did not occur.

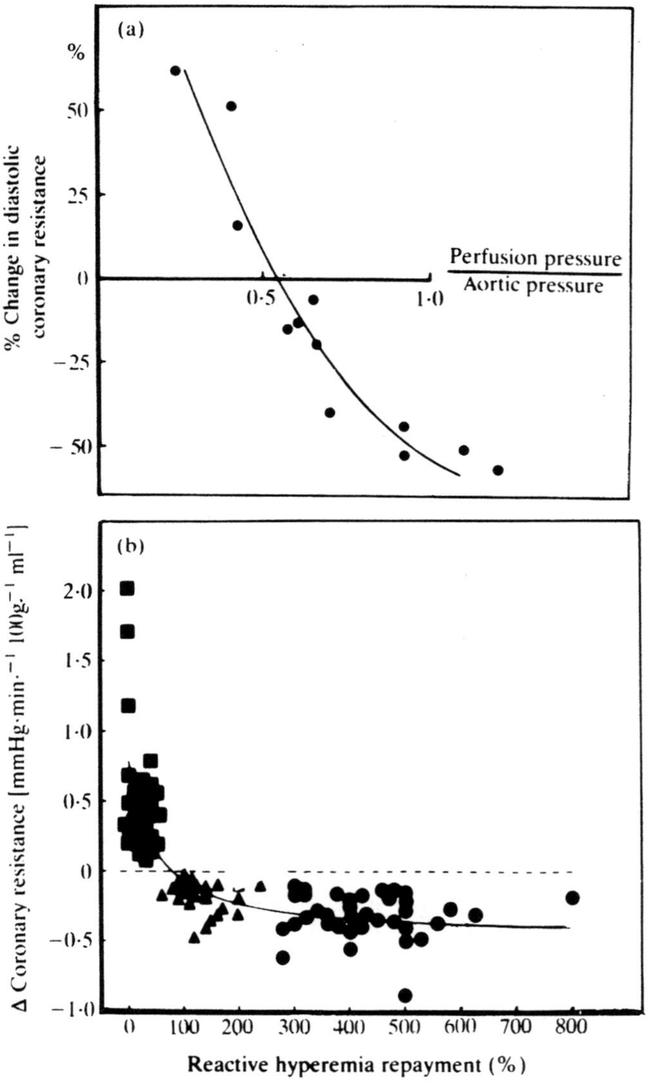

Fig. 1. a) Changes in coronary resistance in response to intracoronary norepinephrine are plotted versus coronary perfusion pressure as a fraction of aortic pressure (From Bassenge et al. (1967)). **b)** Changes in coronary resistance in response to cardiac sympathetic nerve stimulation are plotted versus reactive hyperemia repayment as a measure of coronary dilator reserve (From Heusch and Deussen (1983) by permission of the American Heart Association). In both studies there is a progressive shift from norepinephrine-induced coronary dilation to coronary constriction with progressive coronary hypoperfusion.

During electrical cardiac sympathetic nerve stimulation in anesthetized dogs metabolic coronary dilation was progressively reversed to α-adrenergic coronary constriction when coronary dilator reserve was progressively reduced by an increasing severity of coronary stenosis (Fig. 1) (54). Distal to a severe coronary stenosis which exhausted poststenotic coronary dilator reserve significant α-adrenergic coronary constriction was induced by cardiac sympathetic nerve stimulation, resulting in the precipitation of myocardial ischemia as evidenced by regional contractile dysfunction and net lactate production. The poststenotic coronary constriction and the resulting ischemia were prevented by phentolamine and selective α_2-blockade with rauwolscine in the absence and presence of β-blockade (54). Nifedipine also functionally antagonized the α_2-adrenoceptor mediated poststenotic coronary constriction and prevented the resulting myocardial ischemia (55).

Recently, an enhanced α_2-adrenergic constrictor tone in the hypoperfused canine coronary microcirculation was confirmed by using intravital microscopy (22). The presence of α-adrenergic constrictor tone during coronary hypoperfusion was also confirmed in anesthetized open-chest dogs with a presumably high resting sympathetic tone (59, 68). This α-adrenergic constrictor tone was, however, attenuated by the selective α_1-antagonist prazosin and not by the selective α_2-antagonist yohimbine (69). The different involvement of α_1- (69) or α_2- (54) adrenoceptors in coronary vasoconstriction during myocardial ischemia may be related to the different level of sympathetic activation in these studies.

In contrast to all previously discussed studies which agree on a deleterious role of α-adrenergic coronary constriction during myocardial ischemia, Nathan and Feigl (78) concluded from their data that α-adrenergic coronary constriction exerts a favorable effect on ischemic myocardium by preventing a transmural redistribution of blood flow away from the ischemic subendocardium. In anesthetized dogs they observed during constant inflow coronary hypoperfusion an increase in interpolated subendocardial to subepicardial blood flow ratios in a control, as compared to a phenoxybenzamine-treated region during intracoronary norepinephrine infusion. However, the use of constant inflow coronary hypoperfusion prevented the most significant beneficial effect of α-blockade in the studies described above, i.e., an increase in total coronary blood flow, and absolute data for subendocardial blood flow or measures of regional contractile function and metabolism were not presented to substantiate the aggravation of ischemia in the phenoxybenzamine-treated region. Increased ratios of subendocardial to subepicardial blood flow during α-adrenoceptor activation, however, do not necessarily indicate an attenuation of myocardial ischemia, but may reflect a further decrease in subepicardial blood flow, resulting in a further deterioration of transmural myocardial wall function (73). Under ischemic circumstances, the complete α_1- but incomplete α_2-blockade by phenoxybenzamine (26) is particularly problematic since α_1-adrenergic coronary constriction is attenuated by ischemia (52), whereas α_2-adrenergic coronary constriction is not (31). Thus, phenoxybenzamine may have removed α_1-constrictor tone in the less ischemic subepicardium and left α_2-constrictor tone in the most ischemic subendocardium unopposed, causing an artificial imbalance of transmural blood flow distribution rather than proving a protective role of physiological α-adrenergic coronary constriction. A transmurally nonuniform α_2-adrenergic coronary vasoconstriction contributing to the severity of myocardial ischemia has indeed been demonstrated in conscious β-blocked dogs when, during sympathetic activation by exercise, ischemia was induced by an acute coronary stenosis (93). Intracoronary infusion of the selective α_2-antagonist idazoxan distal to the stenosis resulted in significant increases in ischemic subendocardial and midmyocardial blood flow, whereas subepicardial blood flow was unchanged. Whereas the transmural distribution of coronary vascular α_1- and α_2-adrenoceptors is almost uniform in nonischemic myocardium (17, 73), the preferential α_2-adrenergic coronary constriction in the most ischemic inner myocardial layers (93) may be related to the attenuation of α_1-, but not α_2-adrenergic coronary constriction by ischemia (31, 52), potentially due to the different sensitivity of α_1- and α_2-adrenoceptors to acidosis (71). However, in two recent studies in conscious dogs with either constant pressure coronary hypoperfusion during exercise (65) or exercise-induced ischemia distal to an ameroid occluder (47), the selective α_1-antagonist prazosin also improved regional myocardial blood flow and function.

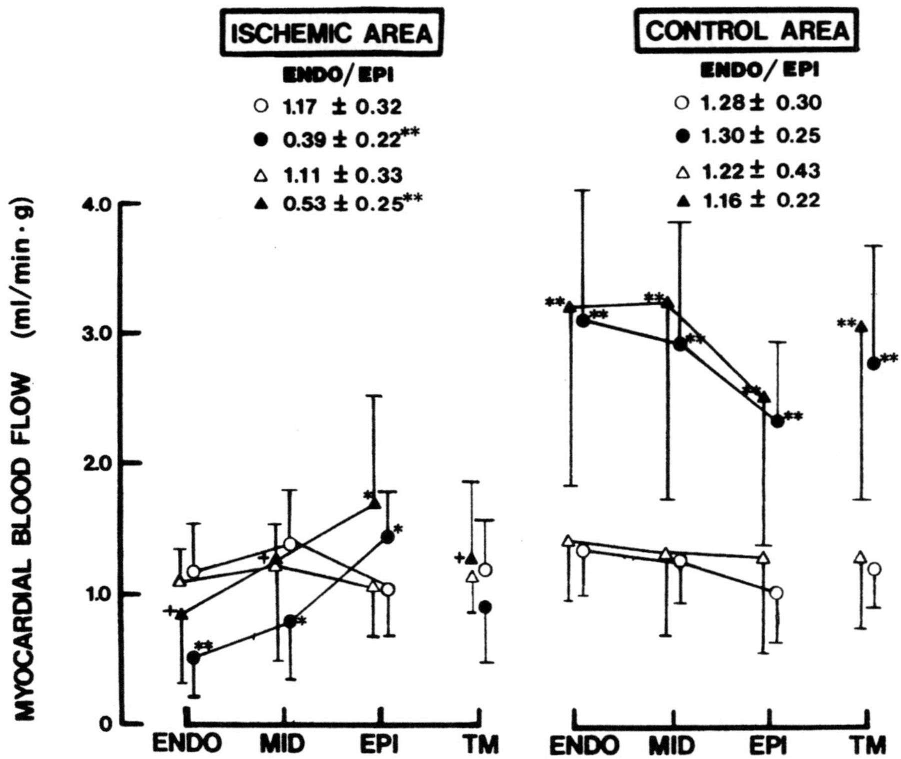

Fig. 2. Transmural distribution of regional myocardial blood flow in the ischemic (left) and control (right) regions at rest and during exercise. At rest, blood flow distribution in the ischemic area was not different from that in the control area. During the control run, however, myocardial blood flow in the control region increased in all transmural layers, whereas in the ischemic region a marked transmural gradient with a decrease in subendocardial blood flow and an increase in subepicardial blood flow developed. Nifedipine did not change myocardial blood flow at rest in either region. However, the decreases in blood flow to the subendocardium and the midmyocardium of the ischemic region during exercise were significantly attenuated. Open circle = control rest; closed circle = control exercise; open triangle = nifedipine rest; closed triangle = nifedipine exercise; ENDO = subendocardium; MID = midmyocardium; EPI = subepicardium; TM = mean transmural myocardial blood flow. Bars indicate 1 SD. *p < .05; ** p < .01 exercise vs rest. $^+p < .05$ nifedipine vs control. (From Heusch et al. (1987) by permission of the American Heart Association).

Recruitment of coronary dilator reserve, presumably through attenuation of α-adrenergic coronary constriction by the Ca-antagonist nifedipine, also improved subendocardial and midmyocardial blood flow and attenuated regional contractile dysfunction during exercise-induced ischemia in conscious dogs (Fig. 2) (53).

A true protective role of cardiac sympathetic nerves in an ischemic myocardial region through preferential subepicardial α-adrenergic coronary constriction was demonstrated in conscious dogs during exercise-induced ischemia, since subendocardial blood flow was higher in the innervated than in a phenol-denervated poststenotic region (21). However, this protective role of subepicardial α-adrenergic coronary constriction was strictly limited to neuronally released norepinephrine whereas, as previously shown by the same authors (20), the coronary vasomotor effects in exercising dogs are essentially exerted by circulating catecholamines. Thus, systemic α-blockade with phentolamine actually increased ischemic subendocardial blood flow in the innervated as well as in the denervated region (21).

The failure to demonstrate any α-adrenergic coronary constriction distal to a severe coronary stenosis with exhausted poststenotic dilator reserve in anesthetized open-chest dogs during cardiac sympathetic nerve stimulation (62) was probably due to the use of pentobarbital-anesthesia which is known to selectively inhibit α-adrenergic coronary vasoconstriction (48, 89). The relatively weak poststenotic coronary vasoconstriction in pigs during intravenous norepinephrine-infusion which did not result in a reduction of regional myocardial blood flow (39) was probably related to the paucity of α-adrenoceptors in the coronary circulation of pigs (92).

Thus, α-adrenergic constrictor tone in ischemic myocardium can be demonstrated in appropriate experimental models. α-adrenergic coronary vasoconstriction acts to initiate or aggravate poststenotic myocardial ischemia. The involvement of α_1- and α_2-adrenoceptors is not clear yet (50).

Clinical myocardial ischemia

There are several more or less anecdotical observations of α-adrenoceptor involvement in coronary vasospasm (67, 85, 98, 104) which may be precipitated by the combined administration of epinephrine and propranolol (104) or the cold pressor test (85) and can be prevented by phenoxybenzamine (67, 104) or prazosin (98). However, in carefully controlled clinical trials an important role of α-adrenergic coronary constriction for the precipitation of vasospasm in epicardial coronary arteries was ruled out (18, 88, 103).

In a stenotic coronary arterial segment with an eccentric atherosclerosis and another wall fraction retaining vasomotion, sympathetic activation by isometric exercise can induce critical narrowing (10, 58) which then results in ischemic myocardial dysfunction and angina pectoris (10). This critical narrowing of an epicardial coronary segment with a preexisting eccentric atherosclerosis is presumably due to α-adrenoceptor activation during isometric exercise (11) and can be prevented by intracoronary nitroglycerin (10) as well as by the Ca-antagonist diltiazem in a dose that does not induce unspecific epicardial coronary dilation (58). A vasoconstriction of stenotic coronary arteries resulting in myocardial ischemia was also induced by dynamic exercise in patients with chronic stable angina and again prevented by intracoronary nitroglycerin (36).

The cold pressor test is used as a provocative intervention to study the effects of reflex sympathetic activation in patients with coronary artery disease (76). Whereas intact coronary arterial segments dilate during the cold pressor test, there is a preferential vasoconstriction of atherosclerotic coronary arterial segments (77, 106). A significant increase in coronary vascular resistance was induced by the cold pressor test in patients with coronary artery disease resulting in the precipitation of angina pectoris in some of them (74, 75, 106). This increase in coronary vascular resistance during the cold pressor test appears to be mediated by activation of α-adrenoceptors since it is prevented by phentolamine (74). Nifedipine also prevents the increase in coronary vascular resistance as well as a net lactate production indicative of myocardial ischemia during the cold pressor test (46). However, caution should be used in interpreting these studies because they were performed either using angiography of epicardial coronary segments (77), which may contribute little to coronary resistance (see above), or using coronary sinus thermodilution techniques (46, 74), which may be unreliable in the presence of flow heterogeneities caused by coronary artery disease. Additional studies on this subject are certainly needed.

There is unequivocal evidence for a significant role of α-adrenergic coronary vasoconstriction in exercise-induced myocardial ischemia in patients with stable angina pectoris (7, 19, 25, 42). The exercise-induced ST-segment depression and angina pectoris in patients with chronic stable angina are reduced by intracoronary phentolamine (7, 19), and exercise duration is prolonged by intravenous phentolamine (42). A reduction in exercise-induced ST-segment depression and an increase in exercise capacity were also achieved in patients with chronic stable angina treated with the selective α_1-antagonist indoramin (25). However, in a recent study the exercise-induced ST-segment depression in patients with chronic stable angina was significantly more attenuated by the nonselective α-antagonist phentolamine than the selective α_1-antagonist indoramin, suggesting an important role for vascular α_2-adrenoceptors in the human coronary circulation (8).

Renin-angiotensin-system in myocardial ischemia

Experimental myocardial ischemia

In anesthetized dogs, intracoronary infusion of 8 μg/min AGT II at constant coronary blood flow induces a constriction of both small and large coronary vessels. In contrast to the large vessels, in which constriction is maintained, small vessels rapidly develop tachyphylaxis (24). It is unclear from these data, however, whether the small-vessel coronary constriction is a transient event, which is initially compensated by an increased myocardial oxygen extraction and then overridden by metabolic vasodilation. In preliminary experiments from our laboratory, intracoronary bolus injection of 1 μg AGT II at a constant coronary perfusion pressure of 100 mmHg induced a marked reduction of coronary blood flow which was reversible within a few minutes. This drop in coronary blood flow could not be compensated by increased myocardial oxygen extraction or metabolic coronary vasodilation. Thus, a pronounced deterioration of regional myocardial wall function resulted, demonstrating that the constrictor effect of AGT II, in principle, is strong enough to evoke ischemic consequences.

Ertl et al. (34) simulated progressive coronary stenoses by stepwise reductions of coronary perfusion pressure in anesthetized dogs. The constrictor response to intracoronary AGT II infusion was not blunted at reduced coronary perfusion pressures, suggesting that AGT II may still be effective when the coronary microcirculation is under the influence of dilator metabolites during myocardial ischemia. However, the validity of these findings is questioned since repeat AGT I and II infusion induced tachyphylaxis, and AGT I surprisingly induced more pronounced coronary constriction than AGT II. Also, the dose range in the above studies was artificially high. The calculated blood concentrations in these studies still surmounted even the pathophysiologic levels in patients with malignant hypertension (38) by 3000- to 20 000-fold. On the other hand, plasma levels do not necessarily reflect local AGT concentrations in the coronary vascular wall.

There are three potential anti-ischemic mechanisms by which ACE-inhibitors may attenuate myocardial ischemia: 1) an improvement of the driving pressure gradient for coronary blood flow, 2) a reduction of myocardial oxygen consumption, and 3) a reduction of coronary vasomotor tone.

Apart from coronary morphology and vasomotor tone, coronary blood flow is determined by the driving pressure, i.e., the gradient between aortic and left-ventricular pressure. The main systemic effect of ACE-inhibitors is a decrease in aortic blood pressure, which is associated with a drop in coronary perfusion pressure and, consequently, in the driving force for coronary blood flow. On the other hand, a reduction in afterload and in left-ventricular diastolic pressure will enhance the driving force for coronary blood flow. The situation becomes more complex in the presence of coronary stenoses when the close relationship between aortic pressure and coronary perfusion pressure is altered, potentially even in a dynamic fashion during changes in stenosis severity (43).

Despite the arterial pressure reduction by ACE-inhibitors, reflex tachycardia does not occur. Consequently, the rate-pressure product — as an index for cardiac work and myocardial oxygen consumption — decreases, and this reduction in metabolic requirements may have a positive impact on myocardial ischemia. The rate-pressure product decreased during 12—60 min of coronary occlusion in anesthetized (6, 33) and conscious (68) dogs treated with different ACE-inhibitors (6, 33, 68). However, despite the reduced myocardial oxygen consumption, myocardial ischemia was not attenuated, since ischemic regional myocardial blood flow (6, 33, 68) and regional myocardial function (68) were not improved. Thus, the potential benefit of the reduced oxygen consumption was probably masked by other mechanisms.

ACE-inhibitors may reduce coronary vasomotor tone by a decrease of local or systemic AGT synthesis, resulting in increased coronary blood flow. Indeed, captopril (33, 100), saralasin (33) (a competitive AGT-receptor antagonist), and zofenoprilate (100) increased coronary arterial inflow during 15—30 min of coronary occlusion in isolated rat hearts (100) and anesthetized dogs (33). The reduction of coronary vasomotor tone in isolated rat hearts by captopril and zofenoprilat is not mediated by prostaglandins (101).

The effect of ACE-inhibitors on regional myocardial blood flow distribution is the result of a complex interaction of these potential anti-ischemic mechanisms, which cannot be separated in the individual setting. In one study using anesthetized dogs, saralasin and captopril increased regional myocardial blood flow in nonischemic- and border-zones during 30 min coronary occlusion (33). However,

ACE-inhibitors did not improve regional blood flow to nonischemic (6, 68) and ischemic subendocardial layers (6, 68) during 12—60 min coronary occlusion in other studies using anesthetized (6) and conscious dogs (68). Even in the study claiming an anti-ischemic action of captopril, a reduction of subendocardial blood flow of the most ischemic zone was apparent (33). The finding that regional myocardial blood flow was improved in the nonischemic zones, but tended to decrease in the most ischemic subendocardial area, is suggestive of a collateral and transmural steal phenomenon. A steal phenomenon was also suggested by the tendency of regional myocardial blood flow to decrease during 3 min of coronary occlusion in dogs treated with captopril (1). Finally, the potential of captopril-induced steal phenomena was recently emphasized by a study in anesthetized dogs where captopril did not change infarct size in dogs with low collateral flow but increased infarct size in dogs with high collateral flow (30).

Exercise-induced myocardial ischemia may be simulated by atrial pacing or cardiac sympathetic nerve stimulation (54) during hypoperfusion of the coronary artery. During pacing-induced myocardial ischemia in anesthetized dogs coronary blood flow and regional myocardial function decreased. Captopril improved coronary arterial blood flow both during resting conditions and pacing-induced myocardial ischemia. However, regional function at rest somewhat deteriorated and even decreased further during pacing-induced myocardial ischemia (34), again suggesting the above-mentioned steal phenomena.

Our own data also do not confirm an anti-ischemic effect of ramiprilat during sympathetic precipitation of acute myocardial ischemia in the anesthetized dog. Cardiac sympathetic nerve stimulation during hypoperfusion of the left circumflex coronary artery resulted in an increase in coronary resistance and a decrease in regional wall thickening, both in the absence and presence of propanolol. Ramiprilat (30 µg/kg i.v.) caused the expected decrease in blood pressure. Ramiprilat did, however, not attenuate the increase in coronary resistance and the decrease in regional contractile function, even when the decrease in coronary perfusion pressure was prevented by inflation of an intraaortic balloon. Ramiprilat also did not prevent the coronary vasoconstriction and ischemic dysfunction induced by intracoronary infusion of the selective α_2-agonist BHT-933.

The coronary vasoconstriction mediated by AGT may be attenuated by an intact endothelium (97, 105), and loss of endothelial function has been reported following ischemia/reperfusion (81, 96). However, when complete coronary occlusion in anesthetized dogs was limited to 15 min and ischemic injury was fully reversible, no augmentation of coronary constrictor responses was observed during reperfusion (Fig. 3) (63).

Zofenopril and captopril did not affect coronary flow before ischemia or during reperfusion, but improved postischemic contractile function and reduced LDH release in isolated rat hearts. Since other ACE-inhibitors in this study exerted no cardioprotective effect, the beneficial effect of zofenopril and captopril was attributed to their sulfhydryl groups (45). Likewise, both zofenopril and enalapril in dogs with 15 min coronary occlusion followed by reperfusion did not change coronary blood flow, but improved contractile function of reperfused myocardium. The beneficial effect of enalaprilat was attenuated by indomethacin and, thus, was dependent on prostaglandin-synthesis, whereas the action of zofenopril was prostaglandin-independent (84).

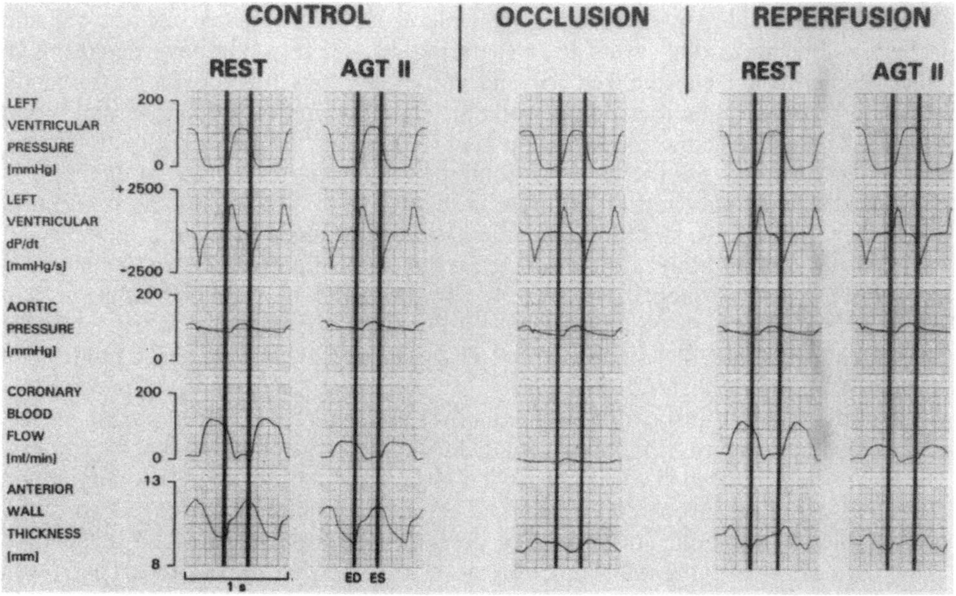

Fig. 3. Representative original recording demonstrating the effects of AGT II (0.01 μg/kg/min i.c.) on systemic hemodynamics, coronary blood flow and regional myocardial wall function. The coronary vasoconstriction induced by AGT II is not augmented during reperfusion following 15 min complete coronary occlusion.

As the renin-angiotensin-system is activated at the early onset of myocardial ischemia (33), AGT may play a role in the extension of irreversible ischemic myocardial damage. A protective role for enalapril in attenuating the development of myocardial infarction was shown within 5 h (66) and 48 h (56) of coronary occlusion in the cat, using ST-segment elevation (66) and creatine kinase (56, 66) as indices of ischemic myocardial damage. Captopril significantly reduced the area at risk and the infarct size (macroscopic enzyme technique) after 6 h of coronary occlusion in anesthetized dogs (32). However, ischemic cell death develops within a time-course of at least 24 h (86). Possibly, captopril (32) and enalapril (66) therefore only delayed cell death, thus pretending a reduction of infarct size at 6 h of coronary occlusion. Conversely, after 24 h of coronary occlusion captopril (29, 68) and teprotide (29) did not reduce infarct size in conscious dogs.

Clinical myocardial ischemia

Findings on the anti-ischemic effects of ACE-inhibitors in patients with coronary artery disease and chronic stable angina are variable (Table 1). As mentioned before, it is difficult to identify the contribution of each of the above potential anti-ischemic mechanisms to the observed clinical results. In several studies reduced oxygen consumption was a common finding. At rest, captopril (16, 27, 28, 49, 72, 90), and teprotide (49) given to patients with ischemic heart disease associated with heart failure (16, 49, 72, 90) or hypertension (27, 72) caused a decrease in coronary blood flow which was significantly correlated to the reduction of the rate-pressure product.

Table 1. Clinical results with different ACE inhibitors in patients with coronary artery disease (CAD).

ACE I	Disease	Rate-pressure product	Coronary blood flow	Exercise duration	ST-segment depression	No. of patients	Authors
REST							
Captopril	CHF, CAD	↓	↓			15	Chatterjee et al. (1982) (16)
Captopril	H, CAD	↓	↓			8	Daly et al. (1984) (27)
Captopril	CAD	↓	↓			14	Daly et al. (1985) (28)
Captopril	CHF, CAD	↓	(↓)			11	Halperin et al. (1982) (49)
Teprotide							
Captopril	CHF, CAD	↓	↓			47	Mettauer et al. (1986) (72)
Captopril	CHF, CAD	↓	↓			14	Rouleau et al. (1982) (90)
EXERCISE							
Captopril	CAD	—		(12↑/5—/5↓)		22	Daly et al. (1985) (28)
Captopril	CAD	—			(8↓/2—/0↑)	10	Keck (1987) (60)
Captopril	CAD	(↓)		(12↑ mean value)	(12↓ mean value)	12	Strozzi et al. (1987) (94)
Captopril	CAD	—	(3↓/6↑)		(8↓ mean value/1↑)	9	Tardieu et al. (1986) (95)
Cilazapril	CAD	—	(1↓/7↑)	(5↑/3—/0↓)	(6↓/2—/0↑)	8	Gasic et al. (1990) (37)
Enalapril	CAD	↓		(8↑/1—/3↓)		12	Gibbs et al. (1989) (40)
Enalapril	CAD	—		(8↑ mean value)	(8↓ mean value)	8	Laj et al. (1987) (64)
Enalapril	CAD	—			(9↑/2—/1↑)	12	Rietbrock et al. (1988) (87)
Quinalapril	CAD	↓			(10↓/0—/0↑)	10	Bussmann et al. (1988) (13)
Quinalapril	CAD	↓			(16↓ mean value)	16	Winkelmann et al. (1991) (102)
Ramipril	CAD	—			(18— mean value)	18	Unterberg et al. (1990) (99)
Benazepril	CAD	—		(23— mean value)	(23— mean value)	23	Klein et al. (1990) (61)
Benazepril	CAD	—		(11— mean value)	(5↓/3—/3↑)	11	Odenthal et al. (1991) (79)

CHF: chronic heart failure, H: hypertension, ACE I: ACE inhibitor

However, despite an improvement of ventricular function, in some patients lactate production occurred (16, 28, 72).

The rate-pressure product was also reduced during exercise-induced ischemia (bicycle, treadmill) in patients treated with captopril (94), enalapril (40), and quinalapril (13). Pooling all data obtained during excercise, captopril (28, 60, 94, 95), cilazapril (37), enalapril (40, 64, 72), and quinalapril (13) significantly prolonged exercise time until myocardial ischemia was precipitated (28, 37, 40, 64, 94) and reduced ST-segment depression (13, 37, 60, 64, 72, 94, 102). However, about 30% of all patients exhibited no increase in excercise time (28, 37, 40) and no attenuation of ST-segment depression (37, 60, 72) or even a deterioration of both parameters (28, 40, 72, 79, 95). Ramipril and benazepril did not attenuate exercise-induced myocardial ischemia (61, 99). Benazeprilat even increased lactate production in four out of six patients with heart failure during pacing-induced ischemia (91). An improvement of myocardial perfusion was detected using myocardial scintigraphy during exercise-induced ischemia in patients treated with captopril (28) and cilazapril (37). However, in 33% of the captopril- and 12% of the cilazapril-treated patients, myocardial perfusion simultaneously deteriorated in another zone, indicating a coronary steal phenomenon.

Thus, ACE-inhibitors may exert an anti-ischemic effect during exercise in patients with coronary artery disease and stable angina. However, despite the positive trend, a significant number of patients does not benefit or even deteriorates when treated with ACE-inhibitors.

In conclusion, although there is some suggestive evidence for an anti-ischemic action of ACE-inhibitors, solid experimental data are still lacking. In particular, it remains unclear to what extent an anti-ischemic action of ACE-inhibitors is through interaction with the bradykinin-prostaglandin-system, through reduction of AGT-mediated coronary vasoconstriction or through a reduction in afterload and myocardial oxygen consumption. Although several clinical studies indicate anti-ischemic actions of ACE-inhibitors, a significant fraction of patients does not benefit or even deteriorates. Unless the mechanisms and determinants of antiischemic action of ACE-inhibitors can be better defined, their use for treatment of myocardial ischemia cannot be recommended at present (70).

Whereas the acute anti-ischemic actions of ACE-inhibition, thus, have to be judged skeptically, a beneficial effect of ACE-inhibition on more chronic sequelae of myocardial ischemia such as infarct expansion, ventricular remodeling and finally mortality are more promissing, both in experimental animals (82) and in man (83).

References

1. Alam S, Rezkalla S, Farkas P, Prcevski P, Figures G, Turi ZG (1989) Does captopril ameliorate myocardial ischemia during coronary balloon occlusion? Circulation 80 (suppl II):II—52 (abstr)
2. Austin RE, Aldea GS, Coggins DL, Flynn AE, Hoffman JIE (1990) Profound spatial heterogeneity of coronary reserve. Discordance between patterns of resting and maximal myocardial blood flow. Circ Res 67:319—331
3. Aversano T, Becker LC (1985) Persistence of coronary vasodilator reserve despite functionally significant flow reduction. Am J Physiol 248:H403—H411

4. Bassenge E, Walter P, Doutheil U (1967) Wirkungsumkehr der adrenergischen Coronargefässreaktion in Abhängigkeit vom Coronargefässtonus. Pfluegers Arch 297: 146—155
5. Bassenge E, Heusch G (1990) Endothelial and neuro-humoral control of coronary blood flow in health and disease. Rev Physiol Biochem Pharmacol 116:77—165
6. Berdeaux A, Bonhenry C, Giudicelli JF (1987) Effects of four angiotensin I converting enzyme inhibitors on regional myocardial blood flow and ischemic injury during coronary artery occlusion in dogs. Fundam Clin Pharmacol 1:201—212
7. Berkenboom GM, Abramowicz M, Vandermoten P, Degre SG (1986) Role of alpha-adrenergic coronary tone in exercise-induced angina pectoris. Am J Cardiol 57: 195—198
8. Berkenboom G, Unger P (1991) Alpha-adrenergic coronary constriction in effort angina. In: Heusch G, Ross J (eds) Adrenergic mechanisms in myocardial ischemia, Darmstadt, Steinkopff, p 359—369
9. Bretschneider HJ (1967) Aktuelle Probleme der Koronardurchblutung und des Myokardstoffwechsels. Regensburger Jbl Aerztl Fortb 15:1—27
10. Brown BG, Lee AB, Bolson EL, Dodge HT (1984) Reflex constriction of significant coronary stenosis as a mechanism contributing to ischemic left ventricular dysfunction during isometric exercise. Circulation 70:18—24
11. Brown BG, Bolson EL, Dodge HT (1984) Dynamic mechanisms in human coronary stenosis. Circulation 70:917—922
12. Buffington CW, Feigl EO (1981) Adrenergic coronary vasoconstriction in the presence of coronary stenosis in the dog. Circ Res 48:416—423
13. Bussman W-D, Goerke S, Schneider W, Kaltenbach M (1988) Angiotensin converting enzyme inhibitor in angina. Dtsch Med Wschr 113:548—550
14. Canty JM, Klocke FJ (1985) Reduced regional myocardial perfusion in the presence of pharmacologic vasodilator reserve. Circulation 71:370—377
15. Canty JM (1992) Barbiturate-anesthesia does not affect coronary autoregulatory responses in closed-chest dogs. Faseb J 6:A1751—(abstr.)
16. Chatterjee K, Rouleau J-L, Parmley WW (1982) Haemodynamic and myocardial metabolic effects of captopril in chronic heart failure. Br Heart J 47:233—238
17. Chen DG, Dai X-Z, Zimmerman BG, Bache RJ (1988) Postsynaptic α1- and α2-adrenergic mechanisms in coronary vasoconstriction. J Cardiovasc Pharmacol 11:61—67
18. Chierchia S, Davies G, Berkenboom G, Crean F, Crean P, Maseri A (1984) α-adrenergic receptors and coronary spasm: an elusive link. Circulation 69:8—14
19. Chierchia S, Pratt T, DeCoster P, Maseri A (1985) Alpha-adrenergic control of collateral flow: another determinant of coronary flow reserve. Circulation 72:(suppl III):190—(abstr.)
20. Chilian WM, Harrison DG, Haws CW, Snyder WD, Marcus ML (1986) Adrenergic coronary tone during submaximal exercise in the dog is produced by circulating catecholamines. Evidence for adrenergic denervation supersensitivity in the myocardium but not in coronary vessels. Circ Res 58:68—82
21. Chilian WM, Ackell PH (1988) Transmural differences in sympathetic coronary constriction during exercise in the presence of coronary stenosis. Circ Res 62:216—225
22. Chilian WM (1991) Functional distribution of α1- and α2-adrenergic receptors in the coronary microcirculation. Circulation 84:2108—2122
23. Coggins DL, Flynn AE, Austin RE Jr, Aldea GS, Muehrcke D, Goto M, Hoffman JIE (1990) Nonuniform loss of regional flow reserve during myocardial ischemia in dogs. Circ Res 67:253—264
24. Cohen MV, Kirk ES (1973) Differential response of large and small coronary arteries to nitroglycerin and angiotensin. Circ Res 33:445—453
25. Collins P, Sheridan D (1985) Improvement in angina pectoris with alpha adrenoceptor blockade. Br Heart J 53:488—492

26. Constantine JW, Lebel W (1980) Complete blockade by phenoxybenzamine of alpha 1- but not of alpha 2-vascular receptors in dogs and the effect of propranolol. Naunyn Schmiedebergs Arch Pharmacol 314:149—156
27. Daly P, Rouleau J-L, Cousineau D, Burgess JH (1984) Acute effects of captopril on the coronary circulation of patients with hypertension and angina. Am J Med 31: 111—115
28. Daly P, Mettauer B, Rouleau J-L, Cousineau D, Burgess JH (1985) Lack of reflex increase in myocardial sympathetic tone after captopril: potential antianginal effect. Circulation 71:317—325
29. Daniell HB, Carson RR, Ballard KD, Thomas GR, Privitera PJ (1984) Effects of captopril on limiting infarct size in conscious dogs. J Cardiovasc Pharmacol 6: 1043—1047
30. de Lorgeril M, Ovize M, Delaye J, Renaud S (1992) Importance of the flow perfusion deficit in the response to captopril in experimental myocardial infarction. J Cardiovasc Pharmacol 19:324—329
31. Deussen A, Heusch G, Thämer V (1985) Alpha 2-adrenoceptor — mediated coronary vasoconstriction persists after exhaustion of coronary dilator reserve. Eur J Pharmacol 115:147-153
32. Ertl G, Kloner RA, Alexander RW, Braunwald E (1982) Limitation of experimental infarct size by an angiotensin-converting enzyme inhibitor. Circulation 65:40—48
33. Ertl G, Alexander RW, Kloner RA (1983) Interactions between coronary occlusion and the renin-angiotensin system in the dog. Basic Res Cardiol 78:518—533
34. Ertl G (1987) Coronary vasoconstriction in experimental myocardial ischemia. J Cardiovasc Pharmacol 9 (suppl 2):S9—S17
35. Feigl EO (1983) Coronary physiology. Physiol Rev 63:1—205
36. Gage JE, Hess OM, Murakami T, Ritter M, Grimm J, Krayenbuehl HP (1986) Vasoconstriction of stenotic coronary arteries during dynamic exercise in patients with classic angina pectoris: reversibility by nitroglycerin. Circulation 73:865—876
37. Gasic S, Dudczak R, Korn A, Kleinbloesem C (1990) ACE inhibition with cilazapril improves myocardial perfusion to the ischemic regions during exercise: a pilot study. J Cardiovasc Pharmacol 15:227—232
38. Gavras H, Kremer D, Brown JJ, Gray B, Lever AF, MacAdam RF, Medina A, Morton JJ, Robertson JIS (1975) Angiotensin- and norepinephrine-induced myocardial lesions: experimental and clinical studies in rabbits and man. Am Heart J 89:321—332
39. Gewirtz H, Most AS, Williams DO (1982) The effect of generalized alpha-receptor stimulation on regional myocardial blood flow distal to a severe coronary artery stenosis. Circulation 65:1329—1336
40. Gibbs JSR, Crean PA, Mockus L, Wright C, Sutton GC, Fox KM (1989) The variable effects of angiotensin converting enzyme inhibition on myocardial ischaemia in chronic stable angina. Br Heart J 62:112—117
41. Gorman MW, Sparks HV Jr (1982) Progressive coronary vasoconstriction during relative ischemia in canine myocardium. Circ Res 51:411—420
42. Gould L, Reddy GV, Gombrecht RF (1973) Oral phentolamine in angina pectoris. Jpn Heart J 14:393—397
43. Gould KL (1980) Dynamic coronary stenosis. Am J Cardiol 45:286—292
44. Gratan MT, Hanley FL, Stevens MB, Hoffman JIE (1986) Transmural coronary flow reserve patterns in dogs. Am J Physiol 250:H276—H283
45. Grover GJ, Sleph PG, Dzwonczyk S, Wang P, Fung W, Tobias D, Cushman DW (1991) Effects of different angiotensin-converting enzyme (ACE) inhibitors on ischemic isolated rat hearts: relationship between cardiac ACE inhibition and cardioprotection. J Pharmacol Exp Ther 257:919—929
46. Gunther S, Green L, Muller JE, Mudge GH, Grossman W (1981) Prevention by nifedipine of abnormal coronary vasoconstriction in patients with coronary artery disease. Circulation 63:849—855

47. Guth BD, Heusch G, Indolfi C, Thaulow E, Ross J Jr (1989) Alphal-adrenergic blockade reduces exercise-induced ischemia and contractile dysfunction in conscious dogs. Circulation 80 Suppl II:II—98
48. Gwirtz PA, Stone HL (1982) Coronary blood flow changes following activation of adrenergic receptors in the conscious dog. Am J Physiol 243:H13—H19
49. Halperin JL, Faxon DP, Creager MA, Bass TA, Melidossian CD, Gavras H, Ryan TJ (1982) Coronary hemodynamic effects of angiotensin inhibition by captopril and teprotide in patients with congestive heart failure. Am J Cardiol 50:967—972
50. Heusch G (1990) α-adrenergic mechanisms in myocardial ischemia. Circulation 81:1—13
51. Heusch G, Deussen A, Thämer V (1985) Cardiac sympathetic nerve activity and progressive vasoconstriction distal to coronary stenoses: feed-back aggravation of myocardial ischemia. J Auton Nerv Syst 13:311—326
52. Heusch G, Yoshimoto N, Heegemann H, Thämer V (1983) Interaction of methoxamine with compensatory vasodilation distal to coronary stenoses. Drug Res 33:1647 to 1650
53. Heusch G, Guth BD, Seitelberger R, Ross J Jr (1987) Attenuation of exercise-induced myocardial ischemia in dogs with recruitment of coronary vasodilator reserve by nifedipine. Circulation 75:482—490
54. Heusch G, Deussen A (1983) The effects of cardiac sympathetic nerve stimulation on the perfusion of stenotic coronary arteries in the dog. Circ Res 53:8—15
55. Heusch G, Deussen A (1984) Nifedipine prevents sympathetic vasoconstriction distal to severe coronary stenoses. J Cardiovasc Pharmacol 6:378—383
56. Hock CE, Ribeiro LGT, Lefer AM (1985) Preservation of ischemic myocardium by a new converting enzyme inhibitor, enalaprilic acid, in acute myocardial infarction. Am Heart J 109:222—228
57. Hoffman JIE (1978) Determinants and prediction of transmural myocardial perfusion. Circulation 58:381—391
58. Hossack KF, Brown BF, Stewart DK, Dodge HT (1984) Diltiazem-induced blockade of sympathetically mediated constriction of normal and diseased coronary arteries: lack of epicardial coronary dilatory effect in humans. Circulation 70:465—471
59. Jones CE, Liang IYS, Maulsby MR (1986) Cardiac and coronary effects of prazosin and phenoxybenzamine during coronary hypotension. J Pharmacol Exp Ther 236: 204—211
60. Keck M (1987) Anti-ischaemic effect of captopril in patients with stable angina pectoris. Herz-Kreisl 19:319—321
61. Klein WW, Khurmi NS, Eber B, Dusleag J (1990) Effects of benazepril and metoprolol OROS alone and in combination on myocardial ischemia in patients with chronic stable angina. J Am Coll Cardiol 16:948—956
62. Kopia GA, Kopaciewicz LJ, Ruffolo RR Jr (1986) Alpha andrenoceptor regulation of coronary artery blood flow in normal and stenotic canine coronary arteries. J Pharmacol Exp Ther 239:641—647
63. Krajcar M, Baumgart D, Heusch G (1992) No augmentation of coronary constrictor responses to angiotensin II in reversibly injured, reperfused myocardium. Eur Heart J (abstract) 13 (suppl):436
64. Laj C, Onnis E, Orani E, Pirasi R, Soro A, Cherchi A (1987) Antiischaemic activity of ACE inhibitor enalapril in normotensive patients with stable effort angina. J Am Coll Cardiol 9:192A—(abstr.)
65. Laxson DD, Dai X-Z, Homans DC, Bache RJ (1989) The role of α1- and α2-adrenergic receptors in mediation of coronary vasoconstriction in hypoperfused ischemic myocardium during exercise. Circ Res 65:1688—1697
66. Lefer AM, Peck RC (1984) Cardioprotective effects of enalapril in acute myocardial ischemia. Pharmacology 29:61—69
67. Levene DL, Freeman MR (1976) α-adrenoceptor-mediated coronary artery spasm. J Am Med Assoc 236:1018—1022

68. Liang C-S, Gavras H, Black J, Sherman LG, Hood WB Jr (1982) Renin-angiotensin system inhibition in acute myocardial infarction in dogs. Effects on systemic hemodynamics, myocardial blood flow, segmental myocardial function and infarct size. Circulation 66:1249—1255
69. Liang IYS, Jones CE (1985) Alpha 1- adrenergic blockade increases coronary blood flow during coronary hypoperfusion. Am J Physiol 249:H1070—H1077
70. Linder C, Heusch G (1990) ACE inhibitors for the treatment of myocardial ischemia? Cardiovasc Drugs Ther 4:1375—1384
71. McGrath JC (1982) Evidence for more than one type of postjunctional alpha-adrenoceptor. Biochem Pharmacol 31:467—484
72. Mettauer B, Rouleau J-L, Daly P (1986) The effect of captopril on the coronary circulation and myocardial metabolism of patients with coronary artery disease. Postgrad Med J 62(suppl 1):54—58
73. Miyamoto MI, Rockman HA, Guth BD, Heusch G, Ross J Jr (1991) Effect of α-adrenergic stimulation on regional contractile function and myocardial blood flow with and without ischemia. Circulation 84:1715—1724
74. Mudge GH, Grossman W, Mills RM Jr, Lesch M, Braunwald E (1976) Reflex increase in coronary vascular resistance in patients with ischemic heart disease. N Engl J Med 295:1333—1337
75. Mudge GH, Goldberg S, Gunther S, Mann T, Grossman W (1979) Comparison of metabolic and vasoconstrictor stimuli on coronary vascular resistance in man. Circulation 59:544—550
76. Mueller HS, Rao PS, Rao PB, Gory DJ, Mudd JG, Ayres SM (1982) Enhanced transcardiac l-norepinephrine response during cold pressor test in obstructive coronary artery disease. Am J Cardiol 50:1223—1228
77. Nabel EG, Ganz P, Gordon JB, Alexander RW, Selwyn AP (1988) Dilation of normal and constriction of atherosclerotic coronary arteries caused by the cold pressor test. Circulation 77:43—52
78. Nathan HJ, Feigl EO (1986) Adrenergic vasoconstriction lessens transmural steal during coronary hypoperfusion. Am J Physiol 250:H645—H653
79. Odenthal HJ, Thürmann P, Wiechmann HW, Josephs W, Lenga P (1991) Treatment of chronic stable angina pectoris with ACE-inhibition. A randomized, placebo-controlled, doubleblind cross-over study. Z Kardiol 80:392—396
80. Pantely GA, Bristow JD, Swenson LJ, Ladley HD, Johnson WB, Anselone CG (1985) Incomplete coronary vasodilation during myocardial ischemia in swine. Am J Physiol 249:H638—H647
81. Pelc LR, Garancis JC, Gross GJ, Warltier DC (1990) Alteration of endothelium-dependent distribution of myocardial blood flow after coronary occlusion and reperfusion. Circulation 81:1928—1937
82. Pfeffer JM (1991) Progressive ventricular dilation in experimental myocardial infarction and its attenuation by angiotensin-converting enzyme inhibition. Am J Cardiol 68:17D-25D
83. Pfeffer MA, Braunwald E, Moyé LA, Basta L, Brown EJ, Cuddy TE, Davis BR, Geltman EM, Goldman S, Flaker GC, Klein M, Lamas GA, Packer M, Rouleau J, Rouleau JL, Rutherford J, Wertheimer JH, Hawkins CM (1992) Effect of captopril on mortality and morbidity in patients with left ventricular dysfunction after myocardial infarction. N Engl J Med 327:669—677
84. Przyklenk K, Kloner RA (1991) Angiotensin converting enzyme inhibitors improve contractile function of stunned myocardium by different mechanisms of action. Am Heart J 121:1319—1330
85. Raizner AE, Chahine RA, Ishimori T, Verani MS, Zacca N, Jamal N, Miller RR, Luchi RJ (1980) Provocation of coronary artery spasm by the cold pressor test. Circulation 62:925—932

86. Reimer KA, Jennings RB, Cobb FR, Murdock RH, Greenfield JC Jr, Becker LC, Bulkley BH, Hutchins GM, Schwartz RP Jr, Bailey KR, Passamani ER (1985) Animal models for protecting ischemic mycoardium: results of the NHLBI cooperative study. Comparison of unconscious and conscious dog models. Circ Res 56: 651—665
87. Rietbrock N, Thürmann P, Kirsten R, Schneider W (1988) Anti-ischaemic effect of enalapril in coronary heart-disease. A randomised, placebo-controlled doubleblind trial on 12 patients. Dtsch Med Wschr 113:300—302
88. Robertson RM, Bernard YD, Carr RK, Robertson D (1983) Alpha-adrenergic blockade in vasotonic angina: lack of efficacy of specific alphal-receptor blockade with prazosin. J Am Coll Cardiol 2:1146—1150
89. Rosendorff C, Hoffman JIE, Verrier ED, Rouleau J, Boerboom LE (1981) Cholesterol potentiates the coronary artery response to norepinephrine in anesthetized and conscious dogs. Circ Res 48:320—329
90. Rouleau J-L, Chatterjee K, Benge W, Parmely WW, Hiramatsu B (1982) Alterations in left ventricular function and coronary hemodynamics with captopril, hydralazine and prazosin in chronic ischemic heart failure: a comparative study. Circulation 65:671—678
91. Rousseau MF, Close P, Pouleur H (1989) Are the angiotensin-converting enzyme inhibitors poor anti-ischemic drugs? Circulation 80(suppl II):II—52—(abstr.)
92. Schulz R, Oudiz RJ, Guth BD, Heusch G (1990) Minimal α1- and α2-adrenoceptor-mediated coronary vasoconstriction in the anaesthetized swine. Naunyn Schmiedebergs Arch Pharmacol 342:422—428
93. Seitelberger R, Guth BD, Heusch G, Lee JD, Katayama K, Ross J Jr (1988) Intracoronary alpha 2- adrenergic receptor blockade attenuates ischemia in conscious dogs during exercise. Circ Res 62:436—442
94. Strozzi C, Cocco G, Portaluppi F, Urso L, Alfiero R, Tasini MT, Montanari L, Al Yassini K, Rizzo A (1987) Effects of captopril on the physical work capacity of normotensive patients with stable-effort angina pectoris. Cardiology 74:226—228
95. Tardieu A, Virot P, Vandroux JC, Vergnoux H, Pinaud D, Chabanier A, Bensaid J (1986) Effects of captopril on myocardial perfusion in patients with coronary insufficiency: evaluation by the exercise test and quantitative myocardial tomoscintigraphy using thallium-201. Postgrad Med J 62(suppl 1):38—41
96. Tsao PS, Aoki N, Lefer DJ, Johnson G, Lefer AM (1990) Time course of endothelial dysfunction and myocardial injury during myocardial ischemia and reperfusion in the cat. Circulation 82:1402—1412
97. Tulenko TN, Constantinescu D, Kikuchi T, Cox RH, Santamore WP (1989) Mutual interaction of vasoconstriction and endothelial damage in stenotic arteries. Am J Physiol 256:H881—H889
98. Tzivoni D, Keren A, Benhorin J, Gottlieb S, Atlas D, Stern S (1983) Prazosin therapy for refractory variant angina. Am Heart J 105:262—266
99. Unterberg C, Buchwald A, Vogt A, Wiegand V (1990) Akute Effekte des Angiotensin-Converting-Enzym-Hemmers Ramipril bei Patienten mit koronarer Herzerkrankung. Med Klin 85:78—81
100. van Gilst WH, Scholtens E, de Graeff PA, de Langen CDJ, Wesseling H (1988) Differential influences of angiotensin converting-enzyme inhibitors on the coronary circulation. Circulation 77(suppl I):I—24—I—29
101. van Wijngaarden J, Tio RA, van Gilst WH, de Graeff PA, de Langen CDJ, Wesseling H (1991) Coronary vasodilation induced by captopril and zofenoprilat: evidence for a prostaglandin-independent mechanism. Naunyn Schmiedebergs Arch Pharmacol 343:491—495
102. Winkelmann BR, Bettinger B, Wittig R, Brunner I, Bahrmann H, Bussmann W-D (1991) Antianginal effects of quinapril in patients with coronary artery disease. Eur Heart J 12(suppl):355

103. Winniford MD, Filipchuk N, Hillis LD (1983) Alpha-adrenergic blockade for variant angina: a long-term, double-blind, randomized trial. Circulation 67:1185—1188
104. Yasue H, Touyama M, Kato H, Tanaka S, Akiyama F (1976) Prinzmetal's variant form of angina as a manifestation of alpha-adrenergic receptor-mediated coronary artery spasm: documentation by coronary arteriography. Am Heart J 91: 148-155
105. Yilmaz G, Aksulu HE, Demirel E, Ercan ZS, Zengil H, Türker RK (1987) Modulation by endothelium of the vascular effects of angiotensin II. Agents Actions 21:184—190
106. Zeiher AM, Drexler H, Wollschlaeger H, Saurbier B, Just H (1989) Coronary vasomotion in response to sympathetic stimulation in humans: importance of the functional integrity of the endothelium. J Am Coll Cardiol 14:1181—1190

Authors' address:
Prof. Dr. Gerd Heusch
Abteilung für Pathophysiologie
Zentrum für Innere Medizin
Universitätsklinikum Essen
Hufelandstraße 55
4300 Essen

ACE-inhibitors in coronary artery disease?

M. Vogt, W. Motz, B. E. Strauer

Department of Medicine, Division of Cardiology, Pneumology and Angiology, Heinrich-Heine-University of Düsseldorf, FRG

Summary: Angiotensin converting enzyme (ACE)-inhibitors are established in the treatment of arterial hypertension and heart failure. In recent years ACE-inhibitors have also been used in the treatment of patients with coronary artery disease (CAD), since from experimental data an antiischemic action of these agents is suggested. Antiischemic effects of ACE-inhibitors may be exerted through a reduction of myocardial oxygen demand, by a reduction of angiotensin-mediated coronary vasoconstriction, by an interaction with bradykinin and the prostaglandin system, by a modulation of endothelial control of vascular tone, and by an interaction with the sympathetic nervous system. However, clinical findings on potential beneficial effects of ACE-inhibitors in patients with CAD are inconsistent and controversial. While in hypertensive patients with CAD ACE-inhibitors generally seem to attenuate myocardial ischemia at rest and during exercise, a significant fraction of about 30% of normotensive patients with CAD does not benefit or even deteriorates. Lowering of coronary perfusion pressure and alteration of transmural blood flow distribution may be responsible for this. In patients with left ventricular dysfunction (SOLVD) or congestive heart failure (CONSENSUS, SOLVD) ACE-inhibitors have been proven to prevent progressive deterioration in left ventricular function and to reduce mortality. In patients with asymptomatic left ventricular dysfunction after myocardial infarction (SAVE), long-term administration of captropril was associated with an improvement in survival and reduced morbidity and mortality due to major cardiovascular events. Therefore, from a prognostic viewpoint patients with CAD and left ventricular dysfunction or congestive heart failure should be treated with ACE-inhibitors, although the clinical use of ACE-inhibitors in patients with ongoing angina pectoris may be limited by an aggravation of angina, presumably due to critically lowering coronary perfusion pressure. Finally, ACE-inhibitors failed to prevent restenosis after successful PTCA. In conclusion, from a prognostic viewpoint patients with CAD and congestive heart failure or left ventricular dysfunction should be treated with ACE-inhibitors. In hypertensive patients ACE-inhibitors generally seem to attenuate myocardial ischemia. In normotensive patients with CAD and angina pectoris but without left ventricular dysfunction ACE-inhibitors cannot generally be recommended at present, unless the patients, which may have benefit from ACE-inhibitor treatment can be better defined.

Key words: ACE-inhibitors; acute myocardial infarction; arterial hypertension; congestive heart failure; coronary artery disease

Introduction

The activated renin-angiotensin-aldosterone system has a variety of actions which may influence systemic and coronary circulatory as well as cardiac function. Apart from the establishment of angiotensin-converting enzyme (ACE) inhibitors in the treatment of hypertension (38, 105, 129, 140) and heart failure (16, 23, 24, 110), these compounds have recieved growing interest with respect to their antiischemic effects and their potential role in the treatment of coronary artery disease. This increasing interest is quite obvious, since arterial hypertension is a major risk factor and often associated with coronary artery disease (58, 59). Furthermore, ischemic heart disease is frequently the underlying cause of chronic congestive heart failure (24, 135). From a theoretical point of view ACE-inhibitors exert favorable effects for their use in patients with coronary artery disease by their vasodilatatory reaction without inducing reflex tachycardia (26, 40). However, the mode of action of ACE-inhibitors is very complex and the findings concerning their use in the treatment of patients with coronary artery disease are controversial.

The purpose of the present paper was to define the potential antiischemic effects of ACE-inhibitors and to discuss the available clinical data concerning the use of ACE-inhibitors in the treatment of coronary artery disease including acute and chronic phase of myocardial infarction.

Physiology of the renin-angiotensin system

The renin-angiotensin system was originally percieved as a classical humoral system, in which the proteolytic enzyme renin is released from the kidneys in response to a decrease in perfusion pressure or upon beta adrenergic stimulation (66). Renin acts on the circulating antiogensinogen, synthesized in the liver, to generate the decapeptide angiotensin I, which is converted to its active form angiotensin II, catalysed by the endothelium-bound angiotensin-converting enzyme. Angiotensin II represents a potent vasoconstrictor, which is rapidly inactivated by angiotensinases with a half-life of about 10 min in humans (96). The carboxypeptidase ACE is identical to the enzyme kininase II and simultaneously inactivates the nonapeptide bradykinin (137, 138). In renal hypertension or in conditions with sodium depletion plasma levels of renin and angiotensin II are elevated and contribute to the blood-pressure regulation (70). Increased plasma levels of renin and angiotensin II have also been found in patients with coronary artery disease, particularly during exercise-induced myocardial ischemia, as well as in myocardial infarction (27, 40, 84). Therefore, a reduction in plasma renin and angiotensin II levels by ACE-inhibitors may become relevant in myocardial ischemia.

During the past decade the view of the renin-angiotensin system has been witnessed by molecular biologic and immunohistochemical studies demonstrating various components of the renin-angiotensin system in various tissues (37, 57). The discovery of expression of renin and angiotensinogen genes and m-RNA, renin-like activity, angiotensin and angiotensin-converting enzyme in the myocardium, the vascular smooth muscle, and the coronary endothelium have accumulated evidence for the existence of a functional cardiac tissue renin-angiotensin system (14, 36, 74, 120). However, the relative contribution of local cardiac angiotensin formation to coronary vasomotor tone and its effects on the coronary vasculature are still under discussion.

Potential antiischemic effects of ACE-inhibitors

Apart from coronary morphology, the overall level of coronary flow is principally determined by the coronary perfusion pressure or, more exactly, the driving pressure gradient for coronary blood flow, myocardial metabolic requirements, coronary vasomotor tone, neural factors (sympathetic and parasympathetic nervous system) and by various humoral factors. ACE-inhibitors can act on each of these determinants to a various degree depending on the state of activation and the relative contribution of these components to coronary vascular resistance (Table 1).

Table 1. ACE-Inhibitors in coronary artery disease: Potential antiischemic effects.

1) Inhibition of systemic and local angiotensin II formation
2) Reduction in left ventricular pre- and afterload
3) Decrease in contractility?
4) Interaction with sympathetic nervous system
5) Lack of reflex-induced tachycardia
6) Interaction with bradykinin metabolism
7) Interaction with prostaglandin synthesis
8) Interaction with endothelium-dependent relaxation (role of sulfhydryl group?)
9) Modulation of endothelin-induced vasoconstriction
10) Alteration of vascular permeability
11) Inhibition of leukocyte chemotaxis

Coronary perfusion pressure

As in any vascular bed, blood flow in the coronary bed depends on the driving pressure and the resistance offered by this bed. Theoretically, the effective coronary driving pressure is the pressure gradient between the aortic pressure and the pressure in either the right atrium or left ventricle in diastole, since coronary flow drains mainly in these two chambers. However, the resistance offered by the coronary bed is influenced importantly by extravascular compressing forces and is not constant throughout the cardiac cycle. Thus, the effective coronary driving pressure is mainly the pressure gradient between aortic and left ventricular pressure. ACE-inhibitors have a dual impact on coronary driving pressure gradient. The main systemic effect of ACE-inhibitors is an arterial vasodilation, which may be accompanied by a drop in aortic pressure and, hence, in coronary perfusion pressure. On the other hand, ACE-inhibitors may enhance the driving pressure gradient for coronary blood flow by reducing the extravascular component of coronary resistance due to a reduction in left ventricular pre- and afterload.

A reduction in aortic pressure following the application of ACE-inhibitors is a common finding, although the degree of aortic-pressure-lowering may vary considerably, depending on the degree of activation of the renin-angiotensin-system and the dosage of ACE-inhibitors used. While in normotensive patients with coronary artery disease and chronic stable angina pectoris, as well as in patients with coronary artery disease and chronic congestive heart failure, the drop in aortic pressure is rather moderate, not exceeding 10 to 15% (13, 20, 25, 26), there may be a dramatic drop in aortic pressure in acute myocardial infarction (118, 131).

Consequently, the clinical use of ACE-inhibitors in the very early phase of acute myocardial infarction may be afflicted with the risk of severe reduction in blood pressure. Since activation of renin-angiotensin system in acute myocardial infarction is quite variable (27, 84), ACE-inhibitors may lead to an unpredictable drop of blood pressure with consecutive deterioration of coronary perfusion. Captopril given orally to patients with subacute myocardial infarction and congestive heart failure resulted in a critical reduction of mean aortic pressure to below 70 mmHg in three out of seven patients (80). This risk of marked reduction in blood pressure was confirmed by others (11, 131).

In patients with coronary artery disease and chronic congestive heart failure, Kiowski et al. (65) studied the acute effects of the ACE-inhibitor cilazapril. In these patients they observed a reduction in blood pressure, in systemic vascular resistance, as well as in coronary vascular resistance, while coronary sinus blood flow remained unchanged. In contrast, Rouleau et al. (101), using captopril in patients with ischemic heart disease, observed a reduction in coronary perfusion pressure and in coronary blood flow. Furthermore, the reduction in coronary blood flow was in parallel with reduced myocardial oxygen consumption and coronary perfusion pressure, suggesting an unaltered coronary vascular resistance. Thus, while a moderate reduction in coronary perfusion pressure could generally be observed also in patients with congestive heart failure due to ischemic heart disease and in normotensive patients with coronary artery disease and chronic stable angina pectoris, the findings on coronary flow response to ACE-inhibitors are quite variable and the differences difficult to explain.

Regional myocardial blood flow distribution

Due to the cyclic action of the heart and its anatomical shape myocardial blood flow is inhomogeneous with respect to the time course, i.e., systolic and diastolic flow, and with respect to the transmural distribution. Regional myocardial blood flow distribution is even more complex when stenosis of the epicardial coronary arteries occur. Since atherosclerotic coronary artery disease is not a homogeneous process, but rather different vascular regions are concerned to a different extent, the effects of ACE-inhibitors on regional myocardial blood flow distribution are of major interest and are the result of a complex interaction of potential anti-ischemic mechanism of these agents. In one study, using anesthetized dogs, captopril and saralasin, a competitive angiotensin-receptor antagonist, increased coronary arterial inflow during 30 min of coronary occlusion (41). However, this increase was mainly due to an increased regional myocardial blood flow in nonischemic and border zones, while a reduction of subendocardial blood flow of the most ischemic zone was apparent. In two other studies using anesthetized and conscious dogs, captopril, trandolapril, enalapril and ramipril (5), as well as teprotide (71), neither improved regional blood flow to nonischemic nor to ischemic subendocardial layers during 12 to 60 min of coronary occlusion. This finding of a tendency towards a decrease in regional myocardial blood flow in the most ischemic subendocardial layer could speak in favour of the occurrence of a collateral and transmural steal phenomenon following ACE-inhibition, although other reasons, i.e., reduced coronary perfusion pressure, may account for a reduced regional myocardial perfusion.

Metabolic factors

The metabolic demand of the myocardium is determined by systolic wall stress, myocardial contractility, and heart rate. By relieving the vasoconstrictor effects of angiotensin II, ACE-inhibitors reduce ventricular afterload. Furthermore, angiotensin II is known to be one of the most potent stimuli for secretion of aldosterone accompanied by a rise in venous pressure due to sodium and fluid retention; it is also known to be a venoconstrictor at high concentrations, causing a rise in venous return (7). Thus, apart from reduction in afterload, ACE-inhibitors can also reduce preload by influencing these two mechanisms. A decrease in left ventricular chamber size would lead to a further decrease in systolic wall stress and, hence, to a reduction in myocardial oxygen consumption. The beneficial metabolic effects of ACE-inhibitors were further supported by reducing blood pressure without causing reflex-induced tachycardia (26, 40). Finally, there may be a minor reduction in myocardial contractility due to blockade of angiotensin II formation. Under experimental conditions angiotensin II has been shown to have direct and indirect positive inotropic effects (34, 46, 67). However, a significant negative inotropic effect of ACE-inhibitors was not observed under clinical conditions (19, 110).

Interactions with the sympathetic nervous system

The interaction between angiotensin II and the sympathetic nervous system may play an essential role in the potential antiischemic effects of ACE-inhibitors. The majority of studies concluded that the facilitation of sympathetic nervous influences on the heart by angiotensin II is based primarily on an increase in the amount of neurotransmitter released from presynaptic nerve terminals (8, 112, 113). Other mechanisms of sympathetic facilitation by angiotensin II that have been demonstrated include attenuation of prejunctional reuptake (63, 113), stimulation of sympathetic ganglia (1, 117), increased catecholamine biosynthesis (9, 100), release of catecholamines from the adrenal medulla (133), and sensitization of postjunctional structures (21, 28).

Stimulation of presynaptic angiotensin II receptors facilitates the release of norepinephrine, while at the postsynaptic site activation of the angiotensin receptors enhances the responses mediated by both vascular alpha1- and alpha2-adrenoceptors (30, 31, 35). Since alpha2-adrenoceptors seem to play a fundamental role in the constriction of coronary resistance vessels distal to coronary stenoses (52) a potentiating effect of angiotension II on alpha2-adrenergic constrictor effects at the postsynaptic site could be of relevance. Therefore, inhibition of angiotensin II formation might result in reduced sympathetic coronary vasoconstriction under certain pathophysiologic conditions, which are accompanied by an activation of both the sympathetic nervous system and the renin-angiotensin system, such as in exercise-induced myocardial ischemia or heart failure. In patients with heart failure captopril suppresses angiotensin II both at rest and during exercise, although antidiuretic hormone and plasma norepinephrine appear only significantly reduced at rest (19). In other studies on patients with heart failure, enalapril (85) and captopril (26) reduced sympathetic activity and, specifically, transmyocardial norepinephrine release during exercise.

Humoral factors

Several humoral factors act on the coronary circulation. In anesthetized dogs, intracoronary infusion of angiotensin II at constant blood flow induced a constriction of both small and large coronary vessels. In contrast to the large vessels, in which constriction was maintained, small vessels rapidly developed tachyphylaxis (22). Intracoronary bolus injection of angiotensin II at a constant coronary perfusion pressure or intracoronary infusion of angiotensin II at stepwise reductions of coronary perfusion pressures, simulating progressive coronary stenosis (42), have demonstrated a preserved coronary constrictor response. This preserved constrictor response suggested that angiotensin II may still be effective when coronary microcirculation is under the influence of dilator metabolites during myocardial ischemia. Catecholamines with alpha-adrenergic properties can cause constriction of both large epicardial arteries and coronary resistance vessels (139). Endothelin, a polypeptide produced by endothelial cells, is another potent coronary vasoconstrictor (136). In addition to angiotensin II, catecholamines and endothelin, vasopressin, thromboxane A2 or serotonin are major humoral coronary vasoconstrictors (12, 33). On the other hand, a number of endogeneous coronary vasodilators is known. These vasodilators include adenosine, nitric oxide ("endothelium-derived relaxing factor", EDRF), acetylcholine, substance P, atrial natriuretic peptide, bradykinin, and prostaglandins (17, 33, 48, 103). A potential antiischemic effect of ACE-inhibitors may result from their interaction with this complex system of humoral vasoactive substances. Apart from blocking angiotensin II formation, interactions with the sympathetic nervous system, the degradation of bradykinin, the synthesis of prostaglandins and the endothelium-dependent relaxation seem to be predominant.

ACE is identical to the enzyme kininase II, which rapidly inactivates bradykinin (137, 138). Bradykinin is an endothelium-dependent vasodilator, acting through the stimulation of EDRF/NO release (61, 88) and prostaglandin synthesis (87). ACE-inhibitors increase bradykinin levels by inhibition of its inactivation and, therefore, also increase prostaglandin synthesis by the endothelium. However, both bradykinin and prostaglandin levels are increased in myocardial ischemia. In anesthetized dogs, bradykinin levels in the coronary sinus blood were increased within a few minutes after onset of myocardial ischemia (64). Similarly, prostaglandin E and F were released during pacing-induced myocardial ischemia in patients with coronary artery disease (6). An angiotensin-induced generation of prostaglandins in the heart, probably mediated via phospholipase C activation, is described (73). However, whether elevated levels of bradykinin and endogeneous prostaglandins have a protective effect in myocardial ischemia remains to be established. Furthermore, it has to be clarified whether ACE-inhibitors might potentiate these protective effects.

Interaction with endothelium-dependent relaxation

Apart from the interaction with inactivation of bradykinin, which itself is an endothelium-dependent coronary vasodilator, ACE-inhibitors can modulate the endothelium-mediated vasodilation. In distinction to other ACE-inhibitors, captopril and zofenoprilat are sulfhydryl-containing agents. In comparison to captopril and zofenoprilat other sulfhydryl-containing agents without ACE-inhibitor properties, such as cysteine and glutathione, have shown similar vasodilating effects (124). This finding suggested an additional sulfhydryl-mediated dilator mechanism. Sulfhydryls are involved in the vasodilator action of nitro compounds, which exert their vasodilator action by activation of guanylate cyclase. This activation requires the presence of heme. By their ability to reduce heme-iron, sulfhydryl groups facilitate the subsequent formation of NO heme, which seems to be the active compound responsible for the activation of guanylate cyclase (54).

However, the sulfhydryl group seems not to be a prerequisite for an interaction between ACE-inhibitors and the endothelium-dependent coronary vasodilation. Bossaller et al. (10) could demonstrate that chronic treatment with enalapril, an ACE-inhibitor without sulfhydryl group, led to an increase of endothelium-dependent relaxation, while endothelium-independent relaxation was unaltered. These findings support the hypothesis that the activity of angiotension converting enzyme is involved in the regulation of the release of endothelial relaxing factors. Furthermore it could be demonstrated in isolated human and bovine coronary arteries that lisinopril, enalapril, and captopril enhanced the bradykinin-induced vasodilation without increasing the concentration of bradykinin in the organ bath (4). Thus, in addition to the inhibition of inactivation of bradykinin, ACE-inhibitors seem to enhance the bradykinin-mediated release of EDRF by a direct action on the endothelium.

ACE-inhibitors and coronary artery disease under clinical conditions

Angina pectoris is a symptom complex brought about by a relative imbalance between nutritional supply and demand of the myocardium. Integrity of the coronary circulation, adequacy of cardiac output, an adequate coronary perfusion or driving pressure, i.e., the gradient between aortic and left ventricular pressure, as well as the presence of normal hemoglobin and plasma viscosity are important factors of a normal supply. On the other hand, metabolic demand is determined by systolic wall stress, which is defined by intraventricular pressure, chamber size and wall thickness, myocardial contractility and heart rate. Antianginal therapy can act on both supply and demand (Fig. 1).

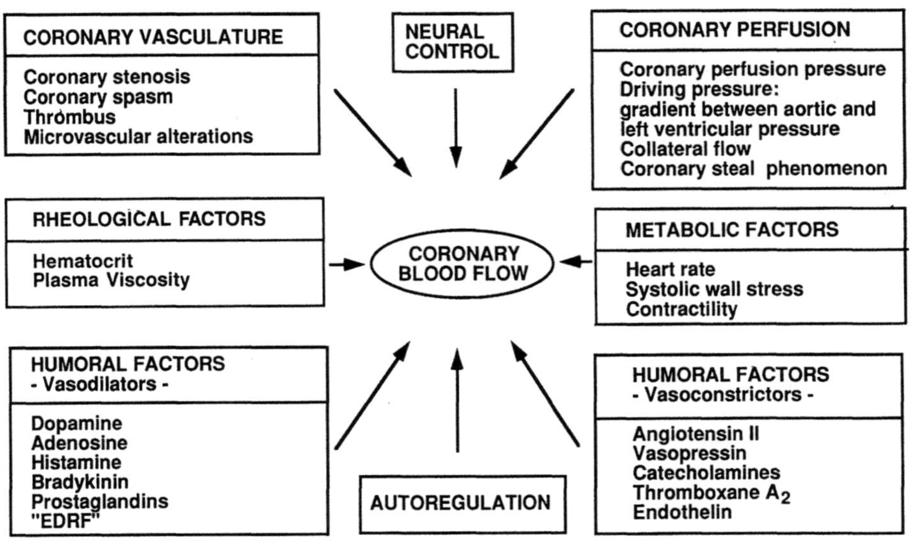

Fig. 1. Schematic presentation of factors involved in the control of the overall level of coronary flow.

Although the body of evidence for potential antiischemic effects of ACE-inhibitors would suggest a beneficial effect in the treatment of angina pectoris, clinical findings on the antiischemic effects of ACE-inhibitors in patients with coronary artery disease and chronic stable angina are variable and inconsistent.

Coronary artery disease and arterial hypertension

Since arterial hypertension is a major risk factor and is often associated with coronary artery disease (58), with the establishment of ACE-inhibitors in the treatment of hypertension the question of an additional antiischemic action of these compounds has prompted interest.

An antiischemic effect of ACE-inhibitors in hypertensive patients with coronary artery disease would be expected through their action on myocardial metabolic demand with a reduction in ventricular pre- and afterload, both contributing to a reduction in systolic wall stress. Furthermore, this antiischemic effect is supported by a lack of reflex-induced tachycardia (26). However, clinical findings were not as convincing as expected. Akhras and Jackson (2) treated hypertensive patients with angina and proven coronary artery disease with captopril. After 2 weeks of treatment captopril increased time to 1 mm ST depression, as well as exercise duration and reduced maximum ST depression in comparison to placebo. In another clinical trial, Strozzi et al. (115) studied 12 hypertensive patients with coronary artery disease during bicycle exercise stress testing. ACE-inhibition by captopril reduced exercise-induced ST segment depression as measured at the maximal rate-pressure product and the incidence of test angina, but did not alter the maximal work load. The number of attacks reported by the patients during normal daily activity was significantly less on the ACE-inhibitor. The authors concluded that ACE-inhibition had an antianginal effect in these hypertensive patients with coronary disease which was not only mediated via its effect on blood pressure or heart rate, but was probably due to coronary vasodilation and increased coronary blood flow. However, at rest captopril given to patients with ischemic heart disease associated with arterial hypertension (25, 83) caused a decrease in coronary blood flow that was mainly due to a reduction in coronary perfusion pressure and was significantly correlated with the reduction of the rate-pressure product and thus a reduced myocardial oxygen consumption. Thus, by reducing coronary blood flow at rest ACE-inhibitors will lead to an increase in coronary reserve in hypertensive patients without any necessary effect on maximal coronary blood flow. Therefore, it can be explained that the exercise time can be increased, but not maximal work load as defined by the rate pressure product.

Regarding the rate-pressure product during exercise a distinction has to be made between the behaviour of heart rate and systolic blood pressure, respectively. An excessive increase in heart rate will lead to a more pronounced deterioration of myocardial oxygen supply than an increase in systolic blood pressure, because an increase in heart rate raises myocardial oxygen demand, while, simultaneously, coronary blood flow was compromised by shortening of diastole and by reduction of the driving pressure due to incomplete relaxation with consecutive increase in left ventricular enddiastolic pressure. On the other hand, an increase in systolic pressure leads to an increase in myocardial oxygen demand, while, simultaneously, the coronary driving pressure was increased and, thus, the balance between demand and supply was less compromised. Furthermore, at the same rate pressure product, which is only an indirect measure of myocardial energy demand, myocardial oxygen demand may be quite different due to alterations in left ventricular geometry and, thus, altered systolic wall stress.

Although beneficial effects of ACE-inhibitors seem to prevail in hypertensive patients with coronary artery disease, in some patients lactate production occurred, suggesting precipitation of myocardial ischemia (83). Finally, in this context it has to be considered that arterial hypertension is often associated with alterations of the coronary microcirculation (114, 127). Hence, in hypertensive patients signs and symptoms of myocardial ischemia may not only result from critical stenoses of epicardial coronary arteries, but may be the consequence of coronary insufficiency due to microvascular alterations. This impaired coronary regulatory capacity at the microvascular level can be attributed to endothelial dysfunction (89) or to structural abnormalities of the coronary resistance vessels, such as medial hypertrophy or perivascular fibrosis (106), both requiring long-term treatment with ACE-inhibitors to improve coronary vasodilating capacity (128).

Coronary artery disease in normotensive patients

While in hypertensive patients with coronary artery disease and stable angina pectoris the beneficial effects of ACE-inhibitors on myocardial ischemia and on angina pectoris seem to be evident and may be attributed to an increase in coronary reserve due to blood pressure control, the question arises of whether ACE-inhibitors develop beneficial effects in normotensive patients with coronary artery disease.

Clinical findings on the anti-ischemic effects of ACE-inhibitors in these patients are variable. The majority of studies has shown that captopril (26, 60, 116, 119), enalapril (50, 68, 98), quinalapril (13), and cilazapril (49) exert an anti-ischemic effect, while some studies could not find such an effect for enalapril (126) and ramipril (121).

However, it is impossible to identify the contribution of each of the above-mentioned potential anti-ischemic mechanisms to the clinical observations. Furthermore to decide whether there is a specific anti-ischemic effect of ACE-inhibitors these studies have to be regarded more detailed. In several studies a reduced oxygen consumption at rest was a common finding. A reduced rate-pressure product was also found during exercise in patients treated with captopril (116), enalapril (50), and quinalapril (13). The assumption of an antiischemic effect was based on the findings that ACE-inhibitors significantly prolonged the exercise time until myocardial ischemia was precipitated (26, 49, 50, 68, 116), reduced the ST segment depression (13, 49, 60, 68, 98, 116, 119), and that these effects could not be related to a reduction in blood pressure. However, as a rule, maximal rate-pressure product was not increased.

Daly et al. (26) reported a decrease in coronary blood flow at rest after captopril given to normotensive paints with coronary artery disease. This decrease in coronary blood flow was significantly correlated with the reduction of the rate-pressure product. Thus, although these patients were normotensive, ACE-inhibition resulted in a reduction in rate-pressure product and presumably in a reduced myocardial oxygen consumption at rest. A further consequence of a reduced resting coronary blood flow is an enhanced coronary flow reserve, which can explain the common finding of an increased exercise time in these patients. The same authors reported a randomized, double-blind, placebo-controlled trial in 22 normotensive patients with chronic stable angina and systolic blood pressure above 120 mmHg. After treatment over 14 days ACE-inhibition by captopril increased exercise time only in those patients with persistent reduction of blood pressure. However, while exercise time was increased, the rate-pressure product at the threshold of angina was not altered (26).

Two other clinical studies questioned a specific antiischemic effect of ACE-inhibitors in normotensive patients with coronary artery disease. For ramipril no attenuation of exercise-induced myocardial ischemia could be detected (121). In our own study on 12 normotensive patients with coronary artery disease, stable angina pectoris and normal left ventricular function enalapril given in addition to preexisting antianginal therapy did not increase exercise time nor attenuate ST segment depression at comparable rate-pressure products. Moreover, in three of the 12 patients therapy had to be discontinued because of severe hypotension and aggravation of angina pectoris (126).

Even in the studies, which derived the result that ACE-inhibitors have an antiischemic effect, about 30% of all patients exhibited no increase in exercise time (26, 49, 50), and no attenuation of ST-segment depression (49, 60, 98), or even showed a deterioration of both parameters (26, 50, 98, 119). The underlying mechanisms for the deterioration in these patients are not clear. Although an improvement of myocardial perfusion was detected using myocardial scintigraphy during exercise in patients treated with captopril (26) and cilazapril (49), in 33% of the captopril- and 12% of the cilazapril-treated patients, myocardial perfusion simultaneously deteriorated in another zone, particularly in the most ischemic subendocardial layers. Critical lowering of coronary perfusion pressure and occurrence of transmural or collateral steal phenomenon, in part due to the interaction between ACE- inhibitors and alpha-adrenergic receptors, may account for this deterioration. Therefore, to decide which normotensive patients may have a benefit from ACE-inhibitor treatment, a further subanalysis of the patients with respect to the coronary status and to a history of myocardial infarction has to be made. In patients with prior myocardial infarction it is of importance whether coronary stenosis is related to the infarcted area or supplies actively contracting regions. In patients with coronary artery disease, angina pectoris, and heart failure, Cleland et al. (20) reported an exacerbation of angina following captopril treatment in those patients with a greater decrease in blood pressure and a stenosis subtending an area of actively contracting regions at rest.

Thus, although ACE-inhibitors exert an antiischemic effect during exercise in normotensive patients with coronary artery disease and stable angina pectoris, a significant number of patients does not benefit or even deteriorates with respect to angina pectoris and myocardial ischemia, when treated with ACE-inhibitors. However, based on the findings of the mentioned clinical studies, the feasibility of a clear statement on the effects of ACE-inhibitors in patients with angina pectoris is limited due to often poor design of the studies, as well as to an often insufficient definition and a limited number of patients. Particularly, chronic effects are difficult to observe, since most of the patients with significant coronary stenosis and angina pectoris undergo interventions.

Coronary artery disease and congestive heart failure

Patients suffering from angina pectoris and heart failure are difficult to manage and have a poor prognosis. Coronary revascularization may be of benefit in carefully selected patients, but the operative morbidity and mortality rates are high because of poor ventricular function, age and other associated problems (62). Furthermore, it is controversial whether successful revascularization can improve severely depressed left ventricular function (3, 47, 53). Patients with heart failure often show markedly elevated preload and afterload which may be due to activation of the sympathetic nervous and the renin angiotensin systems. Thus, the desirable properties of ACE-inhibitors resulting in reduction of pre- and afterload and, possibly, in coronary vasodilation may represent the rationale for treatment of patients with coronary artery disease and congestive heart failure with these agents. Large-scale clinical studies have clearly demonstrated the beneficial effects of ACE-inhibitors, with a prevention of progressive deterioration in left ventricular function, a significant reduction in the rate of heart-failure-related hospitalizations, with a significant reduction in mortality and an improvement in prognosis in the management of patients with left ventricular dysfunction or congestive heart failure (23, 24, 111). Among these patients ischemic heart disease due to coronary artery disease represents a major cause of congestive heart failure and, hence, from a prognostic viewpoint, patients with coronary artery disease and left ventricular dysfunction or congestive heart failure should be treated with ACE-inhibitors.

However, with respect to angina pectoris not all of these patients may have benefit from additional treatment with ACE-inhibitors. In the CONSENSUS Study (24) patients with ongoing chest pain or myocardial infarction in the preceding 3 months were excluded. At rest, captopril given to patients with ischemic heart disease associated with heart failure caused a decrease in coronary blood flow (15, 51, 83, 101). The reduction in coronary blood flow was partially due to a decrease in coronary perfusion pressure. Simultaneously, the decrease in coronary blood flow was significantly correlated with the reduction of the rate-pressure product. However, in some patients lactate production occurred, suggesting myocardial ischemia due to an imbalance between reduction in coronary flow and reduction in myocardial oxygen demand (15, 83, 101). Rousseau et al. (102) demonstrated that benazeprilat increased lactate production, even in four out of six patients with heart failure during pacing-induced ischemia. In a double blind cross-over study, Cleland et al. (20) compared the effects of captopril and placebo in patients with chronic heart failure and angina pectoris. Due to an increase in symptoms of angina with captopril, the patients generally preferred placebo to captopril. The overall exercise performance was not improved, although the rate-pressure product was reduced. Since the reduction in rate-pressure product was largely because of a reduction in blood pressure rather than in heart rate the lack of improvement may be related to a decrease in coronary perfusion pressure.

Thus, the use of ACE-inhibitors in patients with chronic heart failure, coronary artery disease and ongoing angina appears to be ambiguous. However, these studies with a limited number of patients and partially excessive high doses of ACE-inhibitors used can only point out that, in the individual case, patients with coronary artery disease and congestive heart failure may not benefit from ACE-inhibitor treatment with respect to symptoms of angina pectoris, but these findings may not be generalized. In the SAVE trial only about 1% of the patients have to be excluded for associated ischemic discomfort or for symptomatic hypertension (95).

ACE-inhibitors and myocardial infarction

Myocardial infarction is associated with a cascade of compensatory mechanisms, including the activation of the renin-angiotensin system and the sympathetic nervous system, which both act to preserve cardiac pump function. Angiotensin levels have been shown to be high in patients after myocardial infarction with a maximum on the third day (27). After transmural myocardial infarction a series of pathological changes take place that are described by the term "left ventricular remodeling". Left ventricular enlargement as a true remodeling of the ventricle is observed in 40 to 50% of patients following transmural myocardial infarction (56). If the compensatory remodeling is not sufficient to maintain cardiac performance, progressive ventricular dilatation results with ultimate pump failure.

The rationale of ACE-inhibitor treatment after myocardial infarction is based on experimental findings. In a rat model of myocardial infarction, progressive left ventricular dilatation has been shown to occur as a function of the size and age of the infarct (44, 49). In the same infarct model long-term administration of the ACE-inhibitor captopril attenuated this gradual left ventricular enlargement (90) and prolonged survival after myocardial infarction (91). Whereas the CONSENSUS Study excluded patients with ongoing chest pain or myocardial infarction within the preceding 3 months, two preliminary clinical trials in patients with coronary artery disease and myocardial infarction with an ejection fraction less than 45%, but without clinical evidence of heart failure, have shown that captopril significantly reduced the left ventricular end-systolic volume (109) and prevented the progression of left ventricular dilatation in patients with extensive wall motion abnormalities (92).

In this context the question arises about the optimal time interval between myocardial infarction and initiation of ACE-inhibitor treatment, and whether patients with acute myocardial infarction may have benefit from very early ACE-inhibitor treatment.

During the early postinfarction phase, before scar formation, there is an increase in ventricular diastolic volume as a consequence of infarct expansion and an increase in filling pressure (39, 81). This risk period for infarct expansion ranges between 3 and 14 days after infarction (39) and thus coincides with the phase of maximal rises of plasma angiotensin levels (27). Whether these increased plasma levels reflect activation of tissue renin-angiotensin system and its impact on left ventricular remodeling is not yet clarified. After the formation of a scar, the left ventricle may continue to dilate as the result of remodeling of the residual viable myocardium and if the infarct is of sufficient size, the left ventricular volume may continue to increase with a further deterioration in ventricular performance (81, 93). The clinical use of ACE-inhibitors in the very early phase of acute myocardial infarction is afflicted with the risk of severe reduction in blood pressure. Since activation of renin-angiotensin system in acute myocardial infarction is quite variable (27, 84) ACE-inhibitors may lead to an unpredictable drop of blood pressure with consecutive deterioration of coronary perfusion. Captopril given orally to patients with subacute myocardial infarction and congestive heart failure resulted in a critical reduction of mean aortic pressure to below 70 mmHg in three out of seven patients (80). This risk of marked reduction in blood pressure was confirmed by others (11, 131).

The effects of long-term treatment with ACE-inhibitors after myocardial infarction are addressed by two large-scale multicenter trials. In the CONSENSUS II Study, performed in patients with acute myocardial infarction, enalapril therapy started within 24 h after the onset of chest pain. In this study enalapril therapy did not improve survival during the 180 days of observation after infarction (118). In contrast, in the SAVE study, performed in patients with asymptomatic left ventricular dysfunction after myocardial infarction, long-term administration of captopril was associated with an improvement in survival and reduced morbidity and mortality due to major cardiovascular events (95). Reduced morbidity included a reduction of risk for congestive heart failure requiring hospitalization and for recurrent myocardial infarction. In this study therapy with captopril was started within 3 to 16 days after infarction and the patients were followed for an average of 42 months. However, also in this study there was no difference in mortality between the captopril and the placebo group within the first six months of observation. The differences only became apparent in the later follow up. Thus, with respect to the difference in the outcome of these two studies, different effects of captopril and enalapril, the difference in the time interval between infarction and onset of the therapy, differences in the selection of patients and, above all, the different time of observation have to be regarded.

ACE-inhibitors and arrhythmias in myocardial ischemia and reperfusion

Myocardial ischemia and reperfusion injury after the relief of coronary artery spasm or after successful coronary thrombolysis, as well as after percutaneous transluminal coronary angioplasty of evolving myocardial infarction are known to be potent stimuli for ventricular arrhythmias. Therefore, the occurrence of ventricular arrhythmias represents a major problem in the clinical management of patients with coronary artery disease. In this context possible antiarrhythmic effects of ACE-inhibitors would be of interest.

Several investigators have shown that captopril reduces the frequency of ventricular arrhythmias in the reperfusion injured isolated rat heart (29, 72, 122, 123). Since captopril is a sulfhydryl group containing ACE-inhibitor, a direct effect on membrane stabilization via the free radical scavenging properties of the sulfhydryl group were discussed (134). However, several investigators using a variety of converting enzyme inhibitors without a sulfhydryl group, such as ramipril, ramiprilat, enalapril or perindopril have demonstrated a significant reduction of both incidence and mean duration of malignant arrhythmias during reperfusion in experimental models (75, 77, 99, 123). To some extent, arrhythmias may be directly evoked by angiotensin II, since the antiarrhythmic effects of ACE-inhibitors were abolished by simultaneous administration of angiotensin II, but not of angiotensin I (76). Furthermore, bradykinin duplicated and exposure to a bradykinin-inhibitor abolished the antiarrhythmic effects of converting enzyme inhibition (104). The effects of bradykinin, in turn, may involve augmentation of local prostanoid production (125). A relation of the antiarrhythmic effects of ACE-inhibitors to an increased prostaglandin synthesis is supported by the fact that the effects of captopril (123) and enalapril (78) are abolished by indomethacin. Moreover, dramatic reductions in norepinephrine overflow from ischemic hearts after converting enzyme inhibitor treatment imply that the antiarrhythmic effect may in part result from attenuation of angiotensin II-related sympathetic facilitation (123). However, most of the experimental studies were performed in global ischemic isolated rat hearts. Therefore, an extrapolation of these presumed "antiarrhythmic" effects of ACE-inhibitors to clinical conditions in patients with coronary artery disease has to be questioned. Nevertheless, a role for ACE-inhibitors as antiarrhythmics, particularly in ischemia and congestive heart failure has been proclaimed (132), and several authors (20, 130) have observed a reduction of ventricular ectopy in ACE-inhibitor treated patients suffering from heart failure. However, no controlled clinical studies have been reported so far. Furthermore, the SOLVD could not corroborate this hypothesis. In the treatment arm no differences in documented nonfatal cardiac arrest, in arrhythmias recorded by Holter monitoring, and only a slight reduction in presumed arrhythmic deaths could be observed, while in the prevention arm there also was only little difference between the groups in the number of deaths presumed to be due primarily to arrhythmia (110, 111).

Thus, if at all, the antiarrhythmic effects of ACE-inhibitors seem to be the result of a complex interaction of several neurohumoral mediator systems, including changes in the neuroendocrine activation, attenuation of angiotensin II-related sympathetic facilitation, the increase in serum potassium, and changes in the hemodynamics with reduced systolic wall stress and myocardial oxygen demand.

ACE-inhibitors and restenosis after percutaneous transluminal coronary angioplasty

Increased experience and technical advances in percutaneous transluminal coronary angioplasty (PTCA) as an alternative treatment for coronary artery bypass grafting have resulted in a high primary success rate and low complication rate (32). However, the late restenosis rate still limits the long-term benefit of the procedure (69, 108). The cause of restenosis is unclear. Among different factors an intimal proliferation of smooth muscle cells has been implicated (45). Balloon angioplasty extensively damages the medial smooth muscle cells as well as the endothelial lining of the coronary vessel wall (43). Endogeneous growth factors (bFGF, basic fibroblastic growth factor; PDGF, platelet-derived growth factor), released from patelets as well as from damaged endothelial and smooth muscle cells, may regulate the migration of smooth muscle cells from the media into the intima and their proliferative response to balloon injury (55, 57). Several studies have demonstrated that in cultured cells, angiotensin II induces messenger ribonucleic acids to encode important growth factor genes such as PDGF, transforming growth factor-β and thrombospondin (TS) and thus induces cell proliferation (86, 107). Based on the hypothesis that a local renin-angiotensin system may regulate the vascular response to endothelial injury, Powell et al. (97) examined the effects of the ACE-inhibitor cilazapril on neointimal proliferation in the rat balloon-injured carotid artery. They could show that the ACE-inhibitor treatment reduced the proliferative response to balloon injury by 70%. However, these promising data from experimental studies could not be confirmed under clinical conditions. The MERCATOR Study recently came to the disillusioning conclusions that long-term angiotensin converting enzyme inhibition with cilazapril does not prevent restenosis and does not favorably influence the overall clinical outcome after PTCA (82, see Heyndrickx this issue).

In conclusion, due to their potential antiischemic action ACE-inhibitors have been tested in patients with coronary artery disease, including use in stable angina pectoris, chronic heart failure, after myocardial infarction or after PTCA to prevent restenosis. While in hypertensive patients with coronary artery disease a beneficial effect of ACE-inhibitors with improvement of angina pectoris seems to be most convincing, clinical findings in normotensive patients with coronary artery disease but without congestive heart failure are less conclusive. Before ACE-inhibitors can generally be recommended in these patients, a better definition of patients who may benefit is required. Large-scale clinical studies have clearly demonstrated a significant reduction in mortality and an improvement of prognosis along with ACE-inhibitor treatment in patients with congestive heart failure. However, patients with coronary artery disease, congestive heart failure, and ongoing angina pectoris may require additional antianginal therapy. A beneficial role of long-term ACE-inhibitor treatment is furthermore suggested in postinfarction left ventricular remodeling, when started within 3 to 16 days after myocardial infarction. Finally, ACE-inhibitors failed to prevent restenosis after successful PTCA.

References

1. Aiken JW, Reit E (1968) Stimulation of the cat stellate ganglion by angiotensin. J Pharmacol Exp Ther 159:107—114
2. Akhras F, Jackson G (1991) The role of captopril as single therapy in hypertension and angina pectoris. Int J Cardiol. 33:259—266
3. Alderman EL, Fisher LD, Litwin P (1983) Results of coronary artery surgery in patients with poor left ventricular function (CLASS). Circulation 68:785—795
4. Auch-Schwelk W, Bossaller C, Claus M, Graf K, Gräfe M, Schüler S, Fleck E (1992) Mechanismus der Bradykinin-vermittelten vasodilatierenden Wirkung von ACE-Inhibitoren in Koronararterien. Z Kardiol 81 (suppl 1):112
5. Berdeaux A, Bonhenry C, Giudicelli JF (1987) Effects of four angiotensin I converting enzyme inhibitors on regional myocardial blood flow and ischemic injury during coronary artery occlusion in dogs. Fundam Clin Pharmacol 1:201—208
6. Berger HJ, Zaret BJ, Speroff L (1977) Cardiac prostaglandin release during myocardial ischemia induced by atrial pacing in patients with coronary artery disease. Am J Cardiol 39:481—486
7. Bianchi A, de Schaepdryver AF, de Vleeschhouwer GR, Preziosi P (1960) On the pharmacology of synthetic hypertensine. Arch Int Pharmacodyn Ther 124:21—44
8. Boadle MC, Hughes J, Roth RH (1969) Angiotensin accelerates catecholamine biosynthesis in sympathetically innervated tissues. Nature 222:987—988
9. Blumberg AL, Ackerly JA, Peach MJ (1976) Differentiation of neurogenic and myocardial angiotensin II receptors in isolated rabbit atria. Circ Res 36:719—726
10. Bossaller C, Auch-Schwelk W, Götze S, Weber F, Graf K, Gräfe M, Hehlert-Friedrich C, Fleck E (1992) Die chronische Behandlung mit Enalapril führt zu einer Zunahme der endothelabhängigen Relaxation. Z Kardiol 81 (suppl 1):29
11. Brivet F, Deltraissy JF, Gindicelly JF, Richer C, Legrand A, Dormont J (1981) Immediate effects of captopril in acute left ventricular failure secondary to myocardial infarction. Eur J Clin Invest 11:369—374

12. Bush LR, Campbell WB, Kern K (1984) The effects of alpha2-adrenergic and serotonergic receptor antagonists on cyclic blood flow alterations in stenosed canine coronary arteries. Circ Res 55:642—648
13. Bussmann WD, Goerke S, Schneider W, Kaltenbach M (1988) Angiotensin-converting-Enzym-Hemmer bei Angina pectoris. Dtsch Med Wochenschr 113:548—550
14. Campbell DJ, Habener JF (1987) Cellular localization of angiotensin gene expression in brown and adipose tissue and mesentery: Quantification of messenger ribonucleic acid abundance using hybridization in situ. Endocrinology 121:1616—1626
15. Chatterjee K, Rouleau J-L, Parmely WW (1982) Haemodynamic and myocardial metabolic effects of captopril in chronic heart failure. Br Heart J 47:233—238
16. Chatterjee K, Opie LH (1987) Angiotensin inhibitors and other vasodilators with special reference to congestive heart failure. Cardiovasc Drugs Ther 1:1—8
17. Chu A, Morris K, Kuehl WD (1989) Effects of atrial natriuretic peptide on the coronary arterial vasculature in humans. Circulation 80:1627—1632
18. Cleland JGF, Dargie HJ, Hodsman GP (1984) Captopril in heart failure. A double blind controlled trial. Br Heart J 52:530—535
19. Cleland JGF, Dargie HJ, Ball SG (1985) Effects of enalapril in heart failure: a double-blind study of effects on exercise performance, renal function, hormones and metabolic state. Br Heart J 54:305—312
20. Cleland JG, Henderson E, McLenachan J, Findlay TN, Dargie HJ (1991) Effect of captopril, an angiotensin-converting enzyme inhibitor, in patients with angina pectoris and heart failure. J Am Coll Cardiol 17:733—739
21. Clough DP, Mulroy SC, Angell D, Hatton R (1983) Inference by inhibitors of the renin-angiotensin system with neurogenic vasoconstriction. Clin Exp Hypertens 5: 1287—1291
22. Cohen MV, Kirk ES (1973) Differential response of large and small coronary arteries to nitroglycerin and angiotensin. Circ Res 33:445—453
23. Cohn JN (1991) A comparison of enalapril with hydralazine-isosorbide dinitrate in the treatment of chronic congestive heart failure. New Engl J Med 325:303—308
24. The CONSENSUS Trial Study Group (1987) Effects of enalapril on mortality in severe congestive heart failure: results of the Cooperative North Scandinavian Enalapril Survival Study (CONSENSUS). New Engl J Med 316:1429—1435
25. Daly P, Rouleau JL, Cousineau D, Burgess JH (1984) Acute effects of captopril on the coronary circulation of patients with hypertension and angina. Am J Med 31:111—115
26. Daly P, Mettauer B, Rouleau JL, Burgess J (1985) Lack of reflex increase in myocardial sympathetic tone after captopril: Potential antianginal effect. Circulation 71:317—325
27. Dargie HJ, McAlpine HM, Morton JJ (1987) Neuroendocrine activation in acute myocardial infarction. J Cardiovasc Pharmacol 9 (suppl 2):S21—S24
28. Day MD, Moore AF (1976) Interaction of angiotensin II with noradrenaline and other spasmogens in rabbit isolated aortic strips. Arch Int Pharmacodyn Ther 219:29—44
29. De Graeff PA, van Gilst WH, de Langen CDJ (1986) Concentration-dependent protection by captopril against ischemia-reperfusion injury in the isolated rat heart. Arch Int Pharmacodyn 280:181—193
30. De Jonge A, Wilffert B, Kalkman HO (1981) Captopril impairs the vascular smooth muscle contraction mediated by postsynaptic alpha2-adrenoceptors in the pithed rat. Eur J Pharmacol 74:385—386
31. De Jonge A, Thoolen MJ, Timmermans PB (1984) Interaction of angiotensin converting enzyme inhibitors with the sympathetic nervous system. Prog Pharmacol 5/3:25—38
32. Detre K, Holubkov R, Kelsey S, Cowley M, et al. (1988) Percutaneous transluminal coronary angioplasty in 1985—1986 and 1977—1981: The National Heart, Lung, Blood Institute Registry. N Engl J Med 318:265—270
33. Dinerman JL, Mehta JL (1990) Endothelial, platelet and leukocyte interactions in ischemic heart disease: Insights into potential mechanism and their clinical relevance. J Am Coll Cardiol 16:207—211

34. Drimal J, Boska D (1973) Effects of angiotensin II on myocardial mechanics and contractile state of the heart muscle. Eur J Pharmacol 20:130—138
35. Dunn WR, McGrath JC, Wilson VG (1989) Expression of functional postjunctional alpha2-adrenoceptor in rabbit isolated distal saphenous artery-a permissive role for angiotensin II? Br J Pharmacol 96:259—261
36. Dzau VJ (1987) Implications of local angiotensin production in cardiovascular physiology and pharmacology. Am J Cardiol 59:59A—65A
37. Dzau VJ (1988) Circulating versus local-angiotensin system in cardiovascular homeostasis. Circulation 77 (suppl I):14—113
38. Dzau VJ (1989) ACE-inhibitors in hypertension: A US perspective. Cardiology 76 (suppl 2):23—30
39. Eaton LW, Weiss JL, Bulkley BH, Garrison JB, Weisfeldt ML (1979) Regional cardiac dilatation after acute myocardial infarction: recognition by two-dimensional echocardiography. N Engl J Med 300:57—62
40. Ertl G, Gerhards W, Wichmann J, Fauth S, Schweisfurth H (1982) Myokardischämie, Plasma-Renin und Converting-Enzym-Aktivität unter Belastung. Z Kardiol 71:604—611
41. Ertl G, Alexander RW, Kloner RA (1983) Interactions between coronary occlusion and the renin-angiotensin system in the dog. Basic Res Cardiol 78:518—533
42. Ertl G (1987) Coronary vasoconstriction in experimental myocardial ischemia. J Cardiovasc Pharmacol 9 (suppl 2):S9—S17
43. Fingerle J, Au YPT, Clowes AW, Reidy MA (1990) Intimal lesion formation in rat carotid arteries after endothelial denudation in absence of medial injury. Atherosclerosis 10:1082—1087
44. Fletcher PJ, Pfeffer JM, Pfeffer MA, Braunwald E (1981) Left ventricular diastolic pressure-volume relations in rats with healed myocardial infarction: effects on systolic function. Circ Res 49:618—626
45. Forrester JS, Fishbein M, Helfant R, Fagin J (1991) A paradigm for restenosis based on cell biology: Clues for the development of new preventive therapies. J Am Coll Cardiol 17:758—769
46. Freer RJ, Pappano AJ, Peach MJ, Bing KZ, McLean MJ, Vogel S, Sperelakis N (1976) Mechanism for the positive inotropic effect of angiotensin II on isolated cardiac muscle. Circ Res 39:178—183
47. Freeman AP, Walsh WF, Giles BW (1984) Early and long-term results of coronary artery bypass grafting with severely depressed left ventricular performance. Am J Cardiol 54:749—754
48. Furchgott RF, Vanhoutte PM (1989) Endothelium-derived relaxing and contracting factors. FASEB J 3:2007—2010
49. Gasic S, Dudzcak R, Korn A (1990) ACE inhibition with cilazapril improves myocardial perfusion to the ischemic regions during exercise: A pilot study. J Cardiovasc Pharmacol 15:227—232
50. Gibbs JSR, Crean PA, Mockus L, Wright C, Sutton GC, Fox KM (1989) The variable effects of angiotensin converting enzyme inhibition on myocardial ischaemia in chronic stable angina. Br Heart J 62:112—117
51. Halperin JL, Faxon DP, Creager MA (1982) Coronary hemodynamic effects of angiotensin inhibition by captopril and teprotide in patients with congestive heart failure. Am J Cardiol 50:967—972
52. Heusch G (1990) Alpha-adrenergic mechanisms in myocardial ischemia. Circulation 81:1—13
53. Hung J, Kelly DT, Baird DK (1980) Aorto-coronary bypass grafting in patients with severe left ventricular dysfunction. J Thorac Cardiovasc Surg 79:718—723
54. Ignarro LJ (1989) Biological actions and properties of endothelium-derived nitric oxide formed and released from artery and vein. Circ Res 65:1—21
55. Jawien A, Lindner V, Bowen-Pope DF, Schwartz SM, Reidy MA, Clowes AW (1990) Platelet derived groth factor (PDGF) stimulates arterial smooth muscle cell proliferation in vivo. FASEB J 4:342

56. Jeremy RW, Allmann KC, Bautovitch G, Harris PJ (1989) Patterns of left ventricular dilation during the six months after myocardial infarction. J Am Coll Cardiol 13:304—310
57. Jin M, Wilhelm MJ, Lang RE, Unger T, Lindpaintner K, Ganten D (1987) The endogenous tissue renin-angiotensin systems: From molecular biology to therapy. Am J Med 84 (suppl 3A):28—36
58. Kannel WB, Dawber TR (1973) Hypertensive cardiovascular disease. The Framingham Study. In: Onesti G, Kim KE, Maya JH, eds. Hypertension: mechanisms and management. New York: Grune and Stratton:93
59. Kannel WB (1976) Some lessons in cardiovascular epidemiology from Framingham. Am J Cardiol 37:269—282
60. Keck M (1987) Anti-ischemic effect of captopril in patients with stable angina pectoris. Herz Kreisl 19:319—321
61. Kelm M, Schrader J (1988) Nitric oxide release from the isolated guinea pig heart. Eur J Pharmacol 155:317—321
62. Kennedy JW, Kaiser GC, Fisher LD (1981) Clinical and angiographic predictors of operative mortality from the Collaberative Study in Coronary Artery Surgery (CASS). Circulation 63:793—802
63. Khairallah PA (1972) Action of angiotensin on adrenergic nerve endings: Inhibition of norepinephrine uptake. Fed Proc 31:1351—1357
64. Kimura E, Hashimoto K, Furukawa S (1973) Changes in bradykinin level in coronary sinus blood after the experimental occlusion of a coronary artery. Am Heart J 85:635—647
65. Kiowski W, Zuber M, Elsasser S, Erne P, Pfisterer M, Burkart F (1991) Coronary vasodilatation and improved myocardial lactate metabolism after angiotensin converting enzyme inhibition with cilazapril in patients with congestive heart failure. Am Heart J 122:1382—1388
66. Kirchheim HR, Ehmke H, Hackenthal E (1987) Autoregulation of renal blood flow, glomerular filtration rate and renin release in conscious dogs. Pflügers Arch 410:441—449
67. Koch-Weser J (1964) Myocardial actions of angiotensin. Circ Res 14:337—344
68. Lai C, Onnis E, Orani E (1987) Antiischemic activity of ACE inhibitor enalapril in normotensive patients with stable effort angina. J Am Coll Cardiol 9:192A
69. Leimgruber PP, Roubin GS, Hollman J, Cotsonis GA, Meier B, Douglas JS, King SB III, Gruentzig AR (1986) Restenosis after successful angioplasty in patients with single-vessel disease. Circulation 73:710—717
70. Liang CS, Gavras H, Hood B (1978) Renin-angiotensin system inhibition in conscious sodium depleted dogs. Effects on systemic and coronary hemodynamics. J Clin Invest 62:874—881
71. Liang CS, Gavras H, Black J (1982) Renin-angiotensin system inhibition in acute myocardial infarction in dogs. Effects on systemic hemodynamics, myocardial blood flow, segmental myocardial function and infarct size. Circulation 66:1249—1255
72. Li K, Chen X (1987) Protective effects of captopril and enalapril on myocardial ischemia and reperfusion damage of rat. J Mol Cell Cardiol 19:909—915
73. Limas CJ (1974) Stimulation by angiotensin of myocardial prostaglandins. Biochim Biophys Acta 337:417—420
74. Lindpaintner K, Ganten D (1991) The cardiac renin-angiotensin system. An appraisal of present experimental and clinical evidence. Circ Res 68:905—920
75. Linz W, Schölkens BA, Manwen J (1986) The heart as a target for converting enzyme inhibitors: Studies in ischaemic isolated working rat hearts. J Hypertension 4 (suppl 6):S477—S479
76. Linz W, Schölkens BA, Yi-Fan Han (1986) Beneficial effects of the converting enzyme inhibitor ramipril in ischemic hearts. J Hypertens 8 (suppl 10):S91—S99
77. Linz W, Schölkens BA (1987) Influence of local converting enzyme inhibition on angiotensin and bradykinin effects in ischemic rat hearts. J Cardiovasc Pharmacol 10 (suppl 7):S75—S82

78. Linz W, Schölkens BA, Kaiser J (1989) Cardiac arrhythmias are ameliorated by local inhibition of angiotensin formation and bradykinin degradation with the converting-enzyme inhibitor ramipril. Cardiovasc Drugs Ther 3:873—882
79. Majesky MW, Reidy MA, Bowen-Pope DF, Hart CE, Wilcox JN, Schwartz SM (1990) PDGF ligand and receptor gene expression during repair ligand. J Cell Biol 111: 2149—2158
80. McAlpine HM, Morton JJ, Leckie B, Dargie HJ (1987) Use of oral ACE-inhibitors post infarct. J Cardiovasc Pharmacol 9 (suppl 2):S25—S30
81. McKay RG, Pfeffer MA, Pasternak RC (1986) Left ventricular remodeling after myocardial infarction: a corollary to infarct expansion. Circulation 74:693—702
82. MERCATOR Study Group (1992) Does the new angiotensin converting enzyme inhibitor cilazapril prevent restenosis after percutaneous transluminal coronary angioplasty? Circulation 86:100—110
83. Mettauer B, Rouleau J-L, Daly P (1986) The effect of captopril on the coronary circulation and myocardial metabolism of patients with coronary artery disease. Postgrad Med J 62 (suppl 1):54—58
84. Michorowski B, Ceremuzynski L (1983) The renin-angiotensin-aldosterone system and the clinical course of acute myocardial infarction. Eur Heart J 4:259—264
85. Mulligan IP, Fraser AG, Lewis MJ, Henderson AH (1989) Effects of enalapril on myocardial noradrenaline overflow during exercise in patients with chronic heart failure. Br Heart J 61:23—28
86. Naftilan AJ, Pratt RE, Dzau VJ (1989) Induction of platelet derived groth factor A chain and C-myc gene expressions by angiotensin II in culture rat vascular smooth muscle cells. J Clin Invest 83:1419—1424
87. Needleman P, Marshall GR, Sobel BE (1975) Hormone interactions in the isolated rabbit heart. Synthesis and coronary vasomotor effects of prostaglandins, angiotensin and bradykinin. Circ Res 37:802—808
88. Palmer RMJ, Ferrige AG, Moncada S (1987) Nitric oxide release accounts for the biological activity of endothelium-derived relaxing factor. Nature 327:524—526
89. Panza JA, Quyyumi AA, Brush JE Jr, Epstein SE (1990) Abnormal endothelium-dependent vascular relaxation in patients with essential hypertension. N Engl J Med 323:22—27
90. Pfeffer JM, Pfeffer MA, Braunwald E (1985) Influence of chronic captopril therapy on the infarcted left ventricle of the rat. Circ Res 57:84—95
91. Pfeffer MA, Pfeffer JM, Steinberg C, Finn P (1985) Survival after an experimental myocardial infarction: beneficial effects of long-term therapy with captopril. Circulation 72:406—412
92. Pfeffer MA, Lamas GA, Vaughan DE, Parisi AF, Braunwald E (1988) Effect of captopril on progressive ventricular dilatation after myocardial infarction. N Engl J Med 319:80—86
93. Pfeffer MA, Braunwald E (1990) Ventricular remodeling after myocardial infarction: experimental observations and clinical implications. Circulation 81:1161—1172
94. Pfeffer JM, Pfeffer MA, Fletcher PJ, Braunwald E (1991) Progressive ventricular remodeling in rat with myocardial infarction. Am J Physiol 260:H1406—H1414
95. Pfeffer MA, Braunwald E, et al. (1992) Effect of captopril on mortality and morbidity in patients with left ventricular dysfunction after myocardial infarction. N Engl J Med 327:669—677
96. Poulsen K, Poulsen LL (1971) Simultaneous determination of plasma converting enzyme and angiotensinase activity by radioimmunoassay. Clin Sci 40:443—449
97. Powell JS, Clozel JP, Müller RK, Kuhn H, Hefti F, Hosang M, Baumgartner HR (1989) Inhibitors of angiotensin-converting enzyme prevent myointimal proliferation after vascular injury. Science 245:186—188
98. Rietbrock N, Thürmann P, Kirsten R (1988) Anti-ischeamic effect of enalapril in coronary heart disease. A randomized placebo-controlled double blind trial on 12 patients. Dtsch Med Wschr 113:300—302

99. Rochette L, Ribuot C, Belichard P (1987) Protective effect of angiotensin converting enzyme inhibitors (CEI): Captopril and perindopril on vulnerability to ventricular fibrillation during myocardial ischemia and reperfusion in rat. Clin Exp Theory and Practice A9:365—368
100. Roth RH (1972) Action of angiotensin on adrenergic nerve endings: Enhancement of norepinephrine biosynthesis. Fed Proc 31:1358—1364
101. Rouleau J-L, Chatterjee K, Benge W, Parmley WW, Hiramatsu B (1982) Alterations in left ventricular function and coronary hemodynamics with captopril, hydralazine and prazosin in chronic ischemic heart failure: A comparative study. Circulation 65:671—678
102. Rousseau MF, Close P, Pouleur H (1989) Are the angiotensin-converting enzyme inhibitors poor anti-ischemic drugs? Circulation 80 (suppl II):II52
103. Rubio R, Berne RM (1969) Release of adenosine by the normal myocardium and its relationship to the regulation of coronary resistance. Circ Res 25:407—412
104. Schölkens BA, Linz W, Koenig W (1988) Effects of the angiotensin converting enzyme inhibitor ramipril in isolated ischemic rat heart are abolished by a bradykinin antagonist. J Hypertens 6:S25—S28
105. Schoenberger JA (1988) Emerging benefits of angiotensin converting enzyme inhibitors versus other antihypertensive agents. Am J Med 84 (suppl 4A): 30—35
106. Schwartzkopff B, Vogt M, Knauer S, Motz W, Strauer BE (1991) Medial hypertrophy of intramural coronary arteries in patients with reduced coronary reserve in hypertensive heart disease. Circulation 84 (suppl II):II—479
107. Scott-Burden T, Resink TJ, Hahn AW, Bühler FR (1990) Induction of thrombospondin expression in vascular smooth muscle cells by angiotensin II. J Cardiovasc Pharmacol 16 (suppl 7):17—20
108. Serruys PW, Luijten HE, Beatt KJ, Geuskens R, de Feyter PJ, et al. (1988) Incidence of restenosis after successful coronary angioplasty: A time-related phenomenon: A quantitative angiographic study in 342 consecutive patients at 1, 2, 3 and 4 months. Circulation 77:361—371
109. Sharpe N (1991) Angiotensin-converting enzyme inhibitors in heart failure: a role after myocardial infarction. J Cardiovasc Pharmacol 18 (suppl 2):S99—S104
110. The SOLVD Investigators (1990) Studies of left ventricular dysfunction (SOLVD)-rationale, design and methods: two trials that evaluate the effect of enalapril in patients with reduced ejection fraction. Am J Cardiol 66:315—322
111. The SOLVD Investigators (1992) Effect of enalapril on mortality and the development of heart failure in asymptomatic patients with reduced left ventricular ejection fractions. N Engl J Med 327:685—691
112. Starke K, Werner U, Schuermann HJ (1966) Wirkungen von Angiotensin auf Funktion und Noradrenalinabgabe isolierter Kaninchenherzen in Ruhe und bei Sympathikusreizung. Naunyn Schmiedebergs Arch Pharmacol 265:170—186
113. Starke K (1971) Action of angiotensin on uptake, release, and metabolism of 14C NE by isolated rabbit hearts. Eur J Pharmacol 14:112—123
114. Strauer BE (1990) The significance of coronary reserve in clinical heart disease. J Am Coll Cardiol 15:775—782
115. Strozzi C, Cocco G, Portaluppi F, Urso L, Alfrigo R, Rizzo A, Tasini MT, Montanari L, Zannell AH (1987) Ergometric evaluation of the effects of captopril in hypertensive patients with stable angina. Curr Ther Res 41:301—304
116. Strozzi C, Cocco G, Portaluppi F, Urso L, Alfrigo R, Tasini MT, Montanari L, Al Yassini K, Rizzo A (1987) Effects of captopril on the physical work capacity of normotensive patients with stable effort angina. Cardiology 74:226—228
117. Swartz SL, Williams GH, Hollenberg NK, Levine L, Denk JR, Moore TJ (1980) Captopril-induced changes in prostaglandin production. J Clin Invest 65:1257—1264
118. Swedberg K, Held P, Kjekshus J, et al. (1991) Effects of the early administration of enalapril on mortality in patients with acute myocardial infarction. N Engl J Med 327:678—684

119. Tardieu A, Virot P, Vandroux JC (1986) Effects of captopril on myocardial perfusion in patients with coronary insufficiency: Evaluation by the exercise test and quantitative myocardial tomoscintigraphy using thallium-201. Postgrad Med J 62 (suppl 1): 38—41
120. Unger T, Gohlke P, Paul M, Rettig R (1991) Tissue renin-angiotensin system: Fact or fiction? J Cardiovasc Pharmacol 18 (suppl 2):20—28
121. Unterberg C, Buchwald A, Vogt A (1990) Akute Effekte des Angiotensin-Converting-Enzym-Hemmers Ramipril bei Patienten mit koronarer Herzerkrankung. Med Klin 85:78—81
122. van Gilst WH, de Graeff PA, Kingma JH (1984) Captopril reduces purine loss and reperfusion arrhythmias in the rat heart after coronary artery occlusion. Eur J Pharmacol 100:113—117
123. van Gilst WH, de Graeff PA, Wesseling H (1986) Reduction of reperfusion arrhythmias in the ischemic isolated rat heart by angiotensin converting enzyme inhibitors: A comparison of captopril, enalapril, and HOE 498. J Cardiovasc Pharmacol 8: 722—728
124. Van Gilst WH, Scholtens E, de Graeff PA (1988) Differential influences of angiotensin converting-enzyme inhibitors on the coronary circulation. Circulation 77 (suppl I):I24—I29
125. Vanhoutte PM, Auch-Schwelk W, Biondi ML, Lorenz RR, Schini VB, Vidal MJ (1989) Why are converting enzyme inhibitors vasodilators? Br J Clin Pharmacol 28: 95S—104S
126. Vogt M, Ulbricht JU, Motz W (1988) Lack of evidence for antianginal effects of enalapril. Circulation 78 (suppl II):II—328
127. Vogt M, Motz W, Strauer BE (1989) Coronary flow reserve in arterial hypertension. Scand J Clin Lab Invest 49 (suppl):196:7—14
128. Vogt M, Motz W, Pölitz B, Scheler S, Strauer BE (1991) Improvement of coronary reserve by chronic treatment with ACE-inhibitors. Circulation 84 (suppl II): II—136
129. Waeber B, Nussberger J, Brunner HR (1990) Angiotensin converting enzyme inhibition in arterial hypertension. Wien Med Wschr 1/2:22—29
130. Webster WM, Fitzpatrick MA, Nicholls MG, Ikram H, Wells JE (1985) Effect of enalapril on ventricular arrhythmias in congestive heart failure. Am J Cardiol 56:566—569
131. Wenting GJ, Man in't Veld AJ, Woittiez AJ, Derkx FH, Schalekamp AD (1984) Captopril in the treatment of severe acute and chronic heart failure. Progr Pharmacol 5:107—114
132. Wesseling H, De Graeff PA, Van Gilst WH, Kingma JH, de Langen CDJ (1989) Cardiac arrhythmias: A new indication for angiotensin-converting enzyme inhibitors. J Hum Hypertens 3:89—95
133. Westfall TC (1977) Local regulation of adrenergic neurotansmission. Physiol Rev 57:659—729
134. Westlin W, Mullane K (1988) Does captopril attenuate reperfusion-induced myocardial dysfunction by scavenging free radicals? Circulation 77 (suppl I):I—30 — I—34
135. White HD, Norris RM, Brown MA, Brandt PWT, Whitlock RML, Wild CJ (1987) Left ventricular end-systolic as the major determinant of survival after recovery from myocardial infarction. Circulation 76:44—51
136. Yanagisawa M, Kurihara H, Kimura S (1988) A novel potent vasoconstrictor peptide produced by vascular endothelial cells. Nature 331:411—416
137. Yang HYT, Erdös EG (1967) Second kininase in human blood plasma. Nature 215:1402—1403
138. Yang HYT, Erdös EG, Levin Y (1971) Characterization of a dipeptide hydrolase (kininase II: angiotensin I converting enzyme). J Pharmacol Exp Ther 177: 291—300

139. Young MA, Vatner SF (1986) Regulation of large coronary arteries. Circ Res 59:579—585
140. Zannad F, Gilgenkrantz JM (1989) ACE inhibitors in hypertension: A European viewpoint. Cardiology 76 (suppl 12):31—41

Authors' address:
Dr. med. Martin Vogt
Medizinische Klinik und Poliklinik B
Abteilung für Kardiologie, Pneumologie und Angiologie
der Heinrich-Heine-Universität Düsseldorf
Moorenstr. 5
D-4000 Düsseldorf 1, FRG

Molecular mechanisms of cardiac gene expression

B. Nadal-Ginard, V. Mahdavi

Laboratory of Molecular and Cellular Cardiology,
Howard Hughes Medical Institute and Department of Cardiology,
Children's Hospital and Department of Pediatrics,
Harvard Medical School, Boston

Summary: Although the physiological properties of the myocardium and their dynamic character have been the focus of intense research during the past three decades, the biochemical and molecular correlates underlying cardiac development and performance have, until recently, remained poorly understood. The development of modern cellular and molecular biology has provided the necessary tools to undertake the study of the mechanisms involved in cardiac development and to understand the basis for important clinical and experimental problems in cardiovascular physiology. Most of the gene encoding contractile proteins have been cloned and characterized.The availability of molecular probes and the ability to introduce genes into individual cell types and tissues of living animals, are the most important breakthroughs of molecular and cell biology. This permits not only to analyze basic mechanisms of gene expression but has also significant practical applications for gene therapy. It is now possible to analyze the role of different regulatory gene sequences and identify their corresponding trans-active factors. In addition, direct gene injection makes it possible to study gene expression in a natural context, under conditions that are physiologically relevant and controlable.

Key words: Gene regulation; α-, β-myosin heavy chain; transcription factors; cardiac development and hypertrophy; thyroid hormones; in vitro and in vivo gene transfer

The cardiac contractile apparatus

One of the major determinants of long-term outcome for most congenital and acquired cardiac disease is the contractile state of the myocardium. During the past several years significant progress has been made in understanding the developmental and physiological changes of the myocardium that affect cardiac performance. The unit of contraction in the myocardium and in skeletal muscles is the sarcomere (24, 32) (Fig. 1a). The contractile properties of the myocardium, both in terms of force generated and velocity of contraction, are dependent on the number as well as the biochemical composition of its sarcomeres. The sarcomere is constituted by several proteins organized into thin and thick filaments (Fig. 1a). The thick filament contains the molecular motor of contraction, the myosin heavy chain (MHC). During the contraction cycle, the MHC, which carries the ATPase activity required to produce the physical translocation needed for fiber shortening, interacts directly with the actin molecules in the thin filament (Fig. 1a and 1b). The ATPase activity of MHC is modulated by two smaller protein subunits bound to each MHC head — the alkali and essential myosin light chains (MLC). As originally pointed out by Barany (2), there is a direct correlation between the unloaded maximum velocity of shortening of a muscle fiber and the actin-activated ATPase activity of its MHC (Fig. 1b

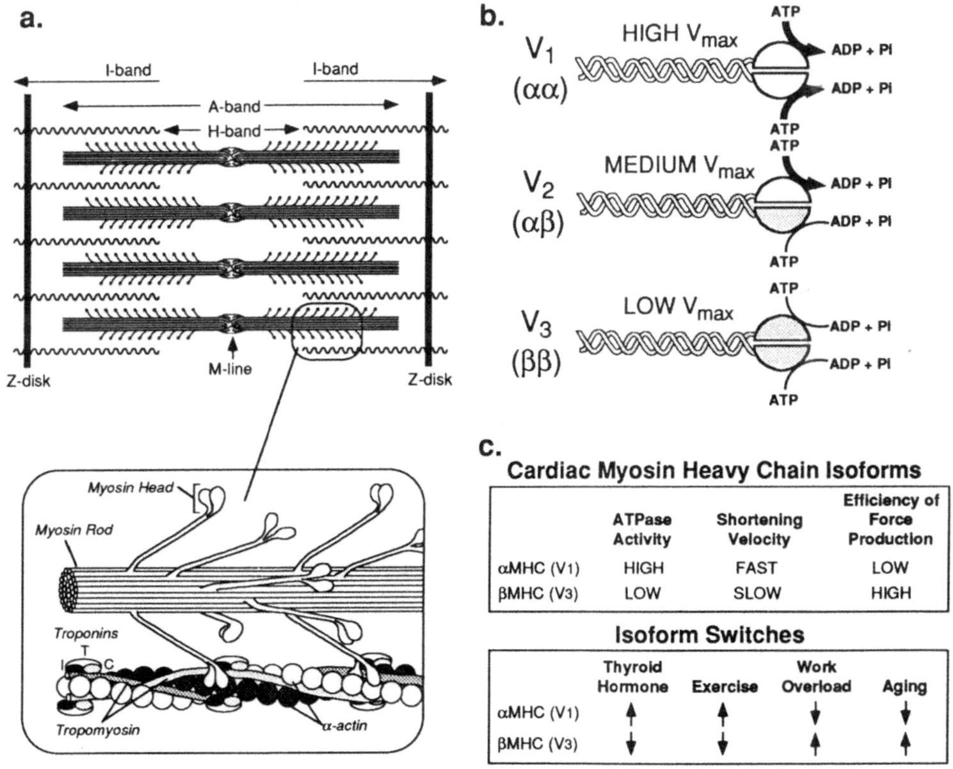

Fig. 1. a) Structural organization of the sarcomere. Each sarcomere (top panel) is constituted by sets of parallel thick and thin filaments (bottom panel) which partially overlap and are interconnected to one another. **b)** The myosin heavy chains α and β have high and low ATPase activity and constitute the V1 and V3 myosins, respectively. **c)** Correlation of the ventricular MHC phenotype with the contractile performance of the myocardium in response to physiological, pathological and developmental stimuli.

and 1c). Although there are some apparent exceptions to this rule, fibers with an MHC with high ATPase activity shorten faster than the ones with a lower enzymatic activity (24). Interestingly, there is an inverse correlation between ATPase activity of the MHC in a fiber and the energetic cost to perform a given workload (2, 24). The faster the fiber, the higher the energetic cost to produce the same amount of work (10). It is clear, therefore, that the type of MHC present in the sarcomeres is physiologically significant and has a profound effect on the contractile properties of the myocardium (Fig. 1c).

In the cardiac ventricles of most mammalian species, including the human, three myosin isoform have been identified based on their electrophoretic mobility — V1, V2, V3 (24). However, these three myosins are composed of only two distinct types of MHCs referred to as α and β. V1 and V3 are composed of αα and ββ homodimers, respectively, while V2 is an αβ heterodimer (Fig. 1b). The two MHC's are produced by two different genes that are closely linked (16, 17) and are located on chromosome 3 in human and 14 in mouse (24). The α-MHC, which has high Ca2+ and actin activated ATPase activity, is associated with an increased shortening velocity of the cardiac fibers. In contrast, the β-MHC, which has lower ATPase activity, is associated with slower shortening velocity (Fig. 1b and 1c), (24). Of note, the ratio of these two different cardiac isoforms is developmentally regulated. In the ventricles of all mammalian species studied so far, β-MHC is the most abundant isoform in utero until late fetal life (16). In small mammals, such as rat and mouse, α-MHC increases immediately prior to birth and becomes the predominant form throughout perinatal and adult life (16). In contrast, in large mammals, such as man, α-MHC is only transiently predominant shortly after birth, with β-MHC becoming the most abundant isoform in the adult (24, 25). The situation is different in the atria where α-MHC is the predominant isoform throughout life in both small and large species (16, 24, 25).

Work overload hypertrophy induces the re-expression of several fetal isoforms in the post-natal myocardium

In all species studied, including man, the distribution of the cardiac MHC isoforms changes during development and in response to certain pathological and experimental conditions such as work overload, (12, 19, 22, 24) and changes in thyroid hormone level (Fig. 2a), (11, 16). In small mammals, in response to a moderate increase in mean aortic pressure (~30 mm Hg) produced by aortic coarctation, there is a rapid induction of ventricular β-MHC mRNA, followed by the appearance of comparable levels of β-MHC protein in parallel with an increase in left ventricular weight (12, 15, 22, 24). A similar change is not detectable in larger mammals, including the human, because β-MHC is the predominant isoform expressed in the normal ventricle. However, in the human atria that normally expresses α-MHC, a switch to β-MHC is readily apparent in response to increased pressure (19). Therefore, in the hypertrophic myocardium, the MHC phenotype is similar to that in the fetal and hypothyroid states, where β-MHC is expressed at high levels (Fig. 2a). Yet, in these animals, the circulating level of thyroid hormone remains normal and their metabolic state argues against hypothyroidism (12). Thus, the MHC isoform switch produced in response to work overload hypertrophy is not regulated through the thyroid hormone pathway.

The isoform switches produced in response to increased afterload are not limited to MHC. In fact, a general myocardial response to work overload occurs rapidly and affects a multitude of cellular compartments (14, 22, 24). This response is characterized by the re-expression of the protein isoforms normally expressed in fetal life, but that are normally suppressed in adulthood (Fig. 2a). To the best of our knowledge this phenomenon has been demonstrated for all the gene phenotypes analyzed so far, including other contractile proteins — such as skeletal α-actin, myosin light chain 1, and β-tropomyosin; membrane proteins like the Na, K ATPase (the cardiac glycoside receptor); secreted molecules such as atrial natriuretic factor (ANF) and those involved in ATP regeneration such as creatine kinase (14, 22, 24). All the above examples represent the re-expression of an isoform normally expressed only during fetal and early post-natal life that is later replaced by the corresponding

a.

Gene Switches in Cardiac Ventricles

<table>
<tr><th></th><th>Fetus & Neonates</th><th>Normal Adult</th><th>Work Overload</th><th>Hypo-thyroid</th><th>Hyper-thyroid</th></tr>
<tr><td>Myosin Heavy Chain</td><td>β</td><td>α</td><td>β, α</td><td>β</td><td>α</td></tr>
<tr><td>α-Actin</td><td>Skeletal Cardiac</td><td>Cardiac</td><td>Cardiac Skeletal</td><td colspan="2" rowspan="4">Same as Normal Adult</td></tr>
<tr><td>Tropomyosin</td><td>α, β</td><td>α</td><td>α, β</td></tr>
<tr><td>Na, K-ATPase</td><td>α_1, β_2</td><td>α_1</td><td>α_1, β_2</td></tr>
<tr><td>ANF</td><td>+</td><td>−</td><td>+ +</td></tr>
</table>

b.

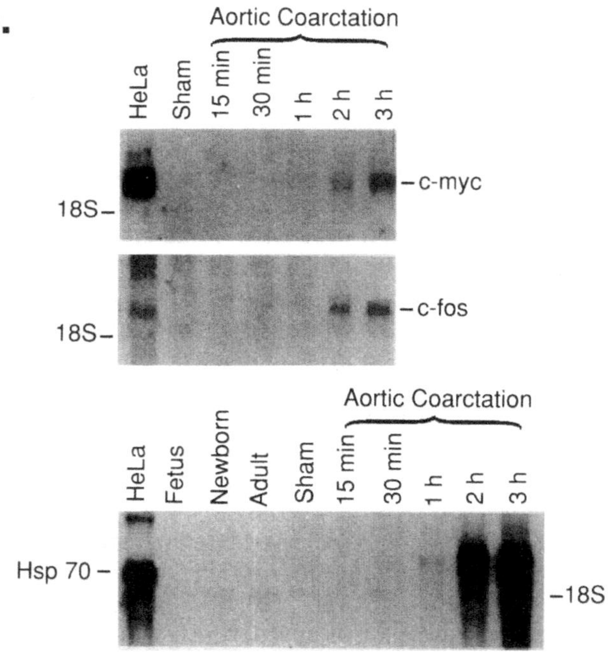

Fig. 2. Reprogramming of cardiac gene expression in response to various stimuli. **a)** Isoforms expressed in the fetal stages are induced in the adult myocardium in response to aortic coarctation. Note that only the α- and β-MHC are regulated by T_3. **b)** and **c)** Induction of proto-oncogenes and heat shock proteins mRNAs in the coarctated animal mimics the response to growth stimuli (12, 14).

adult isoform, except for ANF, whose expression in the ventricles is normally suppressed after birth and it is not replaced by another isoform.

From the above observations it is clear that from this molecular perspective, myocardial hypertrophy is not only a quantitative phenomenon that results in an increase in cardiac mass, but more importantly, results in a significant qualitative change in essential constituents of the myocardium. In general, these changes produce a muscle that has many of the biochemical characteristics of the featal myocardium.

Work overload and stretch produce the rapid expression of a set of proto-oncogenes involved in normal cell growth

The cardiac response to normal growth requirements, as well as to work overload, is dependent on the developmental state of the organ. During fetal and early postnatal life, the demand for an increased cardiac mass is fulfilled mainly by an increase in the number of myocytes (hyperplasia). However, soon after birth, cardiac myocytes loose their ability to divide (32). Later in life, demand for increased mass is fulfilled exclusively through an increase in the size of a fixed number of pre-existing myocytes. To date, there is little insight on the molecular mechanisms responsible for the loss of replicative ability, or terminal differentiation.

What are the mechanisms involved in inducing cell growth and isoform switches in response to work overload? The observed re-expression of fetal isoforms in cardiac hypertrophy is reminiscent of the mitogenic response of many differential cell types, such as hepatocytes, which often involves the suppression of the adult phenotype and re-expression of the fetal pattern, such as the inhibition of albumin and induction of α-protein expression during liver regeneration. In a general biological context, cardiac hypertrophy could be considered the equivalent of the growth response exhibited by most cell types in response to mitogens. In this particular case the growth response is carried out by terminally differentiated cells (myocytes) that are unable to undergo cell division and have only the hypertrophic response open to them. If this hypothesis were correct, it would be expected that the initial response to the hypertrophic stimuli would mimic early events of cell division induced by growth factors in a large variety of cell types.

One of the early responses of stationary cells to growth stimuli is the induction of a series of proto-oncogenes, such as c-fos and c-myc, among others, that directly or indirectly turn on the cascade of events that lead to cell division. Not surprisingly, therefore, c-fos and c-myc mRNAs begin to accumulate within 1 h after the increase in afterload, reach high levels within 3 h, and return to the basal levels in less than 24 h (Fig. 2b), (14, 22). Similarly, the mRNA for one of the major stress proteins, HSP 70, is also increased within 30 min of increasing aortic pressure (Fig. 2c) (14, 22). Thus, similar to the mitogenic response of a variety of cell types, induction of the cellular proto-oncogenes and major stress protein genes reflect early changes occurring in the nuclei of myocardial cells in response to acute pressure overload and appear to play an important role in mediating the hypertrophic response. That these factors play a causative role in the hypertrophic response is suggested by the fact that the overexpression of c-myc in the myocardium of transgenic animals induces cardiac enlargement and cellular hyperplasia (22). Recently, it has been demonstrated that several growth factors, including transforming growth factor β (TGFβ) and basic fibroblast growth factor (bFGF), applied to cardiocytes in culture induce a pattern of contractile protein and proto-oncogenes expression that is very similar to the one produced by work overload in the intact heart (22, 23). These results demonstrate that the lack of mitogenic response by the cardiac myocytes is not due to a loss of receptors for growth factors. They also give further support to the hypothesis that work overload affects gene expression through mechanisms similar or shared by the growth factor receptors.

The inability of the cardiocytes to mount a full mitogenic response in response to work overload or growth factors remains an important challenge that also applies to all other terminally differentiated cells, such as neuron and certain epithelial cells. On one hand, these cells could have irreversibly lost the expression of some of the genes required to traverse the cell cycle. In that case it should be impossible for them to re-enter the cell cycle in response to any stimulus. On the other hand, a part of the terminally differentiated program could induce an inhibitor of the cell cycle. In that case, repression or neutralization of the inhibitor should enable the cells to cycle again. Recently, recessive cellular oncogenes with many of the properties required for this role have been described. One of them, the product of the retinoblastoma (Rb) gene has been shown to belong to this class. The activity of this gene product is neutralized by certain viral oncogenes — SV40 T antigen (4), adenovirus E1A (29). Based on the finding that SV40 T antigene is able to re-induce the ability to cycle to terminally differentiated myotubes (6), it has been possible to re-induce the cell cycle in terminally differentiated myocytes (8).

In physiological terms, the re-expression of the fetal isogenes might be a beneficial adaptation to hemodynamic overload (10). As a consequence of the changes induced in the thin and thick filaments during cardiac hypertrophy, sarcomeres with significantly different functional properties are produced. For the myocardium, the fetal isoform of MHC has been shown to be bioenergetically more efficient than that of the adult. Moreover, because ANF has potent natriuretic, diuretic and vasodilatory effects, the marked induction of this molecule in the ventricle in response to increased blood pressure might be interpreted as an adaptational response to reduce hemodynamic load imposed on the ventricle.

The thyroid receptors are transcriptional regulators of cardiac MHC gene expression

In mammals all the genes of the striated MHC multigene family are, without exception, responsive to T_3 (Fig. 3a), (11). Surprisingly, however, whether T_3 induces or represses the expression of a given MHC gene depends not only on the gene itself, but also on the muscle where it is expressed. Indeed, the same gene can be induced by T_3 in one muscle and repressed in another (11). In the cardiac ventricles, the relative levels of α- and β-MHC are strictly correlated with the T_3 status of the animal and can be manipulated experimentally (11, 16). The expression of α-MHC is dependent on the presence of T_3. The induction of α-MHC at birth is directly correlated with the surge in the circulating T_3 that occurs at this time (16). In hypothyroid animals, the α-MHC gene is not transcribed. The converse is true for β-MHC, which is repressed by T_3. Hyperthyroid states repress the expression of the β-MHC

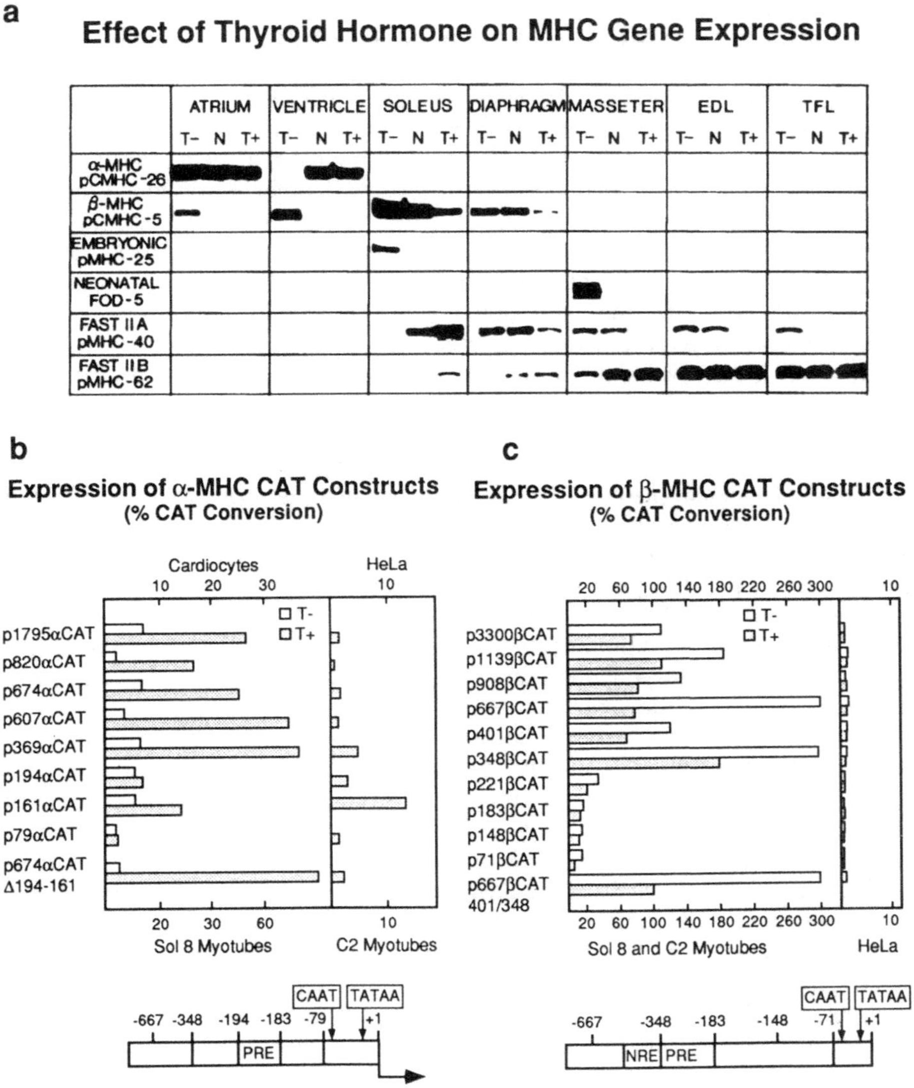

Fig. 3. All sarcomeric MHC genes respond to T_3 in a highly tissue-specific manner. **a)** Pannels of MHC mRNAs analyzed in different muscles of hypo-, eu-, and hyper-thyroid rats. **b)** and **c)** Deletion mapping analysis of the regulatory elements of the α- and β-MHC genes, by transient transfection asssays in different cell types, in the presence or absence of T_3 (11, 18).

gene both at the mRNA and protein levels and produces a myocardium constituted exclusively by α-MHC (Fig. 3a) (11, 16).

The molecular mechanism of thyroid hormone action has been elucidated, at least in part, by the cloning of T_3 receptors (7). The T_3 receptors are hormone-dependent transcriptional factors that exercise their effect through binding to a thyroid hormone responsive element (TRE) in the responsive genes (7, 13). The TRE for the human and rat α-MHC genes has been characterized by a combination of deletion mapping, site-directed mutagenesis, and in vitro and in vivo hormone receptor binding assays (Fig. 3b) (11, 25). These two genes have a TRE with identical sequence of 30 nucleotides, which is able to confer thyroid hormone sensitivity to any heterologous gene (11). Thus, by itself, the TRE of the α-MHC genes constitutes an enhancer element which is required and sufficient to confer T_3 responsiveness.

The mechanism of T_3 repression of MHC gene expression is less well understood. In the human and rat β-MHC genes, homologous sequences to the TRE of the α-MHC genes have not been indentified (Fig. 3c) (18, 25). However, it has been recently demonstrated that inhibition of gene transcription by steroid hormones does not necesseraly require a direct interaction of the receptors with their target genes. Instead, it can involve the formation of heterodimers formed by the hormone receptors and other positive trans-acting factors, such as c-fos and c-jun. The positive regulatory function of these factors becomes inhibited by their heterodimerization with the receptors, thus preventing the expression of the target gene in a hormonally dependent manner (7). Such a mechanism, described for a number of genes that are down-regulated by glucocorticoids and retinoic acid, is likely to be operative for the repression of MHC function by T_3. Indeed, the MEF2-dependent transactivation of β-MHC gene expression (31, and authors, unpublished observations) is inhibited by the T_3 receptors.

Although T_3 plays an important role in regulating cardiac MHC expression, this hormone is not solely responsible for the regulation of these genes. In contrast to its dependence on T_3 in the ventricles, expression of the α-MHC gene is unresponsive to the hormone in the atria of the same heart (Fig. 3a) (11, 16). The different behavior in the two tissues is not due to the lack of functional thyroid hormone receptors in the atria, since other genes in this structure are readily responsive to the hormone. A similar phenomenon is apparent for the β-MHC gene, which is repressed by T_3 in the ventricles, but expressed at almost normal levels in the slow skeletal muscle fibers (Fig. 3b) (11). Because the expression of the cardiac MHC genes is conferred by a combination of several distinct positive and negative cis-regulatory elements (Fig. 3b and 3c) (18, 26), the relative distribution of the corresponding trans-acting factors is likely to vary in the different muscles and in different species. Thus, in addition to T_3 and its receptors, other factors that are specific to different muscle types also play an important role in the regulation of MHC gene expression.

MEF2 (muscle enhancer factor 2) comprises a family of tissue-restricted transcriptional factors

The identification of skeletal-muscle-specific proteins (such as the basic helix-loop-helix (bHLH) of the MyoD family) that activate transcription of a number of gene expressed in skeletal muscle and can convert nonmyogenic cell lines into differentiated skeletal muscle, has provided invaluable clues into events governing myogenesis (21, 28). However, the bHLH protein family is not inclusive because its members have not been identified in cardiac tissues. In addition, a number of genes regulated by MyoD are also expressed in cardiac muscle, where they do not require MyoD for expression. Also, several muscle-specific genes are expressed independently of MyoD in skeletal muscles (21, 26). A plausible model for the activation of the same gene in both skeletal and cardiac muscles would invoke transcription factors common to both muscle types. Candidates for such factors are the transcription regulators called MEF2, which interact with an A/T-rich motif found in the regulatory region of several cardiac and skeletal muscle-specific genes (9, 31). Several distinct MEF2 isoforms, produced by alternative splicing of the transcripts of four distinct but related genes, were cloned in our laboratory (Fig. 4a) (31). These MEF2 proteins belong to the MADS gene superfamily that include the serum response factor (SRF) and transcriptional regulators found in yeast and plants (31).

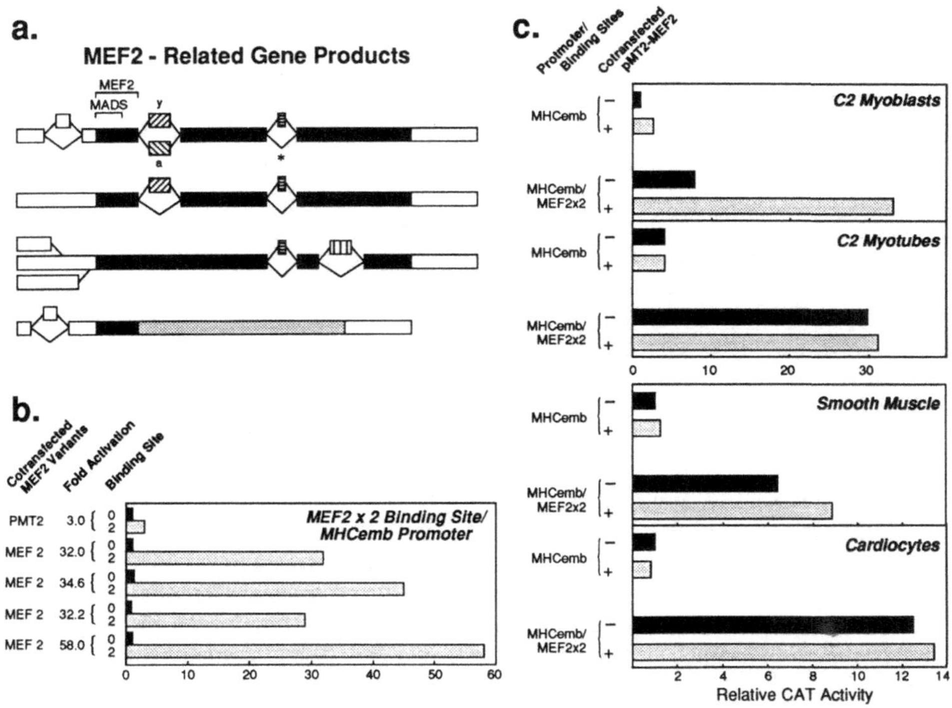

Fig. 4. The human myocyte-specific enhancer factor 2 comprises a group of tissue-restricted MADs box transcription factors. **a)** Schematic representation of the MEF2 isoforms produced by alternative splicing of the transcripts of four different genes. Untranslated sequences are in white. **b)** All four MEF2 genes encode transcription factors that induce expression of MEF2 responsive genes in non-muscle cells (HeLa). **c)** Differentiated muscle cells have endogenous MEF2 activity which is not increased by exogenously transfected MEF2 (31).

Although the MEF2 mRNAs are detected in most tissues, the expression of their corresponding proteins is strictly restricted to cardiac, skeletal and smooth muscles, as well as to the neural cells of the brain (31). These tissues, where different MEF2 isoforms are expressed in a developmentaly regulated manner, display endogenous

MEF2 DNA-binding and transactivating activity (Fig. 4c) (31). In nonmuscle cells, transfection of any of the 13 MEF2 variants is sufficient to induce the expression of promoters under the control of MEF2 regulatory elements, demonstrating that the cloned sequences correspond to positive trans-active factors (Fig. 4b and 4c) (31).

Interestingly, there is a close functional correlation between the bHLH proteins of the MyoD family and the MEF2 proteins. On one hand, expression of MyoD or myogenin in various non-muscle cells is sufficient to induce MEF2 DNA-binding and transcriptional activity (3, 31). MEF2 in turn induces myogenin, another member of the bHLH regulators (5). In addition, MyoD and MEF2 interact in vitro and in vivo, and together activate their target genes in a cooperative fashion (authors, unpublished observations). It is thus tempting to postulate that, similarly to the bHLH regulators in skeletal muscles, novel transcription factors may also be involved in a cross-regulatory loop with MEF2 in cardiac tissues. Such cardiac-specific factors, however, have yet to be identified.

Direct injection of genes in the myocardium of large mammals: a useful model to study gene expression under experimentally controlled physiological conditions

Until recently, regulated gene expression in vivo has been studied by using transfection assays of cultured cells and/or by creating transgenic animals. In the case of terminally differentiated cells, such as the cardiac myocytes, there is lack of phenotypically suitable established cell lines. These problems are further accentuated for the study of genes expressed in the myocardium. Indeed, even in the best of cases, the interpretation and physiological significance of results obtained in primary myocyte cultures is weakened by the fact that the cells are not embedded in their natural environment. These reasons and the paucicity of information on cardiac gene regulation in controlled physiological conditions have stimulated the search for alternative approaches.

Introduction of exogenous DNA into germ cells and creation of transgenic animals has greatly improved the study of gene regulation in a physiologically meaningful environment, as well as during development and organ differentiation. But for practical purposes, this approach is limited to small mammals, the mouse in particular, due to the significant effort and costs related to the creation of transgene carriers and the fact that the vast majority of genetic knowledge in mammals originates from the mouse. Thus, the recent demonstration of gene transfer in vivo by simple injection of pure plasmid DNA into skeletal muscle of living mice (30), was a significant development that provided a convenient approach to study gene regulation that combined many of the advantages of the in vitro transfections and the transgenic models for short term analyses. Variations of this principle for in vivo gene transfer have been used to deliver recombinant DNA, or in vitro genetically altered smooth muscle cells, to vascular endothelium via catheter, resulting in low, but detectable levels of gene expression (1, 20). This model of gene transfer in vivo offers a potential route for gene therapy in human disease.

The potential to take up and express naked DNA introduced by simple injection is not limited to skeletal muscle. In the recent past, several laboratories have demonstrated the expression of naked recombinant DNA injected into the rat heart

(1, 30). In this model, expression of the injected genes, as determined by histochemistry, appears to be localized around the injection channel, with a small number of cells actually expressing the gene product (1, 30).

Rodents differ substantially in their cardiovascular physiology and pathophysiology from humans in the rate of metabolism as reflected in the heart rate, in the pattern of cardiac contractile isoforms, or the induction of isoform switches during development and hypertrophy (12, 13, 19, 22, 24). Moreover, while small mammals have been the model of choice for genetic and molecular analyses, large mammals, and particularly the dog, have been the model of choice for physiological studies. In fact, more experimental data on cardiac performance in a variety of physiological and pathological conditions has been obtained using the dog as a model than from all other species combined, including the human. These facts, together with the closer similarities between canine and human cardiac physiology, make this species the animal of choice for the analysis of gene regulation under experimental conditions that are physiologically meaningful and that could provide relevant insights into expression patterns prevailing in humans.

For all these reasons, we developed a methodology to study gene expression in large mammals by injection of plasmid DNA into canine myocardium (27). The observation that the predominant isoform of contractile proteins in the canine myocardium is (as in humans) the β-MHC further supports the use of this model for studies relevant to human cardiovascular biology. Several important parameters relevant to the expression of injected gene constructs in this model have been characterized (Fig. 5) (27).

Reporter gene constructs under the control of the muscle-specific β-MHC or liver specific (Apo A1) promoters were injected into the canine myocardium. The level of reporter gene expression, which was linear in relation to the amount of DNA injected (Fig. 5a), was not affected by the injection technique employed and did not correlate with the amount of injury imposed upon the cardiac tissue. There was no regional variation in expression of injected reporter genes throughout the left ventricular wall (Fig. 5b). Using the muscle-specific β-MHC promoter, reporter gene expression was one to two orders of magnitude greater in the heart than in skeletal muscle. Expression in the left ventricle was three-fold higher than in the right ventricle and maximal expression was noted at 7 days post injection (27). Furthermore, the pattern of expression of the injected gene constructs with serial deletions of the 5′ flanking region was similar to those transfected in primary cardiocytes, thus proving the utility of this model to map promoter regions in vivo and understand their role under experimental pathophysiological conditions (Figs. 3c and 5c) (18, 26, 27).

Thus, gene injection into canine myocardium is not only a powerful tool to study regulated gene expression in large mammals in vivo, but also provides an experimental model system where the biochemical basis of some important clinical problems prevailing in the human myocardium might be investigated.

Conclusions

The results summarized above constitute a small sample of the insights that the new tools of cellular and molecular biology can provide to further our understanding of the developmental, physiological, and pathological biology of the myocardium.

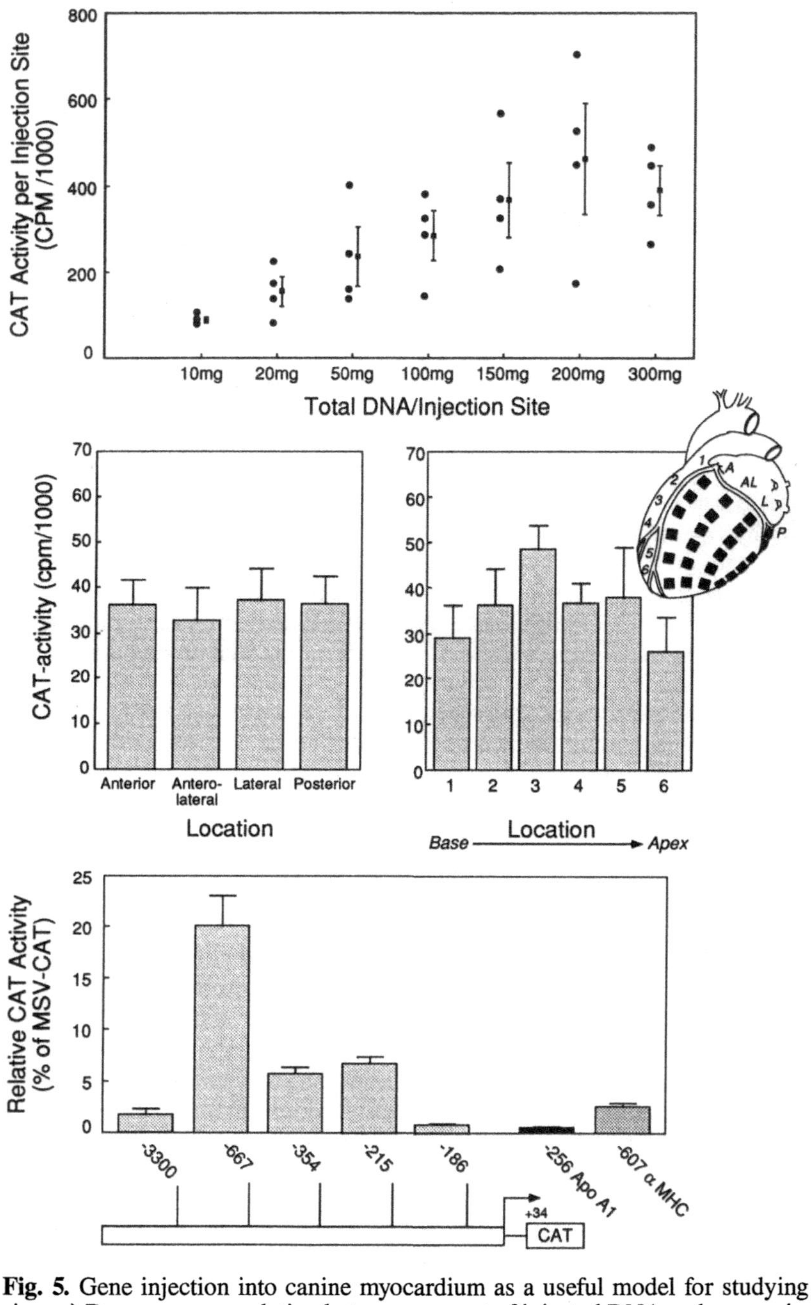

Fig. 5. Gene injection into canine myocardium as a useful model for studying gene expression. **a)** Dose-response relation between amount of injected DNA and expression of gene construct. **b)** Regional expression pattern of injected gene constructs throughout the left ventricular wall, comprising six injection sites ranging from base to apex (see cartoon). **c)** Mapping of the regulatory region of the β-MHC gene in vivo, open bars. Note the lack of activity of injected α-MHC, hatched bar and ApoAI, solid bar, whose corresponding genes are not expressed in the ventricular myocardium.

Despite the limited nature of the survey presented, the examples used are sufficient to demonstrate that the myocardium is biochemically very plastic. In addition, the myocardium can serve as a good experimental model to address some important questions that are relevant, not only to the cardiovascular system, but are also of general biological significance. In addition, it is clear that cardiac development and hypertrophy are not simple quantitative processes leading to an increase in ventricular mass. They are qualitatively different and a heterogeneous process that is highly influenced by the nature of the hypertrophic stimulus and the developmental stage of the myocardium. Further work is needed, however, to elucidate the precise mechanisms by which the hemodynamic and/or mechanic stimuli are converted into biochemical signals that lead to quantitative as well as qualitative changes in gene expression. A better understanding of the genes involved in converting precursor mesenchymal cell into the cardiogenic pathway, the cell specific transcriptional factors responsible for the expression of the cardiac specific genes, as well as the genes involved in blocking these cells in the terminally differentiated phenotype is also required. Without this information it will be very difficult to prevent the development of end stage cardiac failure in patients with long standing congenital cardiac malformations or their sequelae. Therefore, it is imperative to obtain this information in order to manipulate the process of cardiac hypertrophy and changes of contractile state to physiological advantage.

References

1. Acsadi G, Jiao S, Agnes J, Duke D, Williams P, Chong W, Wolff JA (1991) Direct gene transfer and expression into rat heart in vivo. New Biologist 3:71-81
2. Barany M (1967) ATPase activity of myosin correlated with speed of muscle shortening. J Gen Physiol 50:suppl:197—218
3. Cserjesi P, Olson EN (1991) Myogenin induces the myocytes-specific enhancer binding factor MEF-2 independently of other muscle-specific gene products. Mol Cell Biol 11:4854—4862
4. DeCaprio JA, Ludlow JW, Figge J, Shew JY, Huang CM, Lee WH, Marsilio E, Pausha E, Livingston DM (1988) SV40 large tumor antigen forms a specific complex with the product of the retinoblastoma susceptibility gene. Cell 54:275—283
5. Edmondson DG, Cheng T-C, Cserjesi P, Chakraborty T, Olson EN (1992) Analysis of the myogenin promoter reveals an indirect pathway for positive autoregulation mediated by the muscle-specific enhancer factor MEF-2. Mol Cell Biol 12:3665—3677
6. Endo T, Nadal-Ginard B (1989) Sv 40 large T-antigen induces re-entry of terminally differentiated myotubes into the cell cycle. In Kedes LH, Stockdale FE (ed) Cellular and Molecular Biology of Muscle Development, UCLA Symposia on Molecular and Cellular Biology New Series vol 93; AR Liss New York, p 95—104
7. Evans RM (1988) The steroid and thyroid hormone receptor superfamily. Science 240:889—895
8. Field LJ (1988) Atrial natriuretic factor-SV40 T antigen transgenes produce tumors and cardiac arrhythmias in mice. Science 239:1029—1032
9. Gossett LA, Kelvin DJ, Sternberg EA, Olson EN (1989) A new myocyte-specific enhancer-binding factor that recognizes a conserved element associated with multiple muscle-specific genes. Mol Cell Biol 9:5022—5033
10. Grossman W (1980) Cardiac hypertrophy: useful adaptation or pathologic process? Am J Med 69:576—584
11. Izumo S, Mahdavi V, Nadal-Ginard B (1986) All members of the MHC multigene family respond to thyroid hormone in a highly tissue-specific manner. Science 231:597—600

12. Izumo S, Lompre A-M, Matsuoka R, Koren G, Schwartz K, Nadal-Ginard B, Mahdavi V (1987) Myosin heavy chain messenger RNA and protein isoform transitions during cardiac hypertrophy: Interaction between hemodynamic and thryroid hormone-induced signals. J Clin Invest 79:970—977
13. Izumo S, Mahdavi V (1988) Thyroid hormone receptor isoforms generated by alternative splicing differentially activate myosin HC gene transcription. Nature 334: 539—542
14. Izumo S, Mahdavi V, Nadal-Ginard B (1988) Protooncogene induction and reprogramming of cardiac gene expression produced by pressure overload. Proc Natl Acad Sci USA 85:339—343
15. Lompre A-M, Schwartz K, d'Albis A, Lacombe G, Thiem NV, Swynghedauw B (1979) Myosin isoenzyme redistribution in chronic heart overload. Nature 282: 105—107
16. Lompre A-M, Mahdavi V, Nadal-Ginard B (1984) Expression of the cardiac ventricular α and β myosin heavy chain genes is developmentally and hormonally regulated. J Biol Chem 259:6437—6446
17. Mahdavi V, Chambers AP, Nadal-Ginard B (1984) Cardiac α and β myosin heavy chain genes are organized in tandem. Proc Natl Acad Sci USA 81:2626—2630
18. Mahdavi V, Koren G, Michaud S, Pinset C, Izumo S (1989) Identification of the sequences responsible for the tissue-specific and hormonal regulation of the cardiac myosin heavy chain genes. In: Kedes LH, Stockdale FE (ed) Cellular and Molecular Biology of Muscle Development, UCLA Symposia on Molecular and Cellular Biology New Series vol 93; AR Liss New York. pp 369—379
19. Mercadier JJ, Bouveret P, Gorza L, Schiaffino S, Clark WA, Swynghdauw B, Schwartz K (1983) Myosin isoenzymes in normal and hypertrophied human ventricular myocardium. Circ Res 53:52—62
20. O'Brien TX, Hunter JJ, Dyson E, Chien KR (1991) Heart-to-Heart, new approaches for gene transfer in the myocardium. Circulation 86:2133—2136
21. Olson EN (1990) MyoD Family. A paradigm for development? Genes & Dev 4:1454—1461
22. Parker TG, Schneider MD (1991) Growth factors, proto-oncogenes, and plasticity of the cardiac phenotype. Annu rev Physiol 53:179—200
23. Simpson P (1983) Norepinephrine-stimulated hypertrophy of cultured rat myocardial cells is an α1 Adrenergic Response. J Clin Invest 72:732—738
24. Swynghedauw B (1986) Developmental and functional adaptation of contractile proteins in cardiac and skeletal muscles. Physiol Rev 66:710—771
25. Thompson WR, Koren G, Izumo S, Mahdavi V, Nadal-Ginard B (1990) Molecular regulation of myosin heavy chain switches: A model for study of cardiac gene expression. In: Clark EB and Takao A (ed) Developmental Cardiology: Morphogenesis and Function; Mount Kisko NY pp 13—25
26. Thompson WR, Mahdavi V, Nadal-Ginard B (1992) A MyoD1-independent muscle-specific enhancer controls the expression of the beta-myosin heavy chain gene in skeletal and cardiac muscle cells. J Biol Chem 266:22678—22688
27. von Harsdorf R, Schott RJ, Shen Y-T, Vatner SF, Mahdavi V, Nadal-Ginard B (1993) Gene injection onto canine myocardium as a useful model for studying gene expression in the heart of large mammals. Circ Res 72:688—695
28. Weintraub H, Davis RL, Tapscott SJ, Thayer MJ, Krause M, Benezta R, Blackwell TK, Turner D, Rupp R, Hollenberg S, Zhuang Y, Lassar A (1991) The MyoD gene family: Nodal point during specification of the muscle cell lineage. Science 251:761—766
29. White P, Buchkovich KJ, Horowitz JM, Friend SH, Raybuck M, Weinberg RA, Harlow E (1988) Association between a oncogene and anti-oncogene: the adenovirus E1A proteins bind to the retinoblastoma gene product. Nature 334:124—129
30. Wolff JA, Malone RW, Williams P, Chong W, Acsadi G, Jani A, Felgner PL (1990) Direct gene transfer into mouse muscle in vivo. Science 247:1465—1468

31. Yu Y-T, Breitbart RE, Smoot LB, Lee Y, Mahdavi V, Nadal-Ginard B (1992) Human myocyte-specific enhancer factor 2 comprises a group of tissue-restricted MAD box transcription factors. Genes & Dev 6:1783—1798
32. Zak R (1974) Development and proliferative capacity of cardiac muscle cells. Circ Res 35:suppl II:17—26

Authors' address:
Bernardo Nadal-Ginard, M.D., Ph.D.
Department of Cardiology, Children's Hospital
300 Longwood Avenue
Boston, MA 02115 USA

Myocardial perfusion dependent and independent mechanisms of regional myocardial dysfunction in hypertrophy

S. F. Vatner, L. Hittinger*

Departments of Medicine, Harvard Medical School,
Brigham & Women's Hospital, Boston, Massachusetts
and the New England Regional Primate Research Center, Southborough, Massachusetts

Abstract: Reduced coronary reserve is one of the hallmarks of ventricular hypertrophy. Although this reduced coronary reserve may not affect baseline left ventricular (LV) function, it could be of greater importance during periods of stress such as occurs during exercise where increased metabolic demands induced by the stress may not be fully met by increases in coronary blood flow. The impaired subendocardial coronary reserve is caused not only by the hypertrophy but also by the hemodynamic changes, e.g., the LV subendocardial wall stress, which increases markedly upon exercise. In the severely hypertrophied heart during exercise there is impaired subendocardial wall function even after 10 beats, i.e., the first 3 s of exercise, at a time when LV pressures and stresses had not increased, and subendocardial perfusion was still preserved. During more severe exercise, subendocardial dysfunction persisted and was associated with reduced subendocardial perfusion. After β-adrenergic receptor blockade with propanolol, the most intense level of exercise was associated with lesser increases in systolic and diastolic LV wall stresses, heart rate, and LV dP/dt, and the endo/epi blood flow ratio, an index of adequacy of subendocardial perfusion, was no longer reduced below unity, and there were no decreases in subendocardial wall thickening. Thus, the subendocardial dysfunction occurred rapidly, before alterations in LV systolic or diastolic wall stress or an alteration in the endo/epi blood flow ratio. However, the subendocardial hypoperfusion and depression in subendocardial wall thickening observed during more severe exercise in dogs with LV hypertrophy was prevented by pretreatment with β-adrenergic receptor blockade. Therefore, myocardial perfusion dependent and independent mechanisms mediate regional myocardial dysfunction during exercise in the hypertrophied heart.

Key Words: Myocardial hypertrophy; coronary circulation; β-adrenergic receptor blockade; myocardial ischemia; regional wall thickening; transmural function; transmural blood flow

Introduction

Regional left ventricular (LV) function and myocardial perfusion are generally preserved in the presence of severe LV hypertrophy (9, 11—15, 18—21, 23, 27). Blood flow levels per gram of tissue remain normal and the endo/epi ratio is also preserved. Despite the ability of the hypertrophied heart to maintain function and perfusion under baseline conditions, reduced coronary reserve has been shown to be an important feature of right ventricular hypertrophy (19, 20) as well as LV hypertrophy (1—5, 7—9, 11—15, 17, 18, 21, 23, 26, 28). This has been observed in human studies (7,

Supported in part by US Public Health Service grants HL 38070, 33107, 33065, and RR 00168.

* Dr. Hittinger's current address is INSERM U2, Hopital Leon Bernard, 94456 Limeil Brevannes Cedex, France.

8, 17) as well as experimental models. Reduced coronary reserve is evident in response to a potent coronary vasodilator, e.g., adenosine (11, 20), or in response to stress, e.g., pacing (3, 9, 28) or exercise (4, 13, 14, 19). Although this reduced coronary reserve does not impair baseline LV function, it could be of greater importance during periods of stress, such as occurs during exercise, where increased metabolic demands induced by the exercise may not be fully met by increases in coronary blood flow. We hypothesize further that these limitations would be most apparent subendocardially since the increased subendocardial wall stress and compressive forces that occur with severe hypertrophy may be important in mediating the limitation in subendocardial coronary reserve.

Although several studies have examined transmural myocardial perfusion in the hypertrophied heart, relatively few have examined both regional blood flow and regional ventricular function across the wall (13, 14, 26). We have recently had the opportunity to examine the regulation of both regional myocardial perfusion and contraction in the process of severe LV hypertrophy. This review summarizes several of those studies (13, 14, 26).

Methods

The model of severe LV hypertrophy is created by banding the ascending aorta of puppies at 8—10 weeks of age, such that 1 to 2 years later severe LV hypertrophy has developed in response to the increased pressure gradient across the aortic band. Some of these dogs with severe LV hypertrophy progress spontaneously to LV failure (11, 12, 25—27). One of the underlying hypotheses of this review is that the response to stress, e.g., exercise or coronary artery occlusion, in subendocardial layers might be quite different than in subepicardial layers in the presence of compensated severe LV hypertrophy. The techniques used to study the response to exercise and coronary artery occlusion across the myocardial wall in normal dogs and dogs with LV hypertrophy are shown in Fig. 1 and have been described in detail previously (13, 14). Pairs of ultrasonic crystals were implanted in subendocardial and subepicardial layers of the ventricle, as well as transmurally, to complement the normal instrumentation to study global LV function in chronically-instrumented, conscious dogs. At least 2—3 weeks were allowed for the animals to recover from the operation. Using these techniques it was then possible to record instantaneous and continuous measurements of subendocardial and subepicardial wall thickening as well as full wall thickening, LV diameter, pressure, and LV dP/dt. This allowed us to measure global and regional LV function under baseline conditions, and also during exercise and recovery from exercise, as well as during coronary artery occlusion. In order to assess regional myocardial perfusion, radioactive microspheres were injected at baseline and during exercise and recovery. We examined the responses to graded treadmill exercise using three different levels of exercise and followed the recovery from exercise for 1 h. Experiments were conducted in the presence and absence of β-adrenergic receptor blockade with propranolol.

Results and discussion

In normal dogs during graded exercise, there was a gradual increase in subendocardial and subepicardial wall thickening (Fig. 2) along with the expected changes in

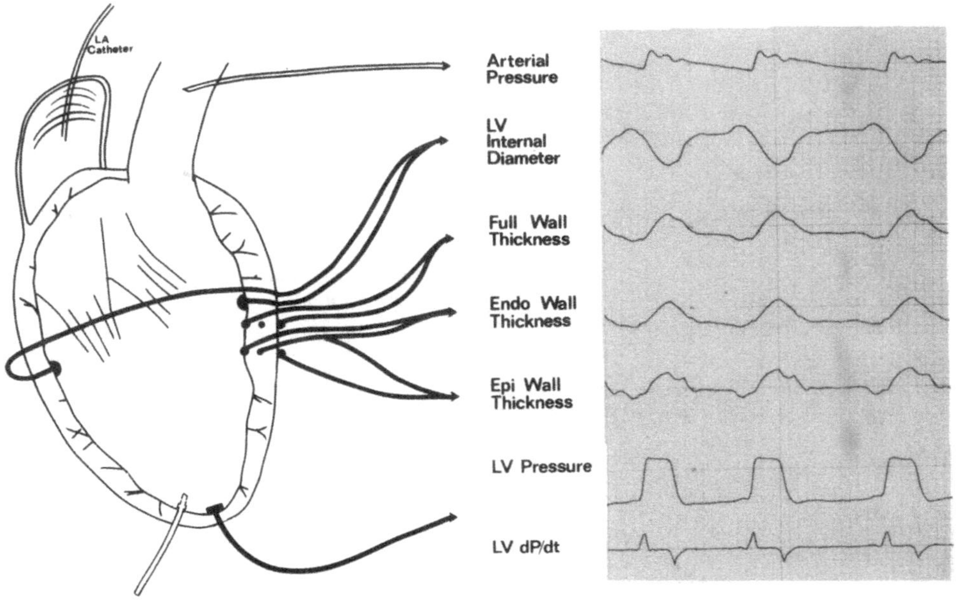

Fig. 1. This figure shows the instrumentation used to measure regional myocardial function across the wall in normal dogs and dogs with severe LV hypertrophy at rest and during exercise. In addition to measurements of arterial and left atrial pressure using catheters, LV internal diameter, full wall thickness, and subendocardial and subepicardial wall thicknesses were measured by using implanted ultrasonic gauges. LV pressure and LV dP/dt were recorded from the implanted LV micromanometer. In addition a catheter was implanted in the left ventricle to calibrate the micromanometer. (Reprinted from Hittinger L, Shannon RP, Kohin S, Manders WT, Kelly P, Vatner SF: Exercise induced subendocardial dysfunction in dogs with left ventricular hypertrophy. Circulation Research 66:329—343, 1990, with permission of The American Heart Association).

global LV dynamics (Fig. 3), i.e., increases in LV dP/dt, heart rate, and systolic and diastolic wall stresses. Increases in subendocardial wall thickening exceeded those for subepicardial wall thickening. In contrast, in dogs with severe LV hypertrophy there was almost an immediate impairment of subendocardial wall thickening as noted in Fig. 4. Within the first 10 beats there was a significant decrease in subendocardial wall thickening which intensified and progressed through the remainder of the exercise protocol. The subendocardial dysfunction persisted into the recovery from exercise (Fig. 2), when other hemodynamic variables returned to control levels.

To assess whether these changes were due to changes in blood flow, radioactive microspheres were administered at control, initially during exercise when the subendocardial dysfunction was observed, later during more severe, steady-state exercise, and during the recovery period at a time when subendocardial dysfunction persisted. Results from those experiments are shown in Fig. 5. At baseline, the endocardial/epicardial (endo/epi) blood flow ratio, an index of adequacy of subendocardial

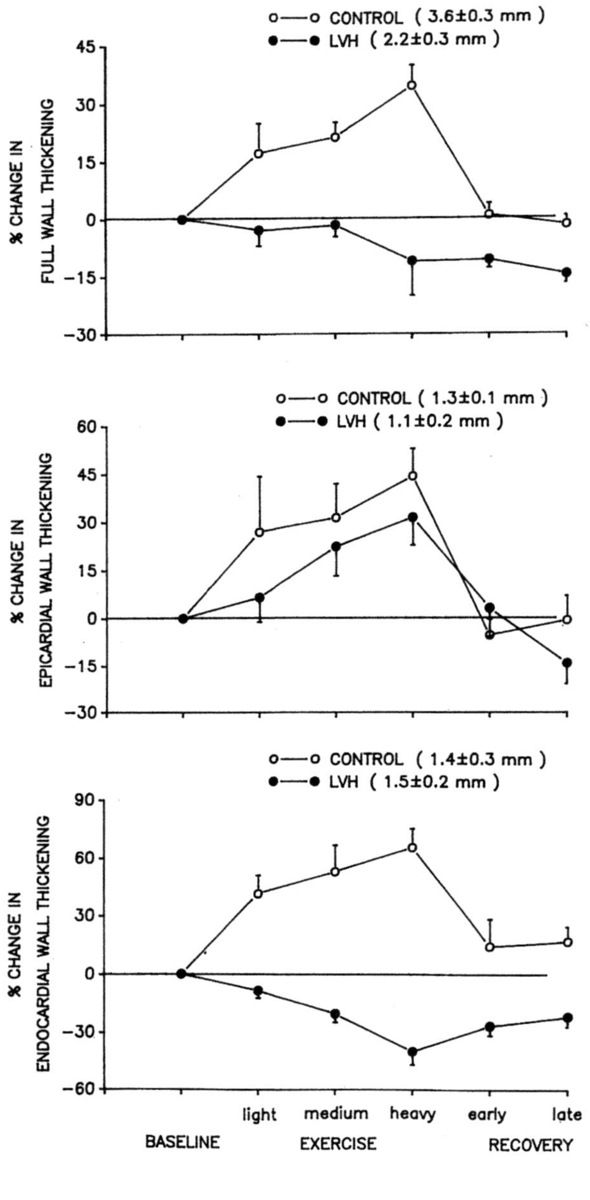

Fig. 2. This figure compares the changes in full wall thickening (top), subepicardial wall thickening (middle) and subendocardial wall thickening (bottom) in both sham-operated controls (open circles) and a group of dogs with severe LV hypertrophy (solid circles). Note that there are no significant differences in responses of subepicardial wall thickening, which increased in both normal dogs and dogs with hypertrophy during exercise and returned to baseline on recovery. In contrast, the subendocardial wall thickening, which increased in normal dogs, actually fell significantly in dogs with severe hypertrophy and remained depressed during the recovery period. (Reprinted from Hittinger L, Shannon RP, Kohin S, Manders WT, Kelly P, Vatner SF: Exercise induced subendocardial dysfunction in dogs with left ventricular hypertrophy. Circulation Research 66:329—343, 1990, with permission of The American Heart Association).

perfusion, was normal in dogs with severe hypertrophy, as has been found by other investigators in the past (1—5, 9, 11—15, 18, 21, 23, 27, 28). However, with more sustained and severe exercise, there was marked impairment of subendocardial flow reserve and a significant reduction in the endo/epi blood flow ratio. This rapidly returned to normal on recovery from exercise such that the subendocardial dysfunction during exercise may in part have been mediated by impaired subendocardial blood flow and the development of subendocardial ischemia. This mechanism could

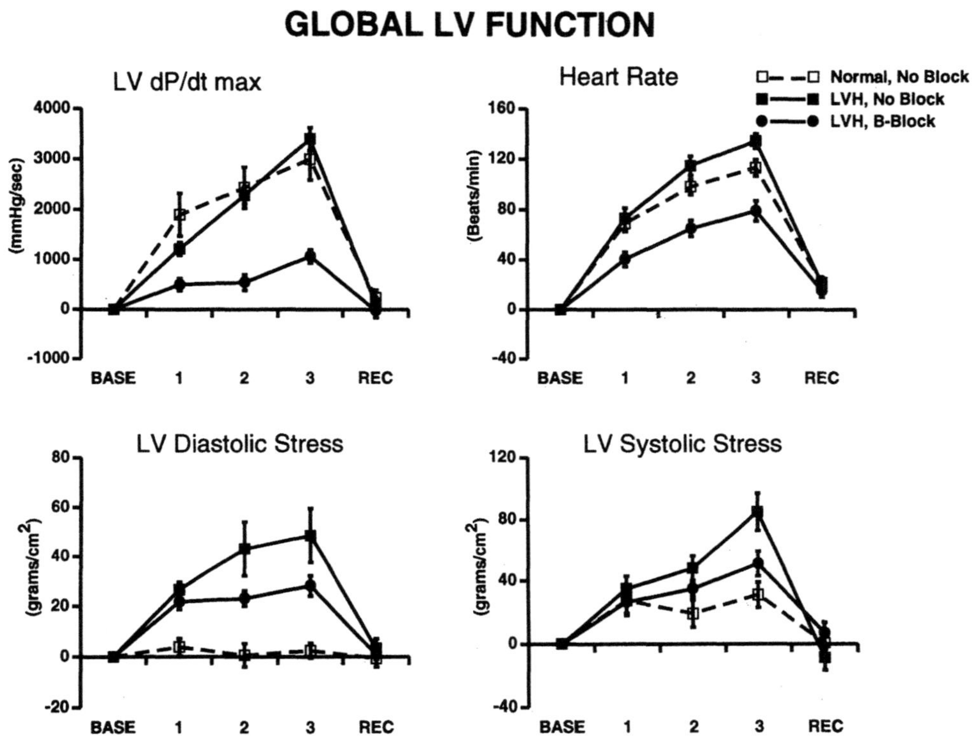

Fig. 3. This figure compares measurements of global LV function, i.e., LV dP/dt (upper left) heart rate (upper right), LV diastolic stress (lower left) and LV systolic stress (lower right) in normal dogs (shown by the open squares) in dogs with severe LV hypertrophy without blockade (shown by solid squares) and with β-adrenergic blockade (shown with the solid circles) in response to three levels of exercise (1, 2, 3) and during recovery (rec). Significantly smaller increases in LV dP/dt and heart rate and diastolic and systolic stresses occurred with exercise in dogs with hypertrophy in the presence of β-adrenergic receptor blockade. (Reprinted from data contained in Hittinger L, Shen Y-T, Patrick TA, Hasebe N, Komamura K, Ihara T, Manders WT, Vatner SF: Mechanisms of subendocardial dysfunction in response to exercise in dogs with left ventricular hypertrophy, Circulation Research 71:423—434, 1992, with permission of The American Heart Association).

not be invoked on recovery from exercise, since perfusion was restored, yet subendocardial dysfunction persisted. Thus, the recovery from exercise was similar to the response to recovery from a brief ischemic episode, i.e., "myocardial stunning" (6, 10). This is the first example of "myocardial stunning" occurring in the absence of any coronary constriction or occlusion, i.e., there is no primary impairment of coronary vascular function in the animals with LV hypertrophy. Myocardial stunning has been demonstrated repeatedly upon recovery from a brief coronary artery occlusion (6, 10) or in response to exercise in the presence of a coronary stenosis (16, 24).

The results from the experiments during severe exercise suggested that subendocardial ischemia developed during exercise, which in turn induced the impaired subendocardial dysfunction. If this were the case, then minimizing the metabolic

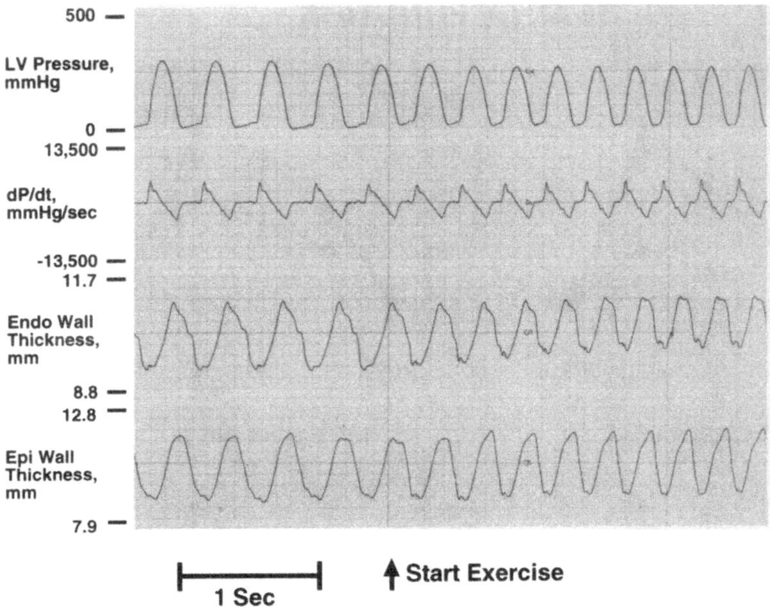

Fig. 4. This figure shows the initial 10 beat response to exercise in dogs with severe LV hypertrophy, on measurements of LV pressure, LV dP/dt and subendocardial and subepicardial wall thicknesses. Note that the subendocardial dysfunction i.e., decreased endo wall thickening, occurred within the first few beats of exercise. (Reprinted from Hittinger L, Shen Y-T, Patrick TA, Hasebe N, Komamura K, Ihara T, Manders WT, Vatner SF: Mechanisms of subendocardial dysfunction in response to exercise in dogs with left ventricular hypertrophy, Circulation Research 71:423—434, 1992, with permission of The American Heart Association).

demands that occur during exercise might alleviate this imbalance between oxygen supply and demand and improve the response of subendocardial wall motion. To test this hypothesis, a further series of experiments was conducted, in which the responses to exercise were compared in the presence and absence of β-adrenergic receptor blockade with propranolol. The working hypothesis was that β adrenergic receptor blockade would limit the increases in heart rate, LV dP/dt, and LV systolic and diastolic wall stresses that occur during exercise, and, therefore, reduce the requirements for oxygen supply and coronary blood flow. Indeed this is what was observed. Figure 3 compares the responses of LV function to exercise in dogs with LV hypertrophy in the presence and absence of β-adrenergic receptor blockade (propranolol, 1 mg/kg). Significantly smaller increases in LV contractility, as reflected by LV dP/dt, heart rate, and systolic and diastolic wall stresses were observed during exercise in the dogs with LV hypertrophy in the presence of β-adrenergic blockade.

The responses of regional myocardial blood flow are shown in Fig. 6. In the presence of β-adrenergic receptor blockade, no longer did the endo/epi blood flow ratio fall significantly. Thus, it appears that there was adequate subendocardial perfusion to meet the demands that occurred during exercise in the presence of β-blockade. In Fig. 7 the responses of regional myocardial function across the wall

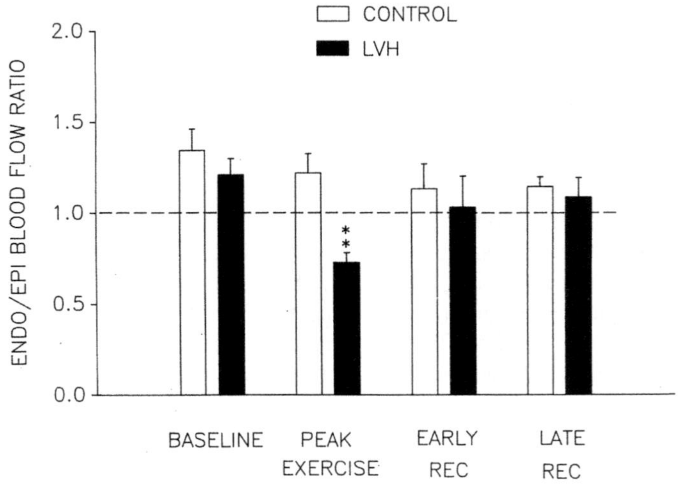

Fig. 5. This figure shows the endo/epi blood flow ratios in sham-operated control dogs (shown by the open bars) and dogs with severe LV hypertrophy (shown by the solid bars) at baseline, during peak exercise and early and late in the recovery period. The endo/epi blood flow ratio was only abnormal during peak exercise and was not abnormal during the recovery period at a time when subendocardial function remained depressed. (Reprinted from Hittinger L, Shannon RP, Kohin S, Manders WT, Kelly P, Vatner SF: Exercise induced subendocardial dysfunction in dogs with left ventricular hypertrophy. Circulation Research 66:329—343, 1990, with permission of The American Heart Association).

are shown. These data are consistent with the responses of blood flow, i.e., there was no longer reduction in subendocardial wall thickening during exercise in the dogs with LV hypertrophy, when they were pretreated with β-adrenergic receptor blockade (Fig. 8). Thus, the regional, subendocardial impairment of function in response to exercise was ameliorated by β blockade, which limited the increases in metabolic demands that occur during exercise and prevented the fall in subendocardial perfusion.

To test further the hypothesis that the subendocardial mechanical dysfunction during exercise in dogs with LVH is due to either enhanced myocardial metabolic demands or relative subendocardial hypoperfusion, regional wall motion was compared in the same dogs with LVH at matched levels of heart rate, LV dP/dt, and wall stress in the presence and absence of β-adrenergic receptor blockade. When data were compared during exercise at equivalent loading conditions (Table 1), the major determinants of myocardial oxygen consumption and coronary perfusion, i.e., heart rate, arterial pressure, LV dP/dt, and systolic and diastolic wall stresses, were not different. However, decreases in subendocardial wall thickening were still observed in the absence of β-adrenergic receptor blockade in LVH dogs exercising at a lower level and were no longer present in LVH dogs exercising at a greater level after β-adrenergic receptor blockade. Surprisingly, the reduced subendocardial wall thickening that occurred at the lower intensity of exercise in dogs with LVH without β-adrenergic receptor blockade was no longer associated with a fall in the endo/epi blood flow ratio during exercise. This was surprising, because neither the enhanced metabolic demands nor the relative subendocardial hypoperfusion (i.e., neither of the two most likely mechanisms of the subendocardial dysfunction) was required for subendocardial dysfunction to occur. The findings that β-adrenergic receptor blockade improved subendocardial wall motion during exercise, even in the face of matched levels of LV systolic and diastolic stresses, heart rate, and LV dP/dt, and that these differences could not be simply attributable to relative subendocardial hypoperfusion suggest that the attenuation of myocardial oxygen demands is not the only mechanism responsible for the salutary effects of β-adrenergic receptor blockade. In fact, it even raises the intriguing possibility that the decreased endo/epi blood flow ratio, which is frequently observed in the hypertrophied heart in response to stress (1—5, 7—9, 11—15, 17—21, 23, 26—28) may under certain circumstances be secondary to reduced subendocardial function rather than a cause of the subendocardial dysfunction.

Keeping in mind that the subendocardial dysfunction occurred very early during exercise, i.e., within the first 10 beats (Fig. 4, Table 2), it was felt important also to examine transmural blood flow early in the response to exercise in dogs with LV hypertrophy to see if the impaired subendocardial perfusion occurred as an initial or later event. To address this question, radioactive microspheres were also injected at stage one of exercise in the dogs with severe LV hypertrophy. The results from those experiments are shown in Fig. 6 for blood flow and in Figs. 2 and 4 for regional function. As noted in Figs. 2 and 4, the subendocardial dysfunction occurred early during exercise and was clearly present during early exercise at a time there was no subendocardial hypoperfusion, as reflected by a normal endo/epi blood flow ratio as shown in Fig. 6. Thus, it is likely that the later episodes of subendocardial dysfunction that occurred during more severe exercise and the subendocardial dysfunction that persisted into recovery, i.e., the myocardial stunning, were due to impaired subendocardial perfusion and the resultant myocardial ischemia that developed. On the other hand, there must be another mechanism that contributes to the subendocardial dysfunction that precedes the derangement in subendocardial perfusion, and is not observed in the presence of β-adrenergic receptor blockade. This mechanism appears independent of blood flow and may be located at any point in the β-adrenergic signalling process from β receptor activation to calcium mobilization to contraction. This mechanism is important in the initial adjustments to exercise in the severely hypertrophied heart and may also be an important mechanism in decompensation from hypertrophy to heart failure.

Comparison of the initial adjustments to exercise with the initial adjustments to coronary artery occlusion is useful to support the concept that the initial subendocardial dysfunction with exercise is not mediated by ischemia. Accordingly, the first 10 beats of exercise (Table 2) are compared with the first 10 beats of coronary artery occlusion in dogs with LV hypertrophy (Table 3). In both instances subendocardial dysfunction was evident as reflected by decrease in extent of subendocardial wall thickening. In both cases there were no major alterations in global LV function. However, there were major differences in the mechanism of subendocardial dysfunction. The response to coronary artery occlusion involved a rapid reduction in systolic wall thickening while end diastolic wall thickness was preserved. In contrast, in response to exercise, end-diastolic subendocardial wall thickness was compromised, with preservation of end-systolic wall thickness. These observations in combi-

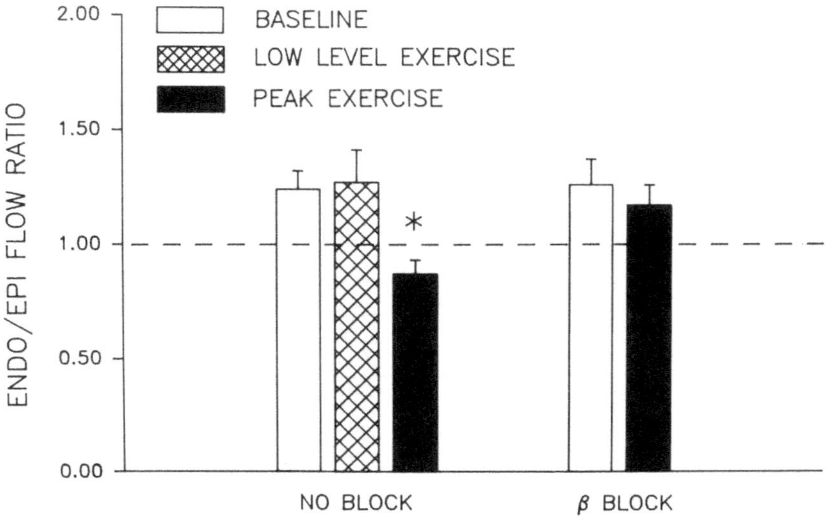

Fig. 6. This figure compares the endo/epi blood flow ratio in dogs with LV hypertrophy in the absence of any blockade on the left and in the presence of β-adrenergic blockade on the right. Measurements prior to exercise (baseline) are shown by the open bars, and responses during peak exercise are shown by the solid bars. The cross hatched bar in the left panel is a measure of blood flow distribution during the initial response to low level exercise. (Reprinted from Hittinger L, Shen Y-T, Patrick TA, Hasebe N, Komamura K, Ihara T, Manders WT, Vatner SF: Mechanisms of subendocardial dysfunction in response to exercise in dogs with left ventricular hypertrophy, Circulation Research 71:423—434, 1992, with permission of The American Heart Association).

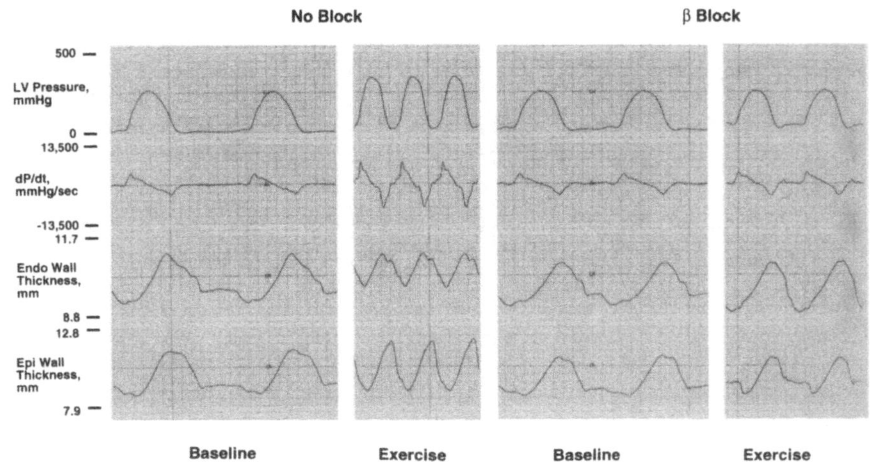

Fig. 7. This figure compares the responses of regional function to exercise in a dog with LV hypertrophy in the absence of β-blockade (left panels) and in the presence of β-blockade (right panels). In the absence of β-blockade, exercise reduced subendocardial wall thickening, i.e., subendocardial dysfunction was observed in the absence of β-adrenergic blockade.

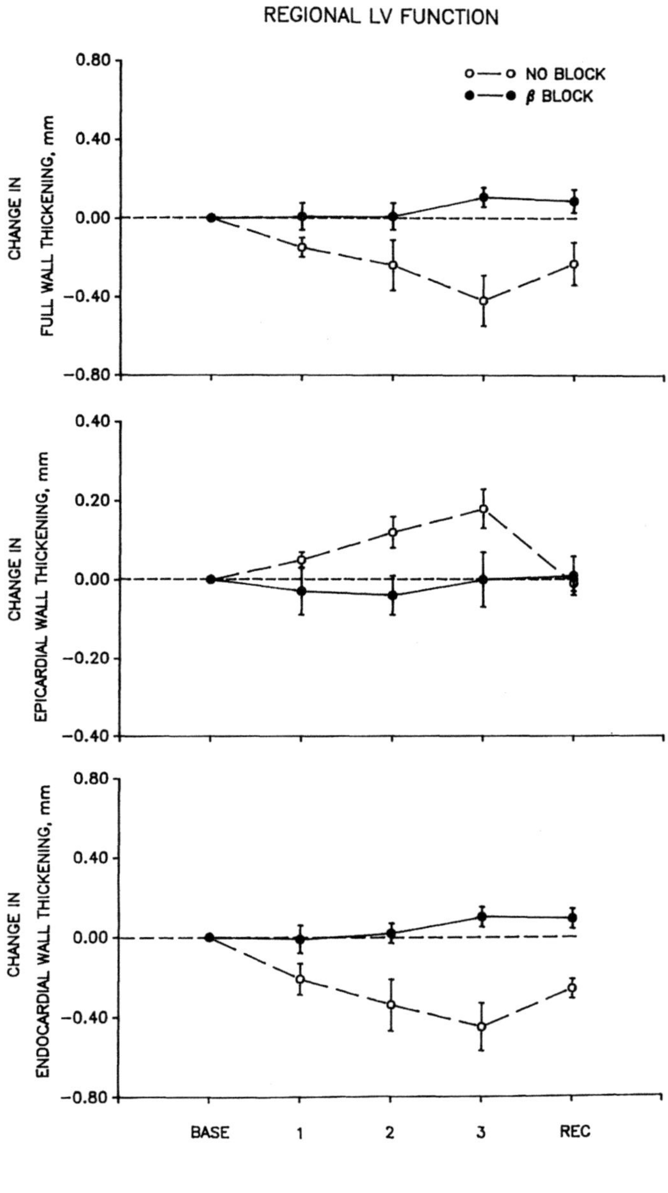

Fig. 8. The changes in regional LV function across the wall are compared in dogs with severe LV hypertrophy without blockade (shown by the open circles) and dogs with hypertrophy in the presence of β-adrenergic receptor blockade (closed circles). Note that the reduced subendocardial wall thickening which occurred in dogs with hypertrophy in the absence of blockade was no longer observed in the presence of β-adrenergic receptor blockade. (Reprinted from Hittinger L, Shen Y-T, Patrick TA, Hasebe N, Komamura K, Ihara T, Manders WT, Vatner SF: Mechanisms of subendocardial dysfunction in response to exercise in dogs with left ventricular hypertrophy, Circulation Research 71:423—434, 1992, with permission of The American Heart Association).

◆
Reduction in subendocardial wall thickening was not observed during exercise in the presence of β-adrenergic blockade. (Reprinted from Hittinger L, Shen Y-T, Patrick TA, Hasebe N, Komamura K, Ihara T, Manders WT, Vatner SF: Mechanisms of subendocardial dysfunction in response to exercise in dogs with left ventricular hypertrophy, Circulation Research 71:423—434, 1992, with permission of The American Heart Association).

Table 1. Effects of exercise with matched loading conditions on global LV function and regional wall motion exercise before and after β-adrenergic receptor blockade in LVH dogs.

	n	No block	n	β-block
Level of exercise	4.8 km/hr 0% grade		6.4 km/hr 16% grade	
Heart rate (beats/min)	10	180 ± 10	10	173 ± 7
Mean arterial pressure (mmHg)	10	96 ± 6	10	91 ± 4
LV systolic wall stress (g/cm²)	7	312 ± 23	7	293 ± 18
End-diastolic stress (g/cm²)	7	47.4 ± 7.3	7	46.5 ± 8.6
LV dP/dt (mmHg/sec)	9	4900 ± 356	9	4133 ± 238
Endocardial myocardial blood flow (ml/min/g)	6	2.75 ± 0.65	6	1.83 ± 0.27
Epicardial myocardial blood flow (ml/min/g)	6	2.07 ± 0.28	6	1.50 ± 0.16
Endo/Epi Ratio	6	1.27 ± 0.14	6	1.21 ± 0.13
Triple Product	7	281 ± 55	7	216 ± 30
Change in full wall thickening (mm)	10	—0.15 ± 0.05	10	0.11 ± 0.05
Change in subendocardial wall thickening (mm)	10	—0.21 ± 0.08	10	0.10 ± 0.04*
Change in subepicardial wall thickening (mm)	10	0.05 ± 0.02	10	0.00 ± 0.07

* $p < 0.05$ β-block different from no block
n = number of animals studied

(Reprinted from Hittinger L, Shen Y-T, Patrick TA, Hasebe N, Komamura K, Ihara T, Manders WT, Vatner SF: Mechanisms of subendocardial dysfunction in response to exercise in dogs with left ventricular hypertrophy, Circulation Research 71:423—434, 1992, with permission of The American Heart Association).

Table 2. Effects of onset of exercise on global LV function and regional wall motion in dogs with LVH.

	n	Baseline	Exercise anticipation	After 10 beats exercise
Heart rate (beats/min)	6	106 ± 7	129 ± 11*	174 ± 11*‡
Mean arterial pressure (mmHg)	6	95 ± 6	105 ± 6*	105 ± 6
LV systolic pressure (mmHg)	6	264 ± 8	283 ± 16	292 ± 6*
LV end-diastolic pressure (mmHg)	6	16.8 ± 1.4	20.5 ± 3.7	20.9 ± 3.7
LV dP/dt (mmHg/sec)	6	3760 ± 368	4665 ± 406*	5308 ± 529*‡
Subendocardial wall thickness (mm)				
End diastolic		9.57 ± 0.72	9.67 ± 0.72	10.10 ± 0.61*‡
End systolic		11.18 ± 0.68	11.19 ± 0.66	11.16 ± 0.65
Wall thickening	6	1.61 ± 0.44	1.52 ± 0.39	1.05 ± 0.29*‡
Subepicardial wall thickness (mm)				
End diastolic		9.95 ± 0.86	9.95 ± 0.84	9.90 ± 0.87
End systolic		11.21 ± 0.91	11.20 ± 0.90	11.24 ± 0.93
Wall thickening	6	1.25 ± 0.19	1.25 ± 0.22	1.34 ± 0.23

* $p < 0.05$, different from baseline
‡ $p < 0.05$, after 10 beats, different from anticipation
n = number of animals studied

(Reprinted from Hittinger L, Shen Y-T, Patrick TA, Hasebe N, Komamura K, Ihara T, Manders WT, Vatner SF: Mechanisms of subendocardial dysfunction in response to exercise in dogs with left ventricular hypertrophy, Circulation Research 71:423—434, 1992, with permission of The American Heart Association).

Table 3. Effects of onset of ischemia induced by coronary artery occlusion (CAO) on global LV function and regional wall motion in dogs with LVH.

	n	Baseline	10 beats after CAO
Heart rate (beats/min)	4	104 ± 9	107 ± 9
Mean arterial pressure (mmHg)	3	94 ± 6	96 ± 6
LV systolic pressure (mmHg)	4	241 ± 20	237 ± 20
LV end-diastolic pressure (mmHg)	4	10.4 ± 1.8	10.4 ± 1.7
LV dP/dt (mmHg/sec)	4	4253 ± 242	4127 ± 196
Subendocardial wall thickness (mm)			
End diastolic	4	7.67 ± 0.66	7.53 ± 0.73
End systolic	4	10.21 ± 0.68	9.32 ± 0.70*
Wall thickening	4	2.55 ± 0.46	1.76 ± 0.40*
Subepicardial wall thickness (mm)			
End diastolic	3	8.74 ± 0.74	8.59 ± 0.76
End systolic	3	10.36 ± 0.57	9.96 ± 0.57*
Wall thickening	3	1.61 ± 0.19	1.37 ± 0.20*

* $p < 0.05$, different from baseline
n = number of animals studied

nation with the regional myocardial blood flow data strongly suggest that ischemia does not mediate the early subendocardial dysfunction that occurs with exercise in the severely hypertrophied heart.

Taking together the data with exercise in the hypertrophied heart in the presence and absence of β-adrenergic receptor blockade and the data with initial adjustment to coronary artery occlusion, several conclusions can be derived. First, the later period of sustained exercise, characterized by impaired subendocardial wall thickening and reduced subendocardial perfusion, is likely the result of an imbalance between myocardial oxygen supply and demand. This results in impaired subendocardial function during exercise and sustained dysfunction after recovery from exercise, i.e., myocardial stunning. The reduced perfusion during exercise most likely results from the impaired coronary reserve in the hypertrophied heart and the enhanced subendocardial wall stress and compressive forces that develop during exercise. β-Adrenergic receptor blockade can alleviate the alterations in regional function and perfusion by reducing the myocardial oxygen demands during exercise and reducing the enhanced wall stress and compressive forces during exercise.

However, β-adrenergic receptor blockade also eliminates the initial subendocardial dysfunction which was not related to subendocardial hypoperfusion. Therefore, activation of β-adrenergic mechanisms and cyclic AMP in the hypertrophied heart also results in impaired function independent of blood flow mechanisms. These alterations could be at the level of β-adrenergic receptor coupling, at the level of the adenylyl cyclase catalytic unit or directly involved in excitation-contraction coupling (22, 25).

References

1. Alyono D, Anderson RW, Parrish DG, Dai XZ, Bache RJ (1986) Alterations of myocardial blood flow associated with experimental canine left ventricular hypertrophy secondary to valvular aortic stenosis. Circ Res 58:47—57
2. Bache RJ, Alyono D, Sublett E, Dai XZ (1986) Myocardial blood flow in left ventricular hypertrophy developing in young and adult dogs. Am J Physiol 251: H949—H956
3. Bache RJ, Arentzen CE, Simon AB, Vrobel TR (1984) Abnormalities in myocardial perfusion during tachycardia in dogs with left ventricular hypertrophy: metabolic evidence for myocardial ischemia. Circulation 69:409—417
4. Bache RJ, Dai X, Alyono D, Vrobel TR, Homans DC (1987) Myocardial blood flow during exercise in dogs with left ventricular hypertrophy produced by aortic banding and perinephritic hypertension. Circulation 76(4):835—842
5. Bache RJ, Vrobel TR, Arentzen CE, Ring WS (1981) Effect of maximal coronary vasodilation on transmural myocardial perfusion during tachycardia in dogs with left ventricular hypertrophy. Circ Res 49:742—750
6. Braunwald E, Kloner RA (1982) The stunned myocardium: Prolonged, postischemic ventricular dysfunction. Circulation 66:1146—1149
7. Cannon III RO, Rosing DR, Maron BJ et al. (1985) Myocardial ischemia in patients with hypertrophic cardiomyopathy: contribution of inadequate vasodilator reserve and elevated left ventricular filling pressures. Circulation 71:234—243
8. Doty DB, Eastham CL, Hiratzka LF, Wright CB, Marcus ML (1982) Determination of coronary reserve in patients with supravalvular aortic stenosis. Circulation 66(Suppl I):I—186—I—192
9. Fujii AM, Gelpi RJ, Mirsky I, Vatner SF (1988) Systolic and diastolic dysfunction during atrial pacing in conscious dogs with left ventricular hypertrophy. Circ Res 62:462—470
10. Heyndrickx GR, Millard RW, McRitchie RJ, Maroko PR, Vatner SF (1975) Regional myocardial functional and electrophysiological alterations after brief coronary artery occlusion in conscious dogs. J Clin Invest 56:978—985
11. Hittinger L, Shannon R, Bishop SP, Gelpi R, Vatner SF (1989) Subendomyocardial exhaustion of blood flow reserve and increased fibrosis in conscious dogs with heart failure. Circ Res 65:971—980
12. Hittinger L, Shannon RP, Kohin S, Lader AS, Manders WT, Patrick TA, Kelly P, Vatner SF (1989) Isoproterenol-induced alterations in myocardial blood flow, systolic and diastolic function in conscious dogs with heart failure. Circulation 80:658—668
13. Hittinger L, Shannon RP, Kohin S, Manders WT, Kelly P, Vatner SF (1990) Exercise induced subendocardial dysfunction in dogs with left ventricular hypertrophy. Circ Res 66:329—343
14. Hittinger L, Shen Y-T, Patrick TA, Hasebe N, Komamura K, Ihara T, Manders WT, Vatner SF (1992) Mechanisms of subendocardial dysfunction in response to exercise in dogs with left ventricular hypertrophy, Circ Res 71:423—434
15. Holtz J, Restorff WV, Bard P, Bassenge E (1977) Transmural distribution of myocardial blood flow and of coronary reserve in canine left ventricular hypertrophy. Basic Res Cardiol 72:286—292
16. Homans DC, Sublett E, Dai X-Z, Bache RJ (1986) Persistence of regional left ventricular dysfunction after exercise induced myocardial ischemia. J Clin Invest 77:66—73
17. Marcus ML, Doty DB, Hiratzka LF, Wright CB, Eastham CL (1982) Decreased coronary reserve: a mechanism for angina pectoris in patients with aortic stenosis and normal coronary artery. N Engl J Med 307:1362—1367
18. Marcus ML, Mueller TM, Eastham CH (1981) Effects of short and long-term left ventricular hypertrophy on coronary circulation. Am J Physiol 241:H358—H362

19. Murray PA, Vatner SF (1981) Abnormal coronary vascular response to exercise in dogs with severe right ventricular hypertrophy. J Clin Invest 67:1314—1323
20. Murray PA, Vatner SF (1981) Reduction of maximal coronary vasodilator capacity in conscious dogs with severe right ventricular hypertrophy. Circ Res 48:25—33
21. O'Keefe DD, Hoffman JIE, Cheitlin R, O'Neill MJ, Allard JR, Shapkin E (1978) Coronary blood flow in experimental canine left ventricular hypertrophy. Circ Res 43:43—51
22. Perreault CL, Shannon RP, Shen Y-T, Hasebe N, Vatner SF, Morgan JP (1992) Excitation-contraction coupling in dogs with compensated hypertrophy. Circulation 86 (Suppl I):I—825, 1992 (Abstract)
23. Rembert JC, Kleinman LH, Fedor JM, Wechsler AS, Greenfield JC Jr (1978) Myocardial blood flow in concentric left ventricular hypertrophy. J Clin Invest 62:379—386
24. Thaulow E, Guth BD, Heusch G, Gilpin E, Schulz R, Kroeger K, Ross J Jr (1989) Characteristics of regional myocardial stunning after exercise in dogs with chronic coronary stenosis. Am J Physiol 257 (Heart Circ Physiol 26):H113—H119
25. Vatner DE, Vatner SF, Fuji AM, Homcy CJ (1985) Loss of high affinity cardiac β-adrenergic receptors in dogs with heart failure. J Clin Invest 76:2259—2264
26. Vatner SF, Hittinger L (1993) Coronary vascular mechanisms involved in decompensation from hypertrophy to heart failure. J Am Coll Cardiol, in press
27. Vatner SF, Shannon R, Hittinger L (1990) Reduced subendocardial coronary reserve, a potential mechanism for impaired diastolic function in the hypertrophied and failing heart. Circulation 81(Suppl III):III—8—III—14
28. Vrobel TR, Ring WS, Anderson RW, Emery RW, Bache RJ (1980) Effect of heart rate on myocardial blood flow in dogs with left ventricular hypertrophy. Am J Physiol 239:H621—H627

Authors' address:
Stephen F. Vatner, M.D.
New England Regional Primate Research Center
One Pine Hill Drive, P.O. Box 9102
Southborough, MA 01772-9102

ACE-inhibitors and coronary microcirculation

B. E. Strauer, M. Vogt, W. Motz

Medizinische Klinik und Poliklinik B der Heinrich-Heine-Universität Düsseldorf

Summary: Arterial hypertension is the most frequent cause of a disturbance of coronary microcirculation. Inspite of having normal epicardial coronary arteries, patients with arterial hypertension often have symptoms of angina pectoris and a positive exercise tolerance test. The angina pectoris-symptoms in patients with arterial hypertension are due to functional and structural alterations of the coronary microcirculation. Consequently, an antihypertensive therapy should not only aim at lowering blood pressure and reversing myocardial hypertrophy, but also improve coronary microcirculation in order to avoid the consequences of chronic ischemia on the myocardium. Until now, only experimental studies have indicated that antihypertensive therapy can improve coronary flow reserve. To determine to what extent under clinical conditions coronary flow reserve can be improved, in hypertensive patients maximal coronary blood flow, minimal coronary resistance, and coronary reserve (Dipyridamol) were studied before and after a long-term antihypertensive treatment (9—12 months) with the ACE-inhibitor enalapril (10—20 mg/d). To assess the chronic effects rather than the acute effects of the antihypertensive pharmacon, the coronary microcirculation was studied after intermission of medical therapy for a period of 1 week. Along with a decrease in LV muscle mass by about 8%, coronary reserve was improved after enalapril by 48%. It is likely that the observed increase in coronary reserve is related to the reversal of structural vascular abnormalities at the level of the coronary microcirculation. Consequently, it seems that reparation of hypertensive remodeling of the coronary microcirculation can be induced by ACE-inhibitor therapy.

Key words: Hypertensive Hypertrophy; Coronary microcirculation; Regression of hypertrophy; myocardial and coronary reparation

Left ventricular hypertrophy is a serious risk factor of cardiovascular complications such as myocardial infarction, stroke and congestive heart failure (14). In contrast to adaptive myocardial hypertrophy due to athletic training, left ventricular hypertrophy due to arterial hypertension is characterized by growth or altered metabolism of non-myocytic cells such as cardiac fibroblasts, smooth muscle cells and endothelial cells (41). These functional and structural activation of non-myocytic cells severely alters the myocardial structure and function. Since an activation of non-myocytic cells can also be present without a concomitant myocardial hypertrophy, its activation is not inevitably linked to the myocytic hypertrophy process.

Consequently, a causative therapy of hypertensive hypertrophy has to aim at a specific reparation of the organ structure of heart and circulation. This can be realized through a specific intervention on the level of the non-myocytic cells such as cardio-fibroblasts in the interstitial space, vascular smooth muscle cells and endothelial cells. A sole therapeutic intervention on the level of the myocytes only leads to echocardiographic regression of myocardial hypertrophy. Accordingly, the decisive reparation of the remodeled organ structure possibly fails to come. Accordingly, the aim of an interventional therapy of the heart in hypertension is not the mere echocardiographic decrement of wall thickness, i.e., reversal of hypertrophy, but the

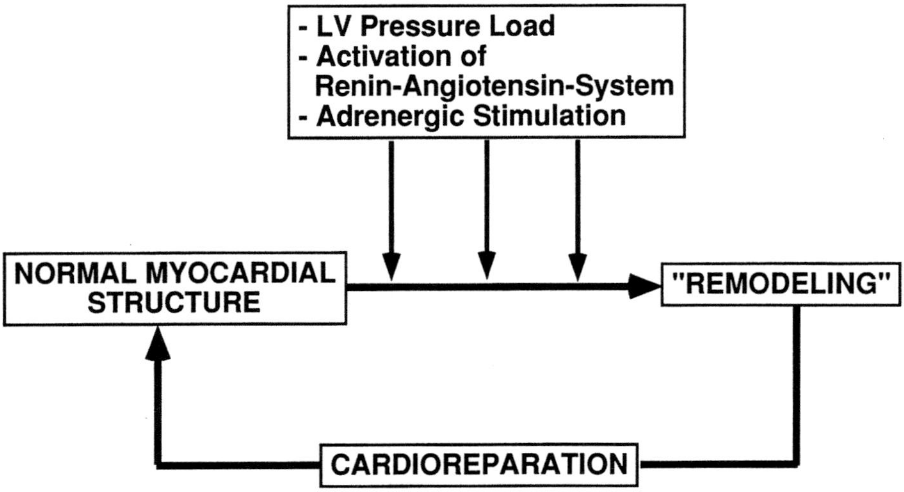

Fig. 1. Concept of cardioreparation of hypertensive remodeling.

basic reparation of the hypertensively remodeled myocardial structure, which comprises, particularly, the myocardial interstitial space, i.e., connective tissue and the coronary microcirculation (41) (Fig. 1).

Patients with arterial hypertension often have symptoms of angina pectoris inspite of a normal coronary angiogram (33—35). About 50% of the hypertensive patients with a normal coronary angiogram who were admitted to the Department of Cardiology of the University of Düsseldorf due to clinically suspected coronary artery disease had a typical exercise-related and nitro-responsive angina. Forty-two percent of these patients showed a clearly pathologic exercise tolerance test inspite of having normal epicardial arteries. Consequently, a normal coronary angiogram does not exclude a disturbance of the coronary circulation. The small coronary arterioles and resistance vessels with a diameter of less than 150 μ of the coronary microcirculation are beyond the resolution of coronary angiography. A normal coronary angiogram only indicates the absence of visible alterations of the great epicardial conductance arteries.

In patients with arterial hypertension maximal coronary blood flow due to dipyridamole is lowered by about 35% compared with healthy normotensive control persons. Accordingly, minimal coronary resistance as the reciprocal paramter of coronary conductance is appropriately elevated and coronary reserve, defined as the quotient of coronary resistance under resting conditions and minimal coronary resistance after dipyridamole, is lowered by about 30% (20, 35, 39). Consequently, patients with arterial hypertension and angina pectoris frequently show a functional impairment of the coronary regulation capacity on the level of the coronary microcirculation. Possible causes of the disturbed coronary flow reserve in arterial hypertension are of vascular, myocardial and metabolic origin (Table 1). Tomanek (37) described a rarefication of the coronary microcirculation as the consequence of an inadequate growth of the capillaries along with the process of hypertrophy in

Table 1. Causes of the disturbed coronary flow reserve in arterial hypertension.

1) *Vascular factors:*
   — Rarefication of coronary microcirculation
   — Wall thickening of coronary resistance arteries
   — Perivascular fibrosis
   — Endothelial dysfunction

2) *Myocardial factors and extravascular compressing forces:*
   — Myocyte hypertrophy
   — Interstitial myocardial fibrosis
   — End-diastolic wall stress (LV filling pressure)

3) *Metabolic factors:*
   — Elevated coronary flow under resting conditions due to increased myocardial oxygen demand

experimental models of arterial hypertension. Furthermore, in experimental studies a wall thickening of resistance arteries in the sense of medial hypertrophy was found (29). Recently, such findings could also be observed in myocardial biopsies of patients in arterial hypertension (31). In addition, perivascular fibrosis as well as a disturbance of coronary endothelial function in the sense of a reduced capacity of EDRF-liberation have to be discussed to be causative for the impaired flow reserve (16, 21).

Besides these vascular factors myocardial hypertrophy as a main determinant of the extravascular component of the coronary resistance remains a further cause of the impaired coronary flow reserve. Qualitative alterations of myocardial structure in the sense of interstitial fibrosis might have an unfavorable impact on the coronary microcirculation. Particularly, a diastolic compression of the endocardial areas of the myocardium through the elevated left ventricular filling pressure might contribute to the impairment of coronary regulatory capacity as well. Due to an elevated instantaneous coronary flow as a consequence of an elevated myocardial energy demand, coronary reserve can be metabolically impaired without the necessary presence of microvascular alterations. Such a metabolically caused limitation of coronary flow reserve is particularly found in hemodynamically decompensated left ventricles due to a prolonged exposure to arterial hypertension and in patients with aortic valve disease (9, 33) (Table 1).

The structural remodeling of the myocardium along with the process of arterial hypertension is not solely caused by the physical pressure load on the cardiac myocytes, but the interrelationship of mechanical stretch, i.e., systolic wall stretch and hormonal stimulation. Besides adrenergic stimulation (13, 28, 36), particularly the renin-angiotensin-system modulates the hypertrophy process of myocytes and smooth muscle cells and induces proto-oncogenes, which induce or reinforce the process of hypertrophy. There is growing evidence that an endogenous renin-angiotensin-system exists in the heart (7, 11, 27). Meanwhile, messenger-RNA (mRNA) of angiotensinogen and renin as well as renin, angiotensin converting enzyme (ACE), angiotensin II as well as its cardiac receptor could be clearly identified by biochemical methods (8). The intracardiac activation of angiotensin I to angiotensin II was also observed recently (15). The physiological significance of the endogeneous cardiac renin-angiotensin-system is not yet completely understood. It could play a role in the regulation of myocardial contractility, coronary vasomotion, as well as in the hypertrophy process of the myocytes and smooth muscle cells. The development of left ventricular hypertrophy due to coarctation of the abdominal aorta in rats could be completely prevented after a pretreatment with an ACE-inhibitor (12). This points to a decisive trophic role of angiotensin II on the myocardium and the antitrophic effect of the therapeutic inhibition of the renin-angiotensin system. During the process of adaptive myocardial hypertrophy due to arterial hypertension, the cardiac endogeneous ACE-activity as well as the messenger-RNA of ACE are elevated. Schunkert and coworkers (30) have found a rise in ACE-mRNA and an increased conversion of angiotensin I to angiotensin II in the pressure-exposed left ventricle. In the non-pressure exposed right ventricle ACE-activity was not different from control animals. Consequently, the stimulus of an increased ACE-expression is locally linked to the muscle fiber stretch as a consequence of the increased systolic wall stress in the pressure loaded left ventricle. The evidence of induction of protooncogenes through angiotensin II supports the assumption that hypertensive remodeling of the heart is modulated through the local and endocrine renin-angiotensin-system (24, 25).

Due to the importance of the renin-angiotensin-system in the process of hypertensive remodeling of the heart and circulation, it is obvious to use ACE-inhibitors in the medical treatment of arterial hypertension. Many experimental and clinical studies have clearly shown that a therapy with ACE-inhibitors induces regression of myocardial hypertrophy (6, 19, 26, 32) (Fig. 2). At least experimentally, in the spontaneously hypertensive rat (SHR), Brilla and coworkers have found a reversal of the interstitial collagen as well as a decrement of the medial wall thickness of coronary resistance vessels after long-term treatment with the ACE-inhibitor lisinopril. Functionally, an improvement of the coronary flow reserve was found in the lisinopril-treated animals (2). A decrement of the vascular wall thickness of the large peripheral conductance arteries was found after an antihypertensive therapy with the ACE-inhibitors enalapril and perindopril in the same experimental model of hypertension. These latter findings were interpreted as an antiproliferative effect of ACE-inhibitors on vascular smooth muscle cells (5, 18).

Until now it has not been clear to what extent a clinical antihypertensive therapy with an ACE-inhibitor can also improve or even normalize the obvious disturbance of coronary microcirculation in arterial hypertension. To answer this question, we studied patients with hypertensive microvascular angina pectoris, i.e., a) a history of arterial hypertension, b) symptoms of angina pectoris and/or c) evidence of myocardial ischemia in the exercise tolerance test or thallium-scan, d) normal epicardial arteries and e) an impaired coronary flow reserve. As an antihypertensive treatment we have chosen the ACE-inhibitor enalapril, because particular antiproliferative effects on the vasculature were expected to occur. After discontinuation of a preexisting antihypertensive therapy for 1 week, the coronary circulation and left ventricle muscle mass were studied initially. Then the patients were treated with enalapril (10—20 mg/d) for a period of 9 to 12 months. To assess the chronic effect of antihypertensive treatment on coronary microcirculation rather than the acute effect of enalapril, the coronary circulation was studied after the medical therapy had been discontinued for a period of 1 week. The objective of the study

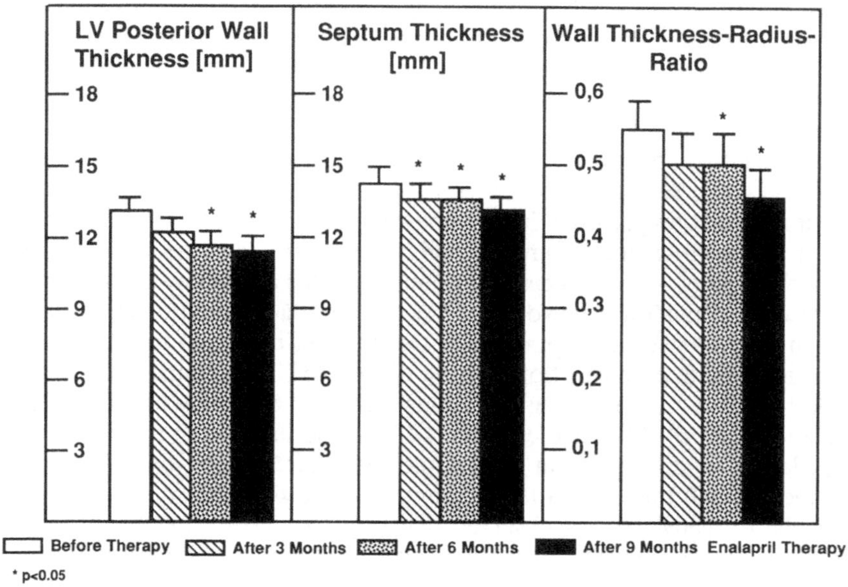

Fig. 2. Left ventricular posterior wall thickness, septum thickness, as well as wall thickness radius-ratio before and after 3, 6 and 9 months therapy with enalapril (19).

was to assess the chronic effect of an antihypertensive long-term treatment with enalapril on the coronary microcirculation and not the acute effect of the antihypertensive substance (22, 40).

During antihypertensive treatment with enalapril systolic and diastolic blood pressure values were within the normotensive range. The reduction of systolic blood pressure was about 20 mmHg and the reduction of the diastolic blood pressure about 8—10 mmHg. Left ventricular muscle mass decreased from 268 ± 58 g to 247 ± 50 g ($p < 0.05$). It is noteable that in all patients no marked LV hypertrophy existed initially (22, 40).

Before and after discontinuation of enalapril therapy coronary perfusion pressure, heart rate, myocardial oxygen consumption and pulmonary capillary wedge pressure were similar. Consequently, measurement of coronary regulatory capacity was measured under identical perfusion pressures before and after therapy and there were also no obvious differences with respect to myocardial energy consumption and heart rate as well as in the end-diastolic compressing forces under both conditions. After the treatment period maximal coronary blood flow after dipyridamole increased from 181 ± 69 to 258 ± 116 ml/min · 100 g ($p < 0.001$) by 43%. Minimal coronary resistance as the reciprocal parameter of coronary conductance decreased from 0.66 ± 0.23 to 0.47 ± 0.24 mmHg/min · 100 g · ml^{-1} ($p < 0.001$) by 29%. Coronary reserve was improved by 48% compared with its initial value (22, 40).

Since coronary reserve has improved chronically, i.e., independent from the acute effect of the antihypertensive agent, regression of structural alterations on the level of the myocardium and the coronary resistance vessels are likely to have occurred. For example, a decrease in medial wall thickness, an increase in capillary density, as well as a decrease in perivascular fibrosis are possible. On the myocardial level a decrease in myocytic hypertrophy as well as a possible decrease in the amount of the interstitial collagen concentration have to be considered. Until now the influence of a chronic medical therapy on the coronary microcirculation has been studied experimentally in the model of the spontaneously hypertensive rat (SHR) only. Anderson and coworkers (1) found an increase in coronary flow reserve without a concomitant reversal of myocardial hypertrophy along with a chronic antihypertensive treatment with hydralazine. From this study it was concluded that an alteration of the myocardial factor is not a necessary prerequisite for an improvement of coronary flow reserve. Strauer and coworkers (34) showed that a chronic therapy with the calcium channel blocker felodipine led to a decrement in medial wall thickness along with an increase in coronary flow reserve. Others (3, 17, 38) found an increase in the capillary density of the myocardium after a chronic therapy with nifedipine, moxonidine and captopril. Mall and coworkers (17) found in addition to an increase in capillary density a decrement in LV-muscle mass of the left ventricle and a decrease in medial wall thickness after nifedipine and moxonidine. An increase in coronary regulatory capacity was observed due to a treatment with the ACE-inhibitors captopril (3) and lisinopril (2). Canby and coworkers (3) attributed the increase in coronary regulatory capacity to the increase in capillary density and Brilla and coworkers (2) to both reversal of left ventricular muscle mass and decrease in medial wall thickness of the coronary resistance arteries. In conclusion, these experimental studies have demonstrated that a chronic therapy with various antihypertensive drugs will lead to reversal of myocytic hypertrophy on the level of the myocardium as well as to a decrease in medial wall thickness and an increase in the capillary density on the level of the coronary microcirculation. Functionally, an increase in the coronary regulatory capacity of the coronary microcirculation results (Table 2).

Through the concomitant reversal of hypertrophy along with blood pressure reduction a decrease of the myocardial component of the coronary resistance inevitably occurs. Consequently, it is difficult to differentiate between the influence of the myocardial factors such as hypertrophy and fibrosis and the vascular factors such as medial wall thickening and capillary density on the coronary flow reserve

Table 2. Experimental findings regarding therapy of coronary microcirculation (state of the art).

Substance	LV muscle mass	Medial wall thickness	Capillary density	Coronary reserve	Author
Hydralazine	=			↑	Anderson, 1989
Felodipine	↓	↓		↑	Strauer, 1990
Nifedipine			↑		Turek, 1987
Nifedipine	↓	↓	↑		Mall, 1991
Moxonidine	↓	↓	↑		Mall, 1991
Captopril	↓		↑	↑	Canby, 1989
Lisinopril	↓	↓		↑	Brilla, 1991

in experimental as well as in clinical conditions. Under clinical conditions a distinct decrease in minimal coronary resistance as the reciprocal parameter of coronary conductance by 29% occurred along with a moderate amount of reversal of myocardial hypertrophy due to enalapril treatment (22, 40). On the contrary, inspite of a distinct reversal of myocardial hypertrophy a non-significant decrease in minimal coronary resistance by 11% only was found after chronic treatment with the beta receptor blocker bisoprolol (22, 23). These findings indicate that a sole influence on the myocardial factor "left ventricular hypertrophy" does not necessarily lead to a distinct improvement of conductance of the coronary microcirculation, and that improvement of coronary conductance due to enalapril therapy cannot be solely caused by regression of myocardial hypertrophy. Furthermore, additional vascular effects of the ACE-inhibitor enalapril are likely (Fig. 3). This interpretation is also

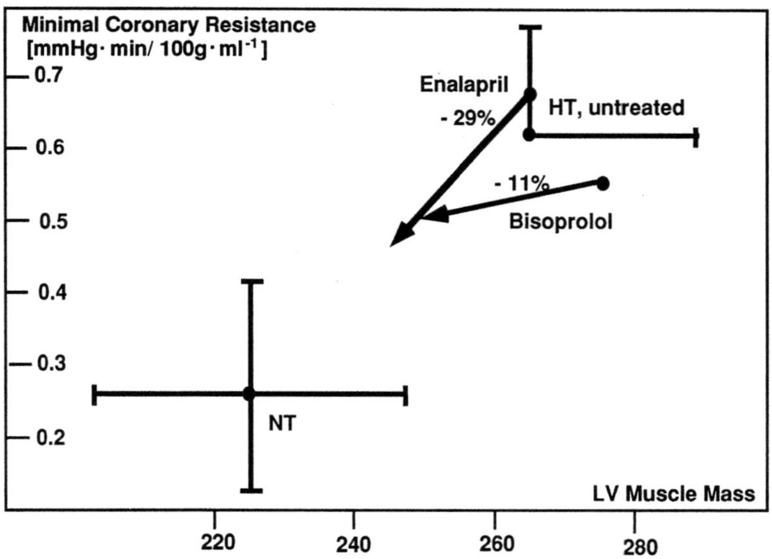

Fig. 3. Depicted is left ventricular muscle mass on the abscissa and the minimal coronary resistance on the ordinate. In normotensive control persons (NT) a normal minimal coronary resistance exists in the presence of a normal left ventricular muscle mass. In hypertensive patients (HT) minimal coronary vascular resistance is significantly increased along with the presence of left ventricular hypertrophy. After therapy with enalapril (arrow) a distinct decrease in minimal coronary resistance occurs inspite of a only moderate decrease in myocardial hypertrophy. Under treatment with the beta-receptor-blocker bisoprolol (arrow) a moderate non-significant decrease in minimal coronary resistance occurs inspite of clear reversal of myocardial hypertrophy. Consequently, a) an influence on the myocardial factor "left ventricular hypertrophy" does not automatically lead to an improvement of conductance of the coronary microcirculation and b) an improvement of coronary conductance after enalapril cannot be the sole consequence of reversal of hypertrophy. Accordingly, additional vascular effects of the enalapril treatment seem to be responsible for the improvement in coronary flow reserve.

supported by experimental findings of Christensen and coworkers (4). They could demonstrate that the media-lumen-ratio of mesenteric resistance arteries was distinctly lower after treatment with the vasodilators captopril, hydralazine, and isradipine than after the beta-receptor blocker metoprolol. The only study on human coronary resistance vessels was published by Heagerty and coworkers (10). They found a clear decrement of the ratio between medial wall thickness and lumen diameter in subcutaneous resistance vessels after an antihypertensive combination therapy. Due to these studies of the peripheral circulation (4, 10) and the experimental studies (2, 5, 18) which have shown an antiproliferative effect of ACE-inhibitors on the vessel wall, it is likely that the improved coronary flow reserve under enalapril is caused by reparation of structural vascular alterations of the coronary microcirculation such as a decrease in medial wall thickness and perivascular fibrosis. Furthermore, a quantitative decrement in interstitial myocardial fibrosis might have also contributed in the sense of a decrement in the myocardial component of coronary resistance (Table 3).

Table 3. Possible causes for an improvement in coronary flow reserve after treatment with an ACE-inhibitor.

1. *Coronary microcirculation*	2. *Myocardium*
Reversal of structural changes	Decrease of myocyte hypertrophy
— Decrease of medial wall thickness	Reduction of interstitial fibrosis
— Increase in capillary density	
— Decrease of perivascular fibrosis	

Accordingly, a chronic therapy with the ACE-inhibitor enalapril has to be considered as a cardioreparative treatment. It restores the structural integrity in hypertensive heart disease, because reversal of myocytic hypertrophy, a decrease in myocardial fibrosis as well as an almost normalization of the coronary microcirculation can be realized.

References

1. Anderson PG, Bishop SP, Digerness SB (1989) Vascular remodeling and improvement of coronary reserve after hydralazine treatment in spontaneously hypertensive rats. Circ Res 64:1127—1136
2. Brilla CG, Janicki JS, Weber KT (1991) Cardioreparative effects of lisinopril in rats with genetic hypertension and left ventricular hypertrophy. Circulation 83:1771—1779
3. Canby CA, Tomanek RJ (1989) Role of lowering arterial pressure on maximal coronary flow with and without regression of cardiac hypertrophy. Am J Physiol 257 (Heart Circ Physiol 26):H1110—H1118
4. Christensen KL, Jespersen LT, Mulvany MJ (1989) Development of blood pressure in spontaneously hypertensive rats after withdrawal of long-term treatment related to resistance vessel structure. J Hypertens 7:83—90
5. Clozel JP, Kuhn H, Hefti F (1989) Effects of chronic ACE inhibition on cardiac hypertrophy and coronary vascular reserve in spontaneously hypertensive rats with developed hypertension. J Hypertens 7:267—275

6. Cruickshank JM (1992) Reversibility of left ventricular hypertrophy (LVH) by differing types of antihypertensive therapy. J Hum Hypertension 6:85—90
7. Dzau VJ, Ellison KE, Brody T, Ingelfinger J, Pratt RE (1987) A comparative study of the distributions of renin and angiotensin messenger ribonucleic acids in rat and mouse tissues. Endocrinology 120:2334—2338
8. Dzau VJ (1984) Cardiac renin-angiotensin system. Molecular and functional aspects. Am J Med 22—27
9. Eberli FR, Ritter M, Schwitter J, Bortone A, Schneider J, Hess OM, Krayenbühl HP (1991) Coronary reserve in patients with aortic valve disease before and after successful aortic valve replacement. Europ Heart J 12:127—138
10. Heagerty AM, Bund SJ, Aalkjaer C (1988) Effects of drug treatment on human resistance arteriole morphology in essential hypertension: direct evidence for structural remodelling of resistance vessels. Lancet 1209—1212
11. Jin M, Markus JW, Lang RE, Unger T, Lindpaintner K, Ganten D (1988) Endogenous tissue renin-angiotensin system. Am J Med 84:28—36
12. Kromer EP, Riegger GAJ (1988) Effects of long-term angiotensin converting enzyme inhibition on myocardial hypertrophy in experimental aortic stenosis in the rat. Am J Cardiol 62:161—163
13. Laks MMN (1976) Norepinephrine — the myocardial hypertrophy hormone? Am Heart J 91:674—675
14. Levy D, Garrison RJ, Savage DD, Kannel WB, Castelli WP (1990) Prognostic implications of echocardiographically determined left ventricular mass in the Framingham Heart Study. N Engl J Med 322:1561—1566
15. Lindpaintner K, Jin M, Wilhelm MJ, Suzuki WF, Linz W, Schoelkens BA, Ganten D (1988) Intracardiac generation of angiotensin and its physiologic role. Circulation 77 (Suppl I):1—18
16. Lüscher TF, Raij L, Vanhoutte PM (1987) Endothelium-dependent vascular responses in normotensive and hypertensive Dahl rats. Hypertension 9:157—163
17. Mall G, Greber D, Gharebhagi H, Wiest G, Mattfeldt T, Ganten U (1991) Myokardprotektion und Hypertrophieregression bei spontan hypertensiven Ratten durch Nifedipin und Moxonidin. Stereologische Untersuchungen. In: Ganten D, Wall G, Hrsg. Herz-Kreislauf-Regulation, Organprotektion und Organschaden. Stuttgart — New York: Schattauer, 91—106
18. Michel JB, Levy BI (1990) Vascular effects of ACE inhibition by perindopril. Drugs (Suppl 1) 39:39—42
19. Motz W, Strauer BE (1988) Rückbildung der hypertensiven Herzhypertrophie durch chronische Angiotensin-Konversionsenzymhemmung. Z Kardiol 77:53—60
20. Motz W, Vogt M, Scheler S, Schwartzkopff B, Strauer BE (1991) Coronary circulation in arterial hypertension. J Cardiovasc Pharmacol 17 (Suppl 23):S35—S39
21. Motz W, Vogt M, Rabenau O, Scheler S, Lückhoff A, Strauer BE (1991) Evidence of endothelial dysfunction in coronary resistance vessels in patients with angina pectoris and normal coronary angiograms. Am J Cardiol 68:996—1003
22. Motz W, Vogt M, Scheler S, Schwartzkopff BE, Kelm M, Strauer BE (1992) Prophylaxe mit gefäßaktiven Substanzen. Z Kardiol (im Druck)
23. Motz W, Vogt M, Scheler S, Schwartzkopff B, Strauer BE. Verbesserung der Koronarreserve nach Hypertrophieregression durch antihypertensive Therapie mit einem Beta-Rezeptorenblocker. Dt Med Wochenschr (zur Publikation eingereicht)
24. Naftilan AJ, Pratt RE, Eldrige CS, Lin HL, Dzau VJ (1989) Angiotensin II induces c-fos expression in smooth muscle via transcriptional control. Hypertension 13:706—711
25. Naftilan AJ, Pratt RE, Dzau VJ (1989) Induction of platelet-derived growth factor A chain and c-myc gene expressions by angiotensin II in cultured rat vascular smooth muscle cells. J Clin Invest 83:1419—1424
26. Nakashima Y, Fouad FM, Tarazi RC (1984) Regression of left ventricular hypertrophy from systemic hypertension by enalapril. Am J Cardiol 53:1044—1049

27. Ohkuber H, Nakayama K, Tanaka T, Nahanishi S (1986) Tissue distribution of rat angiotensinogen mRNA and structural analysis of its heterogeneity. J Biol Chem 261:319—323
28. Östman-Smith I (1981) Cardiac sympathetic nerves as the final common pathway in the induction of adaptive cardiac hypertrophy. Clin Sci 61:265—272
29. Plunkett WG, Overbeck HW (1988) Arteriolar wall thickening in hypertensive rats unrelated to pressure or sympathoadrenergic influences. Circ Res 63:937—943
30. Schunkert H, Dzau VJ, Tang SS, Hirsch AT, Apstein CS, Correll BH (1990) Increased rat cardiac angiotensin converting enzyme activity and mRNA expression in pressure overload left ventricular hypertrophy. J Clin Invest 86:1913—1920
31. Schwartzkopff B, Motz W, Knauer S, Frenzel H, Strauer BE (1992) Morphometrische Untersuchung intramyokardialer Arteriolen aus Endomyokardbiopsien des rechtsventrikulären Septums bei Patienten mit arterieller Hypertonie und Linksherzhypertrophie. In: Ganten D, Mall G, Hrsg. Gefäß- und Herzhypertrophie. Schattauer, Stuttgart — New York:33—43
32. Sen S, Tarazi RC, Bumpus FM (1981) Reversal of cardiac hypertrophy in renal hypertensive rats: medical vs. surgical therapy. AM J Physiol 270:H408—412
33. Strauer BE (1979) Myocardial oxygen consumption in chronic heart disease: role of wall stress, hypertrophy and coronary reserve. Am J Cardiol 44:730—740
34. Strauer BE (1990) The significance of coronary reserve in clinical heart disease. J Am Coll Cardiol 15:775—783
35. Strauer BE (1983) Hypertensive heart disease. Springer, Berlin — New York — Heidelberg — Tokyo
36. Tarazi RC, Sen S, Saragoca M, Kairallah P (1982) The multifactorial role of catecholamines in hypertensive cardiac hypertrophy. Eur Heart J (Suppl 3):A103—A110
37. Tomanek RJ, Palmer PJ, Pfeiffer GL, Schreiber KL, Eastham GL, Marcus ML (1986) Morphometry of canine coronary arteries, arterioles and capillaries during hypertension and left ventricular hypertrophy. Circ Res 58:38—46
38. Turek Z, Kubat K, Kazda S, Hoofd V, Rahnsan K (1987) Improved myocardial capillarisation in spontaneously hypertensive rats treated with nifedipine. Cardiovasc Res 21:725—729
39. Vogt M, Motz W, Strauer BE (1989) Coronary flow reserve in arterial hypertension. Scand J Clin Lab Invest 49:Suppl 196:7—15
40. Vogt M, Motz W, Pölitz B, Scheler S, Strauer BE (1991) Improvement of coronary reserve by chronic treatment with ACE inhibitors. Circulation 84:III—136 (Abstr)
41. Weber KT, Anversa P, Armstrong PW, Brilla CG, Burnett JC, Crnickshank JM, Devereux RB, Giles TD, Korsgaard N, Leier CV, Mendelsohn FAO, Motz WH, Mulvany MJ, Strauer BE (1992) Remodeling and reparation of the cardiovascular system. J Am Coll Cardiol 20:3—16

Authors' address:
Prof. Dr. B. E. Strauer
Medizinische Klinik und Poliklinik B
der Heinrich-Heine-Universität Düsseldorf
Moorenstr. 5
D-4000 Düsseldorf 1, FRG

Myocardial fibrosis: role of angiotensin II and aldosterone

K. T. Weber, C. G. Brilla, S. E. Campbell, E. Guarda, G. Zhou, K. Sriram

Division of Cardiology, Department of Internal Medicine,
University of Missouri-Columbia, Columbia, Missouri, USA

Summary: In this report we review the replacement (i.e., scarring) and reactive (i.e., perivascular and interstitial fibrosis) fibrous tissue responses found in the myocardium in response to effector hormones of the renin-angiotensin-aldosterone system. Experimental data are presented to indicate: a) endogenous or exogenous elevations in plasma angiotensin II are associated with acute cardiac myocyte necrosis and subsequent microscopic scarring; b) chronic elevations in plasma aldosterone (ALDO), relative to Na^+ intake, are associated with a perivascular and interstitial fibrosis of the coronary and systemic circulations and are also seen in response to chronic administration of the mineralocorticoid hormone deoxycorticosterone (DOC); and c) chronic mineralocorticoid excess, due to ALDO or DOC, is associated with enhanced urinary K^+ excretion, cardiac myocyte necrosis and scarring. Pharmacologic agents which interfere with these effector hormones (e.g., ACE inhibition and ALDO receptor antagonism) protect the myocardium against this pathologic structural remodeling created by the reactive and replacement (reparative) fibrosis. Evidence is also presented to indicate that chronic ACE inhibition is associated with a regression in reactive myocardial fibrosis. Based on these experimental findings we would suggest that clinical trials are indicated to address the prevention and regression of myocardial fibrosis — an important determinant of pathologic structural remodeling and abnormal myocardial stiffness.

Key words: Left-ventricular hypertrophy; collagen; angiotensin II; aldosterone; mineralocorticoids

Introduction

Left-ventricular hypertrophy (LVH), detected by echocardiography as an increment in left-ventricular mass, is a primary risk factor associated with the appearance of myocardial failure in both the general population and patients with uncomplicated essential hypertension (18, 20, 44, 49). The increment in mass itself, mediated by the hypertrophic growth of myocytes, need not be responsible for pathologic LVH, however. Instead, an associated abnormality in myocardial structure may be responsible. For example, an increased concentration of fibrillar collagen, which we define as fibrosis, may represent a structural basis for myocardial failure. Such an abnormal fibrous tissue response will impair the mechanical and/or electrical behavior of the myocardium (69, 71) and is the result of altered metabolic behavior and/or growth of cardiac fibroblasts (70). Myocardial fibrosis is commonly observed in hypertensive heart disease (2, 38, 43, 57). Thus, a nonmycyte cell, the cardiac fibroblast, and not hypertrophied myocytes would determine whether tissue homogeneity is preserved in LVH. When homogeneity of the hypertrophied myocardium is preserved, as in the athlete or patient with atrial septal defect, anemia or compensated arterio-venous fistula, the hypertrophic process is adaptive. When tissue homogen-

This work was supported in part by NIH grant #RO1-HL-31701

ity is lost, as may occur in the hypertensive patient, LVH is pathologic. Heterogeneity is based on disproportionate fibroblast collagen synthesis, relative to collagen degradation. Such an abnormal fibrous tissue response can occur at any time: it may accompany myocyte growth; it may present after myocyte hypertrophy is established; or it may occur independent of myocyte hypertrophy.

Morphologic features of fibrillar collagen remodeling, as well as its functional consequences, have been recently reported (67—69). Mechanisms responsible for myocardial fibrosis have likewise been reviewed (68, 70) and the following identified: a) the signals mediating fibrosis and myocyte hypertrophy are largely independent of each other; b) the fibrous tissue response occurs on either a reactive or a reparative basis, based on whether there is associated myocyte loss; and c) elevations in plasma angiotensin II (AII), aldosterone (ALDO), or deoxycorticosterone (DOC) are closely associated with these fibrous tissue responses. Specifically, a role for AII and chronic mineralocorticoid excess (relative to dietary sodium intake) was identified in promoting a *reparative (replacement) fibrosis,* or scarring, because of cardiac myocyte necrosis. In addition, ALDO and DOC each contributed to a *reactive fibrosis,* or disproportionate accumulation of fibrillar collagen which appears within the adventitia of intramyocardial coronary arteries and neighboring interstitial spaces, in the absence of myocyte loss. This reactive fibrosis is also seen in systemic organs with chronic mineralocorticoid excess (35, 63). Based on these findings the potential exists to prevent this pathologic structural remodeling of the myocardium and its intramural coronary circulation using angiotensin converting enzyme (ACE) inhibition or antagonism of ALDO receptors. Experimental findings indicate the feasibility of achieving the same and are reviewed below, together with recent evidence concerning the regression of myocardial fibrosis by ACE inhibition. The purpose of this report will be to review each of these findings and to present a theoretical framework that would explain the pathogenesis of myocardial fibrosis that appears with mineralocorticoid excess.

Angiotensin II and myocardial fibrosis

Reparative fibrosis

In vivo antimyosin antibody labeling was used to detect abnormal sarcolemmal permeability, an early marker of impending myocyte death, that could occur in response to exogenous AII administration. A nonhypertensive, intraperitoneal dose of AII was found to be associated with a labeling of individual cardiac myocytes wthin 24 h of its administration (65). Pretreatment with phenoxybenzamine and propranolol did not prevent this necrosis; antagonists to AII receptors have not yet been examined. Fibroblast proliferation and microscopic scarring followed myocyte loss, but the scars involved only a small portion of the myocardium.

Plasma AII was significantly increased in rats with surgically induced unilateral renal ischemia (8). A similar pattern of antimyosin labeling was found in these rats within 24 h of induction and could be prevented by the ACE inhibitor captopril (65). In this model of secondary hyperaldosteronism, microscopic scarring was found in both the hypertensive, hypertrophied left ventricle (8, 65) and the normotensive, nonhypertrophied right ventricle (8) and could be prevented by captopril (65). Antimyosin labeling was not observed when hypertension of comparable severity was induced by constricting the abdominal aorta below the renal arteries, and in which case an elevation of plasma AII did not occur (8).

Thus, acute elevations in plasma AII, whether induced by exogenous administration or which occurred endogenously secondary to renal ischemia, were associated with cardiac myocyte necrosis and a subsequent reparative fibrosis of the ventricles. However, the degree of scarring, and by implication the extent of cell loss, was modest. A typical morphologic presentation of a microscopic scar that has replaced lost myocytes is shown in the upper panel of Fig. 1.

Reactive fibrosis

Previous *in vitro* studies (30), using a cultured fibroblast-like cell line, suggested that AII (0.5—50 μg/ml culture medium) promoted cell growth. Zhou et al. (74) recently found that high concentrations (10^{-7} M) of AII increased collagen synthesis in cultured adult rat cardiac fibroblasts and this response appeared to be mediated via type I and type II AII receptors. In cultured fibroblasts obtained from the adult myocardium of spontaneously hypertensive rats (SHR) a dose-dependent (10^{-10} to 10^{-6} M) rise in collagen synthesis was observed which exceeded that seen in cardiac fibroblasts of normotensive genetic controls (WKY) (60).

A disporportionate accumulation of fibrillar collagen, expressed as an interstitial and perivascular fibrosis of the myocardium (see lower panel, Fig. 1), appears in renovascular hypertension (68) of diverse etiology and where circulating AII and ALDO are each increased. This fibrous tissue response is discrete from microscopic scarring (53, 65). Fibroblast proliferation and enhanced collagen synthesis per fibroblast are each contributory to this reactive fibrous tissue response. For example, experimental models of *bilateral* renal artery ischemia, ^{3}H-thymidine labeling and radioautography, identified fibroblast proliferation within both the normotensive right ventricle and the pressure overloaded left ventricle during postoperative week one (54). These rapidly growing fibroblasts were located within the adventitia and perivascular space of intramyocardial coronary arteries. Inflammatory cells were not seen at these sites. Proliferating fibroblasts were also observed at sites distant to these vessels, where myocyte necrosis had occurred, presumably due to AII-induced myocyte toxicity (53). Collagen synthesis (^{3}H-proline incorporation) is increased in the left ventricle during this interval; the right ventricle was not examined (50). An increased expression of mRNAs for type I and III collagens has been observed on postoperative day 3 after surgically induced *unilateral* renal ischemia (19). During this same time frame fibroblast proliferation is observed within interstitial spaces adjacent to intramyocardial coronary arterioles, in the absence of an inflammatory cell response (17), and at distant discrete sites of cardiac myocyte necrosis (65).

The mechanisms responsible for fibroblast growth in perivascular and neighboring interstitial spaces, and which is independent of myocyte necrosis, remain to be identified. The involvement of both ventricles, however, suggests the importance of a circulating substance and not ventricular loading in these models of renovascular hypertension. Subcutaneous administration of AII in rats (41.7 μg/h/kg) is associated with arterial hypertension, LVH and an increase in collagen synthesis observed on day 10 and which was present throughout the left ventricle (48). This contrasted to a smaller dose of AII (12.5 μg/h/kg) which produced less severe hypertension and

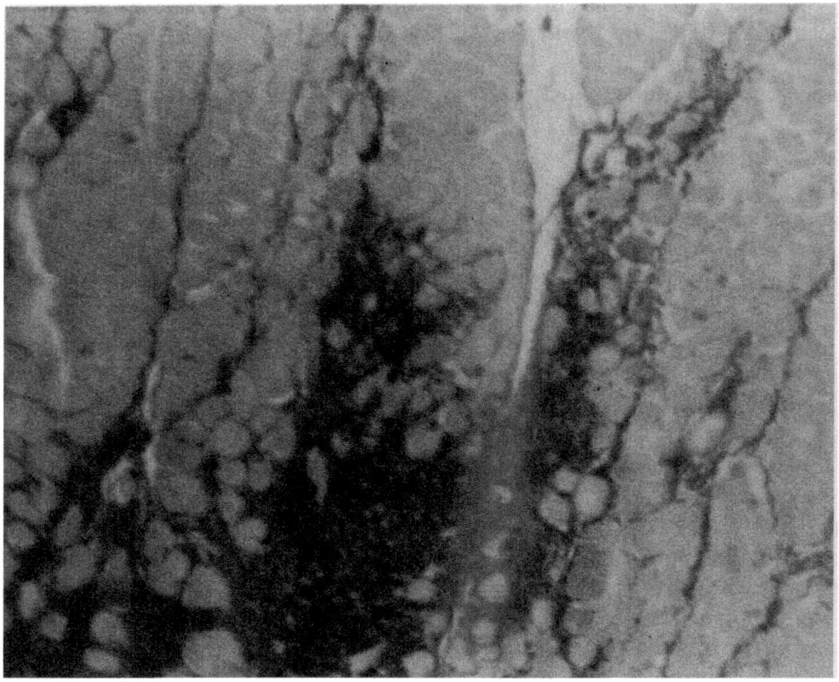

Fig. 1a

LVH, but no alteration in collagen metabolism. Collagen synthesis in the right ventricle was not examined and the response in plasma ALDO was not reported.

In addition to the potential direct interaction of AII on cardiac fibroblast growth and collagen synthesis, abnormalities in intramural coronary artery permeability may be associated with elevations in plasma AII and could permit the escape of growth promoting substances (e.g., PDGF) into or the activation of in-residence growth factors (e.g., TGF-β) within the interstitial space. These growth factors could be involved in the subsequent perivascular and interstitial fibrosis that appears as a secondary event. In rats receiving a hypertensive dose of AII for several hours, abnormalities in coronary and mesenteric macromolecular permeability have been observed (32, 33, 72). Bhan et al. (4) concluded that AII was responsible for alterations in endothelial cell permeability and insudative changes that appeared within the coronary vasculature independent of arterial hypertension or released catecholamines. In this connection, Reddy et al. (58) found that acute elevations in arterial pressure created by intravenous AII were associated with increased coronary permeability to macromolecules that appeared in cardiac lymph. This contrasted to comparable arterial hypertension created by the intravenous sympathomimetic amine methoxamine alone or methoxamine in combination with ALDO, where lymph protein concentration was not increased in either case. Abnormalities in intramural coronary permeability have also been observed with chronic unilateral renal ischemia

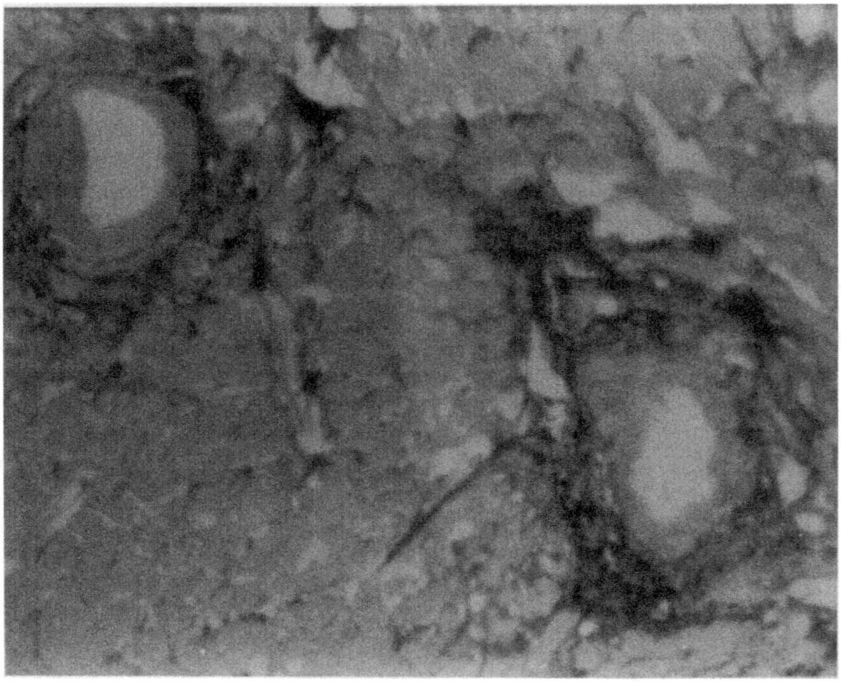

Fig. 1b

Fig. 1. Photomicrographs of the rat myocardium depicting the reparative (**a**) and reactive (**b**) fibrosis that accompanies mineralocorticoid excess. (×40). In the upper panel fibrous tissue replaces lost myocytes to form a scar, while in the lower panel it presents as a perivascular/interstitial fibrosis (a reactive process). (See text).

in the rat (3) and dog with a one kidney/one clip model of renovascular hypertension (47). Thus, elevations in plasma AII, which are accompanied by increased ALDO secretion by the adrenal glands and therefore increased plasma ALDO, promote abnormal permeability of the intramural coronary vasculature. The mechanism by which either or both these hormones alter coronary endothelial cell permeability remains to be examined.

Mineralocorticoids and myocardial fibrosis

Reparative fibrosis

Early antimyosin labeling, such as that observed following AII administration, has not been seen with ALDO administration (unpublished data). However, a reparative fibrosis has been observed in both ventricles in uninephrectomized rats receiving either ALDO (10) or DOC acetate (DOCA) (21) on a chronic basis (weeks), together with enhanced dietary sodium. In either of these models of mineralocorticoid excess circulating AII would be suppressed. In pretreating rats prior to the induction of primary hyperaldosteronism with spironolactone, an ALDO receptor antagonist, myocardial scarring was not observed (10). These findings, however, did not distinguish between the role of enhanced urinary potassium excretion with reduced myocardial potassium stores from a direct cytotoxic effect of ALDO. In this connection, Darrow et al. (22) had previously observed that chronic mineralocorticoid excess due to DOCA administration was associated with myocardial potassium depletion and cardiac myocyte necrosis and that resultant scarring could be prevented by potassium chloride supplementation to the diet. To further distinguish between such primary and secondary effects of ALDO in causing myocyte necrosis, Campbell et al. (16) compared two groups of uninephrectomized rats receiving ALDO and enhanced dietary sodium — one received amiloride, a potassium-sparing diuretic and sodium-proton antiport inhibitor, the other did not. Unlike spironolactone, amiloride is not an ALDO receptor antagonist. Microscopic scarring of the myocardium was found 8 weeks later in animals with untreated primary hyperaldosteronism, while there was no evidence of scarring in animals that received amiloride. These results support the role of enhanced urinary potassium excretion in causing cell loss in chronic hyperaldosteronism. They further suggest that ALDO does not have a direct cytotoxic effect on cardiac myocytes. Amiloride, on the other hand, did not prevent the reactive fibrosis of the ventricles.

Aldosterone and reactive fibrosis

Jalil et al. (39) found that captopril pretreatment in the rat with unilateral renal ischemia prevented the perivascular and interstitial fibrosis of the myocardium in this model of secondary hyperaldosteronism. This observation, however, did not distinguish between the relative importance of either AII or ALDO in mediating the fibrous tissue response. Additional *in vivo* studies were therefore needed. In a model of primary hyperaldosteronism, Brilla et al. (5) demonstrated that reactive myocardial fibrosis was found in the pressure overloaded hypertrophied left ventricle, as well as the normotensive nonhypertrophied right ventricle, while it was absent in either ventricle in nonhypertensive rats receiving ALDO with dietary sodium restriction or in rats with infrarenal aorta banding, where the renin-angiotensin-aldosterone system is not activated. Myocardial fibrosis was also not observed in uninephrectomized animals receiving a high sodium diet without ALDO administration (8). Thus, *in vivo* studies have shown the following regarding the regulation of the reactive myocardial fibrosis: a) ventricular systolic loading is not a determinant of this fibrous tissue response; b) arterial hypertension itself, representing an increase in coronary perfusion pressure in each ventricle, is also not responsible; c) elevations in plasma ALDO without sodium loading are not associated with fibrosis; and d) dietary sodium loading in uninemphrectomized animals without ALDO administration is also not contributory. The evidence obtained to date therefore supports the role of a chronic mineralocorticoid excess state attributed to elevated plasma ALDO (or DOC), together with enhanced dietary sodium intake relative to sodium excretion, in mediating the reactive myocardial fibrosis of the ventricles.

Additional support of this hypoethesis was obtained in rats with either renovascular hypertension or primary hyperaldosteronism, who were pretreated with either a small or a large dose of spironolactone. In this study Brilla et al. (9) found that the smaller dose of spironolactone did not prevent hypertension or LVH, while the larger dose had these effects. With either dose of spironolactone, however, the interstitial and perivascular fibrosis was not seen and this was true in both primary or secondary hyperaldosteronism. Not unexpectedly, captopril was unable to prevent this reactive fibrosis of the ventricles in rats with primary hyperaldosteronism, even though it did prevent arterial hypertension. As noted earlier, captopril was indeed cardioprotective in rats with unilateral renal ischemia. Each of these findings further demonstrate that arterial hypertension itself is not a determinant of the fibrous tissue response.

Findings of a morphologic study designed to address the fibrous tissue response present in postmortem systemic organs and myocardium in patients with autopsy proven adrenal adenoma was recently reported (15). A perivascular and interstitial fibrosis of intramural arteries and arterioles was found not only in the heart, but in systemic organs, such as the pancreas and adrenal glands, as well. Microscopic scarring was also found in the myocardium. These findings are in keeping with experimental studies of chronic ALDO administration in uninephrectomized rats receiving a high sodium diet (8, 35). They underscore the importance of circulating ALDO, together with sodium loading, in contributing to the reactive and reparative fibrous tissue responses.

The fact that fibrosis appears in the nonhypertrophied right ventricle emphasizes that the fibrous tissue response can occur in the absence of myocyte growth. It also clarifies why myocardial collagen concentration is increased in secondary hyperaldosteronism seen with myocardial failure due to rapid pacing, where arterial pressure remains normal or declines (68) while fibrosis is absent in the hypertrophied myocardium when plasma ALDO remains normal, such as occurs with chronic anemia, compensated arteriovenous fistula, hyperthyroidism, acromegaly, atrial septal defect, or exercise training (69).

The short- (e.g., collagen metabolism) and long- (e.g., mitosis) term effects of ALDO on cardiac fibroblasts have recently been examined. Brilla et al. (11) observed that collagen synthesis in confluent adult rat cardiac fibroblasts was increased by ALDO in concentrations (10^{-9} M) found in patients with primary or secondary hyperaldosteronism. ALDO was not found to promote cell division. Whether or not cardiac fibroblasts contain type-I corticoid receptors (for mineralocorticoids) remains to be elucidated. Fibroblasts of the aorta, however, are known to contain such corticoid receptors (51). Moreover, a heterogeneity in corticoid receptor affinity for steroid hormones has been demonstrated within the cardiovascular system: small arteries have a greater affinity than the aorta, while veins do not contain these receptors (45).

Deoxycorticosterone and reactive fibrosis

DOC is another mineralocorticoid hormone. It is less potent than ALDO due to its higher plasma protein binding, but like ALDO (35) its chronic administration in uninephrectomized rats receiving high dietary sodium is associated with arterial hypertension and a reactive fibrous tissue remodeling of the coronary and systemic vasculatures (63). In recent studies, Brilla et al. (5) have shown that the reactive myocardial fibrosis seen in either ventricle in association with chronic DOCA administration is less extensive than that found with ALDO, while the mineralocorticoid-like substance glycyrrhizic acid did not elicit the fibrous tissue response despite comparable hypertension and LVH to that found with DOCA and ALDO treatment. The presumed absence of 11β-hydroxy steroid dehydrogenase (11β-HSD) in the myocardium (28) may explain why this derivative of the licorice root did not promote fibrosis. Alternatively, glycyrrhizic acid-mediated inhibition of any 11β-HSD present, would remove the mineralocorticoid specificity it confers to type-I corticoid receptors, thereby negating the role of this steroid hormone on fibroblast-mediated collagen synthesis. This issue requires further investigation.

In the rat receiving DOCA for 6 weeks, increased DNA activity was found in the heart at two sites (21). The first included intramural arteries and arterioles, where nuclei of smooth muscle cells, endothelial cells and fibroblasts were labeled with thymidine. Similar findings were observed in the mesenteric circulation. The second discrete site consisted of focal collections of labeled fibroblasts together with collagen fibers, where myocyte necrosis had occurred. These findings with chronic DOCA administration are in keeping with the persistent and progressive nature of the reactive perivascular fibrosis that occurs with chronic mineralocorticoid excess (64) and the separate issue of cardiac myocyte necrosis that accompanies increased potassium excretion in this setting (vide supra).

Thus, the vascular remodeling of the coronary and systemic circulations seen in the setting of arterial hypertension due to chronic DOCA or ALDO administration is related to excess mineralocorticoid hormones, relative to dietary sodium loading, and not hypertension per se. The importance of mineralocorticoids to vascular remodeling clarifies the uncertainty related to the vasculotoxicity of AII or plasma renin activity, each of which is suppressed with chronic DOCA or ALDO administration. Mineralocorticoids, not AII, are most relevant to the reactive fibrous tissue response. Recognition of the major contribution of these steroid hormones to cardiovascular remodeling explains the increased risk of morbid and mortal events that occur, not only in patients having arterial hypertension in association with high plasma renin activity, but low renin activity as well (1, 13, 24, 26), where plasma ALDO or other mineralocorticoid hormones may be increased.

Mineralocorticoids and sodium permeability

The mechanism responsible for mineralocorticoid-enhanced collagen synthesis in the myocardium is unknown. Previous studies indicate that vascular smooth muscle permeability to sodium, potassium and chloride is increased in the aorta and femoral artery of either DOCA- (41) or ALDO- (31) treated rats and that this increase in ion turnover is evident before hypertension has appeared. In both excised arteries and vascular smooth muscle cell preparations (25, 27), obtained from animals treated with DOCA, sodium permeability is substantially increased within 18—24 h of treatment. Increased sodium permeability may be related to increased expression of sodium-potassium ATPase isoforms when DOCA administration is associated with sodium loading vis a vis DOCA alone (36). Whether such a response would occur in fibroblasts or whether a change in fibroblast membrane properties would augment collagen synthesis remains to be elucidated although preliminary data (K. Sriram unpublished observations) suggests that a membrane bound, ouabain sensitive Na^+-K^+-ATPase may indeed be involved.

In DOCA-salt treated, uninephrectomized rats, collagen synthesis is increased in both the aorta and myocardium (56). This is also true of mesenteric arteries, but not mesenteric veins or the vena cava (42). These findings could be explained by differences in intraluminal pressure between the arterial and venous circulations. However, given the information presented above, which suggests that arterial pressure itself is not a determinant of fibrosis, we would propose that these findings are in keeping with the heterogeneity in steroid receptor distribution which favors systemic arteries and aorta while they are absent in veins (45). In this connection, the sodium-potassium ATPase inhibitor digitoxin prevented the expected rise in myocardial collagen synthesis that occurs within the first week of secondary hyperaldosteronism due to bilateral renal ischemia (66).

Pathogenesis of perivascular/interstitial fibrosis: theoretical possibilities

In response to parenchymal cell necrosis, collagen metabolism is increased as part of a necessary wound healing response that serves to restore the structural integrity of any tissue. Collagen deposition in the form of scarring is a known outcome to cardiac myocyte loss. Should alterations in collagen synthesis and degradation be evoked and proceed to fibrillar collagen accumulation in the absence of myocyte necrosis, however, one would have an inappropriate fibrosis or wound-healing response gone awry. In order to prevent such a reactive fibrous tissue response in the myocardium, we must understand the factors which regulate its wound-healing response in the absence of myocyte injury. Toward this end, we briefly present several theoretical scenarios.

Angiotensin and aldosterone as components of a wound healing response

An emerging body of information implicates steroid and peptide hormones in the regulation of fibroblast growth, collagen metabolism and the expression of various growth factors. In addition to its important influences on cardiovascular and renal homeostasis, the RAAS may also represent an integral component of a wound healing response that eventuates in fibrous tissue formation. Several lines of evidence can be cited in support of this viewpoint: a) mRNA for angiotensinogen, identified by in situ hybridization, has been localized in loose connective cells, such as brown adipocytes and fibroblasts, in the adventitia of the cardiovascular system (14); b) autoradiographic detection of angiotensin converting enzyme reveals that it is found in the endothelium and adventitia of intramyocardial coronary arteries, as well as valve leaflets, which consist of fibroblasts, fibrillar collagen and endothelial cells (73); c) 4 weeks after myocardial infarction, ACE was largely localized in the scar tissue that had formed at the site of myocyte loss (40); d) myofibroblasts, transformed fibroblasts that play an integral part in wound healing, contract in response to AII (29) while their connexons, or intracellular connections, are responsive to mineralocorticoids (23), and e) cardiac fibroblast collagen synthesis, as noted earlier, is augmented by ALDO and AII although the concentrations of each which elicited this response (10^{-9} vs 10^{-7} M, respectively) were considerably different (11, 74). The presence of these effector hormone of the RAAS within the interstitial space, generated either locally or from blood-borne sources, appear to be involved in the fibrous tissue response of the myocardium.

Recent evidence also implicates endothelin (ET) in the wound-healing response that involves AII and ALDO. This peptide hormone is produced by vascular endothelial cells, as well as epithelial cells (59, 62). ET stimulates cardiac fibroblast collagen synthesis (E. Guarda, unpublished observations) and mitosis of fibroblast-like cells (12, 46). In addition to these paracrine properties, ET has autocrine properties that promote the generation of ALDO in cultured bovine aorta endothelial cells through a mechanism that involves ACE and AII (34). ET expression is regulated by a variety of hormones and regulatory polypetides (55), including AII (59). A theoretical model involving AII, ALDO, and ET as components of a wound-healing response is depicted in Fig. 2, where endothelial cells recognize peptide hormones while fibroblasts are responsive to both peptide and steroid hormones.

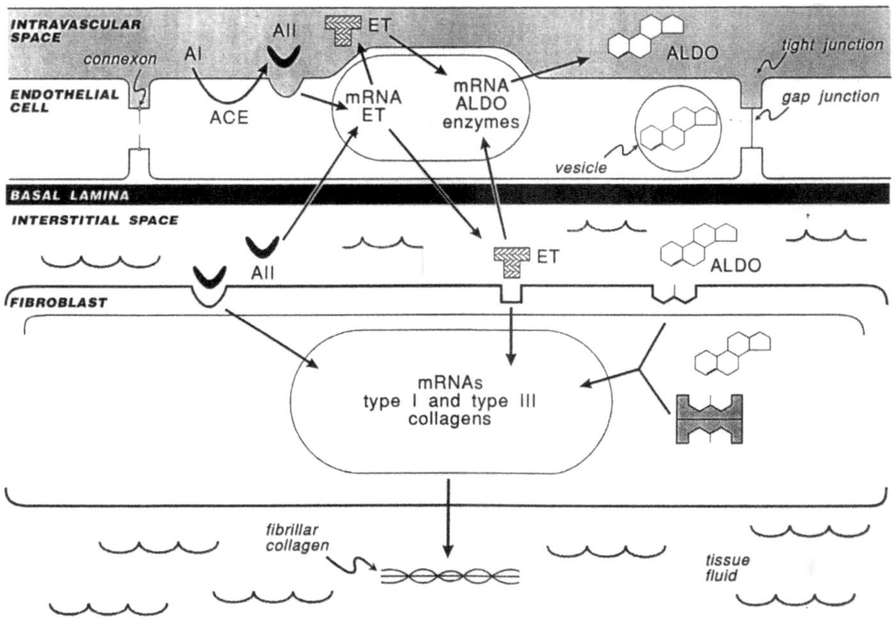

Fig. 2. A theoretical model that depicts angiotensin II (AII), aldosterone (ALDO), and endothelin (ET) as components of a wound-healing system that promotes the synthesis and deposition of fibrillar type I and type III collagens in the interstitial space. Circulating angiotensin I (AI) is converted to AII by angiotensin converting enzyme (ACE) of vascular endothelial cells. AII, which binds to its type-I or type-II receptors, has paracrine properties that promote collagen synthesis of fibroblasts and autocrine properties that induce ET synthesis by endothelial cells. ET, in turn, also promotes fibroblast collagen synthesis via an ACE dependent pathway. ET may also induce cell division as well. In addition to these paracrine effects, ET has autocrine properties that stimulate ALDO synthesis by endothelial cells. Circulating and AII and ALDO gain access to the interstitial space through tight junctions and perhaps by vesicular transport as well. ALDO, bound to corticoid receptors located in fibroblast cell membrane or cytosol, stimulates collagen synthesis. Intercellular communication through connexons or gap junctions may also represent an important component of this system. (See text for further details.).

Abnormal coronary macromolecular permeability

The endothelium of the vasculature is normally impermeable to macromolecules. The appearance of albumin in the urine, for example, heralds an abnormality in glomerular endothelial permeability which could be initiated by a host of factors, including endothelial cell injury, antigen-antibody complexes, or endothelial cell contraction in response to various stimuli. Endothelial cells contain actin filaments that

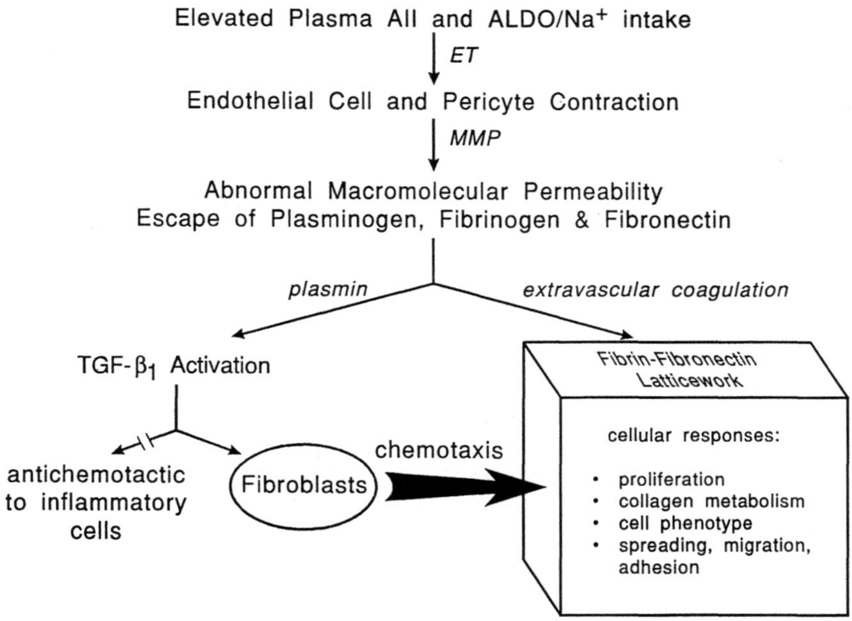

Fig. 3. A theoretical model that depicts a series of events that eventuate in a perivascular and interstitial accumulation of fibrillar collagen — a reactive fibrosis that occurs in the absence of cardiac myocyte necrosis. Elevations in circulating angiotensin II and aldosterone, relative to dietary Na^+ intake, are associated with endothelial cell and/or pericyte contraction mediated by angiotension II itself and/or its stimulation of endothelin (ET) production. ET, in turn, could also stimulate the release of matrix metalloproteinase (MMP) from endothelial cells or fibroblasts. This protease degrades type-IV collagen of basal lamina, thereby creating the final pathway for the escape of macromolecules from the intravascular space into the interstitium.Two events follow: first, the activation of various growth factors; and second, the formation of a fibrin-fibronectin gel as a result of extravascular coagulation. This gel serves as a three-dimensional lattice for invading and proliferating fibroblasts governed by chemoattractant factors. Growth factors (e.g., PDGF, IL series) typically involved in promoting leukocyte, monocyte or lymphocyte invasion are not likely participatory, while TGF-β_1 is contributory to the suppression of such an inflammatory cell response. Within the interstitices of this gel, fibroblasts undergo various responses that include enhanced growth, altered metabolic behavior and cell phenotype, and spreading, migration and adhesion within the fibronectin fibril assembly. Ultimately, there is an accumulation of fibrillar type I and III collagens which presents morphologically as a perivascular fibrosis of intramyocardial coronary arteries and arterioles with extensions into neighboring interstitial spaces. (See text for further details.)

foster their contraction in response to vasoactive peptides, such as AII and ET (52). Pericytes, or fibroblast-like cells that reside within arterioles, capillaries and venules, also contain actin filaments. They contract in response to these peptide hormones (52) and thereby may also promote the entry of macromolecules into the interstitial space (see Fig. 3). In order to create the remaining path for intravascular protein escape through the basal lamina, matrix metalloproteinase production by endothelial cells (37) or fibroblasts is needed to degrade type IV collagen. The appearance of plasminogen, fibrinogen and fibronectin in the interstitium leads to extravascular coagulation and the formation of a fibrin-fibronectin gel into which fibroblasts and inflammatory cells could migrate, as dictated by chemoattractant factors.

At this juncture, growth factors are also activated to modulate the growth, behavior and cytodifferentiation of mesenchymal cells. TGF-β_1, for example, whose expression is increased in DOCA hypertension (61), may be activated by protease digestion (e.g., plasmin). Once activated, TGF-β_1 can serve as a chemotactic signal to fibroblast migration and evoke a host of cellular responses that modulate fibroblast collagen synthesis and promote their transformation to myofibroblasts, as well as foster the growth of fibroblasts that express TGF-β (autoinduction). TGF-β_1 may also be antichemotactic to inflammatory cells and explain why leukocytes and monocytes are not found around intramyocardial coronary arteries in states of mineralocorticoid excess.

Fibronectin fibrils form the structural network that guides the movement of invading fibroblasts (see Fig. 4). Activated, less differentiated fibroblasts proliferate and migrate within the interstitices of this network. Migratory cells have an altered secretory phenotype, particularly with respect to their elaboration of glycosaminoglycans. Their production of hydrophilic hyaluronic acid creates local swelling and distention of interstitices to facilitate fibroblast migration. More mature cells become stationary by virtue of their integrin attachments to fibronectin; these cells secrete dermatan sulfate and heparan sulfate which serve to shrink the size of these interstitices. Mature cells also synthesize and deposit type I and III fibrillar collagens. Type-III collagen is first laid down on fibronectin fibrils followed by type-I collagen. Within 2 weeks this series of events presents itself as morphologically distinct perivascular and interstitial fibrosis.

Prevention and regression of myocardial fibrosis

Prevention of fibrosis

In demonstrating the contribution of circulating AII and ALDO in mediating a structural remodeling of the myocardium through the appearance of a reactive and a reparative fibrosis, evidence has been presented to indicate that ACE inhibition and ALDO receptor antagonism can prevent this pathologic process (9, 68), as well as its adverse consequences on myocardial stiffness (69). These cardioprotective properties were evident in experimental models of primary and secondary hyperaldosteronism.

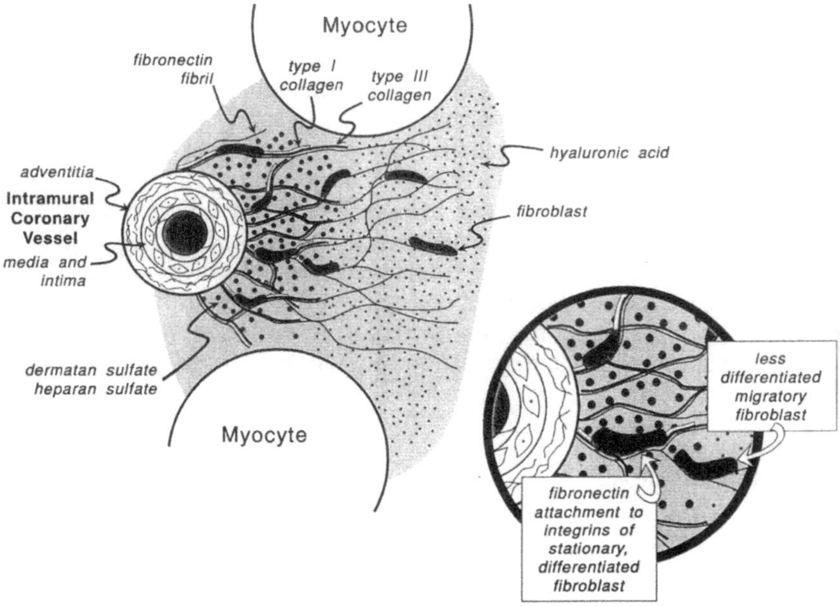

Fig. 4. A theoretical model further depicting the course of events that lead to the development of perivascular and interstitial fibrosis. Fibronectin fibrils form a latticework around vessels having abnormal macromolecular permeability. Fibroblasts proliferate and migrate within this network. Fibroblast motility is fostered by their lack of attachment to fibronectin fibrils. The density of fibroblasts is greatest around vessels. Those closest to the vessel are more mature and stationary, while those more remote are less differentiated and mobile. Hyaluronic acid, a hydrophilic glycosaminoglycan produced by migrating and proliferating fibroblasts, appears first. This creates hydrated, swollen spaces within the lattice that facilitate fibrobast movement. Subsequently, sulfated glycosaminoglycans are formed (e.g., dermatan sulfate, chondroitin sulfate). They polymerize monomers and serve to reduce the size of spaces between fibronectin fibrils. Mature fibroblasts initially synthesize fibrillar type III collagen that is deposited on fibronectin fibrils. Thereafter, type I collagen fibers appear. These fibers surround the fibronectin-type III fibrillar collagen assembly. (See text for further details.)

Regression of fibrosis

Brilla et al. (6, 7) recently examined whether it would be possible to reverse the adverse structural remodeling of the myocardium and its intramyocardial coronary arteries due to fibrosis with the ACE inhibitor lisinopril. Given the importance of AII and ALDO in promoting fibrosis, the hypothesis tested was whether such an agent would reduce collagen synthesis while collagen degradation would proceed at its normal rate. A 12 week period of treatment was used to normalize collagen concentration and reduce collagen content. Whether this ACE inhibitor would accelerate collagen degradation is unknown. Oral lisinopril administration was accompanied by a regression of the perivascular and interstitial fibrosis that was present in 14-week-old male rats with genetic hypertension. The reduction in collagen concentration to normal was confirmed using both a morphometric determination of collagen volume fraction and a biochemical assay for hydroxyproline concentration in the myocardium. In removing the reactive myocardial fibrosis, left ventricular stiffness returned to levels found in age/sex matched genetic controls. The regression in fibrosis was observed with either a small dose of lisinopril that did not reduce arterial pressure or regress LVH, or a large dose that normalized arterial pressure and LV mass. The mechanism by which lisinopril removed collagen from the myocardium remains to be established. A theoretical argument, however, could be offered based on our cell culture studies: AII reduces collagenase activity while AII and ALDO each increase cardiac fibroblast collagen synthesis. ACE inhibition may therefore promote a regression in fibrosis by removing each stimulus to fibrosis while permitting enhanced collagen degradation through uninhibited collagenolytic activity.

Summary and future directions

An abnormal fibrous tissue response that appears within the interstitial space of the myocardium in certain expressions of cardiovascular disease represents a structural basis for its failure and propensity for arrhythmia. The importance of fibrosis suggests a cellular basis for pathologic structural remodeling involving cardiac fibroblasts and the regulation of collagen metabolism by effector hormones of the RAAS. This view broadens our perspective of myocardial disease in that it suggests cardiac myocytes and abnormalities in their biochemical behavior may not be the sole mechanism responsible for ventricular dysfunction and arrhythmias.

The pathophysiologic and pathogenic mechanisms involved in mediating the fibrous tissue response remain to be more fully elucidated. The exciting new technologies of the cellular and molecularly biology laboratory need to be further integrated into the next phase of experimental investigation. Notwithstanding the remaining gaps in our knowledge, the proposition that elevation in circulating AII and ALDO have paracrine and autocrine properties that modulate the behavior of fibroblasts and thereby tissue structure extends their importance beyond the traditional role involving physiologic control of vascular resistance and sodium homeostasis.

Finally, clinical trials that would address the cardioprotective and cardioreparative properties of pharmacologic strategies in various clinical disorders, where fibrosis is an important component of the adverse structural remodeling of the myocardium and systemic circulation, should be initiated. This includes systemic hypertension with pathologic LVH, chronic myocardial failure, and acute myocardial infarction with ventricular dysfunction. In each of these circumstances renin-dependent and renin-independent mechanisms serve to alter the AII and mineralocorticoid profile of the plasma and cardiovascular tissues.

References

1. Alderman MH, Madhaven S, Ooi WL, Cohen H, Sealey JE, Laragh JH (1991) Association of the renin-sodium profile with the risk of myocardial infarction in patients with hypertension. N Engl J Med 324:1098—1104

2. Anderson KR, St. John Sutton MG, Lie JT (1979) Histopathological types of cardiac fibrosis in myocardial disease. J Pathol 128:79—85
3. Bhan RD, Giacomelli F, Wiener J (1978) Ultrastructure of coronary arteries and myocardium in experimental hypertension. Exp Mol Pathol 29:66—81
4. Bhan RD, Giacomelli F, Wiener J (1982) Adrenoreceptor blockade in angiotensin-induced hypertension: effect on rat coronary arteries and myocardium. Am J Pathol 108:60—71
5. Brilla CG, Weber KT (1990) Mineralocorticoid excess, dietary sodium and myocardial fibrosis. J Lab Clin Med (in press)
6. Brilla CG, Janicki JS, Weber KT (1991) Cardioreparative effects of lisinopril in rats with genetic hypertension and left ventricular hypertrophy. Circulation 83:1771—1779
7. Brilla CG, Janicki JS, Weber KT (1991) Impaired diastolic function and coronary reserve in genetic hypertension: role of interstitial fibrosis and medial thickening of intramyocardial coronary arteries. Circ Res 69:107—115
8. Brilla CG, Pick R, Tan LB, Janicki JS, Weber KT (1990) Remodeling of the rat right and left ventricle in experimental hypertension. Circ Res 67:1355—1364
9. Brilla CG, Weber KT (1991) Prevention of myocardial fibrosis in renovascular hypertension and hyperaldosteronism: anti-fibrotic effects of spironolactone [Abstract]. In: 17th International Aldosterone Conference. Meetings & Events Communications, Evansville, Ind, pp 56—57
10. Brilla CG, Weber KT (1992) Reactive and reparative myocardial fibrosis in arterial hypertension in the rat. Cardiovasc Res 26:671—677
11. Brilla CG, Zhou G, Weber KT (1992) Aldosterone and collagen synthesis in cultured adult rat cardiac fibroblasts [Abstract]. FASEB J 6:A1914
12. Brown KD, Littlewood CJ (1989) Endothelin stimulates DNA synthesis in Swiss 3T3 cells. Biochem J 263:977—980
13. Brunner HR, Laragh JH, Baer L, Newton MA, Goodwin FT, Krakoff LR, Bard RH, Bühler FR (1972) Essential hypertension: renin and aldosterone, heart attack and stroke. N Engl J Med 286:441—449
14. Campbell DJ, Habener JF (1987) Cellular localization of angiotensinogen gene expression in brown adipose tissue and mesentery: quantification of messenger ribonucleic acid abundance using hybridization in situ. Endocrinology 121:1616—1626
15. Campbell SE, Diaz-Arias AA, Weber KT (1992) Fibrosis of the human heart and systemic organs in adrenal adenoma. Blood Pressure (in press)
16. Campbell SE, Janicki JS, Matsubara BB, Weber KT (1992) Myocardial fibrosis in the rat with primary hyperaldosteronism: prevention of scarring by amiloride. Am J Hypertens (in press)
17. Campbell SE, Matsubara BB, Janicki JS, Weber KT (1991) Myocardial fibroblast response in renovascular hypertension: temporal and distribution patterns [Abstract]. Clin Res 39:691A
18. Casale PN, Devereux RB, Milner M, Zullo G, Harshfield GA, Pickering TG, Laragh JH (1986) Value of echocardiographic measurement of left ventricular mass in predicting cardiovascular morbid events in hypertensive men. Ann Intern Med 105:173—178
19. Chapman D, Weber KT, Eghbali M (1990) Regulation of fibrillar collagen types I and III and basement membrane type IV collagen gene expression in pressure overloaded rat myocardium. Circ Res 67:787—794
20. Cooper RS,Simmons BE, Castaner A, Santhanam V, Ghali J, Mar M (1990) Left ventricular hypertrophy is associated with worse survival independent of ventricular function and number of coronary arteries severely narrowed. Am J Cardiol 65:441—445
21. Crane WAJ, Dutta LP (1963) The utilisation of tritiated thymidine for deoxyribonucleic acid synthesis by the lesions of experimental hypertension in rats. J Path Bact 86:83—97
22. Darrow DC, Miller HC (1942) The production of cardiac lesions by repeated injections of desoxycorticosterone acetate. J Clin Invest 21:601—611
23. Davidson JS, Baumgarten IM (1988) Glycyrrhetinic acid derivatives: a novel class of inhibitors of gap-junctional intercellular communication. Structure-activity relationship. J Pharmacol Exp Ther 245:1104—1107

24. Davis BA, Crook JE, Vestal RE, Oates JA (1979) Prevalence of renovascular hypertension in patients with grade III or IV hypertensive retinopathy. N Engl J Med 301: 1273—1276
25. Davis JPL, Chipperfield AR, Harper AA (1991) Comparison of the electrical properties of arterial smooth muscle in normotensive rats and rats with deoxycorticosterone acetate-salt-induced hypertension: possible involvement of (Na^+-K^+-Cl^-) co-transport. Clin Sci 81:73—78
26. Dunn MJ, Tannen RL (1974) Low-renin hypertension. Kidney Int 5:317—325
27. Friedman SM, Tanaka M (1987) Increased sodium permeability and transport as primary events in the hypertensive response to deoxycorticosterone acetate (DOCA) in the rat. J Hypertens 5:341—345
28. Funder JW, Pearce PT, Smith R, Smith AI (1988) Mineralocorticoid action: target tissue specificity is enzyme, not receptor, mediated. Science 242:583—585
29. Gabbiani G (1981) The myofibroblast: a key cell for wound healing and fibrocontractive diseases. In: Deyl Z, Adam M (eds) Connective Tissue Research: Chemistry, Biology, and Physiology. Liss, New york, pp 183—194
30. Ganten D, Schelling P, Flugel RM, Ganten U (1975) Effect of angiotensin and an angiotensin antagonist on iso-renin and cell growth in 3T3 mouse cells. IRCS J Med Sci 3:327—332
31. Garwitz ET, Jones AW (1982) Aldosterone infusion into the rat and dose-dependent changes in blood pressure and arterial ionic transport. Hypertension 4:374—381
32. Giacomelli F, Anversa P, Wiener J (1976) Effect of angiotensin-induced hypertension on rat coronary arteries and myocardium. Am J Pathol 84:111—125
33. Giese J (1964) Acute hypertensive vascular disease. 2. Studies on vascular reaction patterns and permeability changes by means of vital microscopy and colloidal tracer technique. Acta Pathol Microbiol Scand 62:497—515
34. Guarda E, Myers P, Zhou G, Brilla C, Weber K (1992) Endothelin-1 elicits aldosterone (ALDO) release from cultured endothelial cells [Abstract]. FASEB J 6:A1811
35. Hall CE, Hall O (1965) Hypertension and hypersalimentation. I. Aldosterone hypertension. Lab Invest 14:285—294
36. Herrera VLM, Chobanian AV, Ruiz-Opazo N (1988) Isoform-specific modulation of Na^+, K^+-ATPase α-subunit gene expression in hypertension. Science 241:221—233
37. Herron GS, Werb Z, Dwyer K, Banda MJ (1986) Secretion of metalloproteinases by stimulated capillary endothelial cells. J Biol Chem. 261:2810—2813
38. Huysman JAN, Vliegen HW, VanderLaarse A, Euldering F (1989) Changes in non-myocyte tissue composition associated with pressure overload of hypertrophic human hearts. Pathol Res Pract 184:577—581
39. Jalil JE, Janicki JS, Pick R, Weber KT (1991) Coronary vascular remodeling and myocardial fibrosis in the rat with renovascular hypertension: response to captopril. Am J Hypertens 4:51—55
40. Johnston CI, Mooser V, Sun Y, Fabris B (1991) Changes in cardiac angiotensin converting enzyme (ACE) after myocardial infarction and hypertrophy in rats. Clin Exp Pharmacol Physiol 18:107—110
41. Jones AW, Hart RG (1975) Altered ion transport in aortic smooth muscle during deoxycorticosterone acetate hypertension in the rat. Circ Res 37:333—341
42. Jwatsuki K, Cardinale GJ, Spector S, Udenfriend S (1977) Hypertension: increase of collagen biosynthesis in arteries but not veins. Science 198:403—405
43. Karsner HT (1955) Human Pathology. JB Lippincott, Philadelphia
44. Koren MJ, Devereux RB, Casale PN, Savage DD, Laragh JH (1990) Relation of left ventricular mass and geometry to morbidity and mortality in uncomplicated essential hypertension. Ann Intern Med 115:345—352
45. Kornel L, Kanamarlapudi N, Ramsay C, Travers T, Kamath S, Taff DJ, Patel N, Packer W, Raynor WJ (1983) Arterial steroid receptors and their putative role in the mechanism of hypertension. J Steroid Biochem 19:333—344

46. Kusuhara M, Yamaguchi K, Ohnishi A, Abe K, Kimura S, Oono H, Hori S, Nakamura Y (1989) Endothelin potentiates growth factor-stimulated DNA synthesis in Swiss 3T3 cells. Jpn J Cancer Res 80:302—305
47. Laine GA (1988) Microvascular changes in the heart during chronic arterial hypertension. Circ Res 62:953—960
48. Leipälä JA, Takala TES, Ruskoaho H, Myllylä R, Kainulainen H, Hassinen IE, Anttinen H, Vihko V (1988) Transmural distribution of biochemical markers of total protein and collagen synthesis, myocardial contraction speed and capillary density in the rat left ventricle in angiotensin II-induced hypertension. Acta Physiol Scand 133: 325—333
49. Levy D, Garrison RJ, Savage DD, Kannel WB, Castelli WP (1990) Prognostic implications of echocardiographically determined left ventricular mass in the Framingham Heart Study. N Engl J Med 322:1561—1566
50. Lindy S, Turto H, Uitto J (1972) Protocollagen proline hydroxylase activity in rat heart during experimental cardiac hypertrophy. Circ Res 30:205—209
51. Meyer WJ III, Nichols NR (1981) Mineralocorticoid binding in cultured smooth muscle cells and fibroblasts from rat aorta. J Steroid Biochem 14:1157—1168
52. Miller FN, Sims DE (1986) Contractile elements in the regulation of macromolecular permeability. Fed Proc 45:84—88
53. Moore RD, Schienberg MD, Koletsky S (1963) Cardiac lesions in experimental hypertension. Arch Pathol 75:28—44
54. Morkin E, Ashford TP (1968) Myocardial DNA synthesis in experimental cardiac hypertrophy. Am J Physiol 215:1409—1413
55. Ohta K, Hirata Y, Imai T, Kanno K, Emori T, Shichiri M, Marumo F (1990) Cytokine-induced release of endothelin-1 from porcine renal epithelial cell line. Biochem Biophys Res Commun 169:578—584
56. Ooshima A, Fuller GC, Cardinale GJ, Spector S, Udenfried S (1974) Increased collagen synthesis in blood vessels of hypertensive rats and its reversal by antihypertensive agents. Proc Natl Acad Sci USA 71:3019—3023
57. Pearlman ES, Weber KT, Janicki JS, Pietra G, Fishman AP (1982) Muscle fiber orientation and connective tissue content in the hypertrophied human heart. Lab Invest 46:158—164
58. Reddy HK, Campbell SE, Janicki JS, Zhou G, Weber KT (1992) Coronary microvascular fluid flux and permeability: influence of angiotensin II, aldosterone and acute arterial hypertension. J Lab Clin Med (in press)
59. Resink TJ, Hahn AWA, Scott-Burden T, Powell J, Weber E, Bühler FR (1990) Inducible endothelin mRNA expression and peptide secretion in cultured human vascular smooth muscle cells. Biochem Biophys Res Commun 168:1303—1310
60. Sano H, Okada H, Kawaguchi H, Yasuda H (1991) Increased angiotensin II-stimulated collagen synthesis in cultured cardiac fibroblasts from spontaneously hypertensive rats [Abstract]. Circulation 84(Suppl. II):II—48
61. Sarzani R, Brecher P, Chobanian AV (1989) Growth factor expression in aorta of normotensive and hypertensive rats. J Clin Invest 83:1404—1408
62. Schrey MP, Patel KV, Tezapsidis N (1992) Bombesin and glucocorticoids stimulate human breast cancer cells to produce endothelin, a paracrine mitogen for breast stromal cells. Cancer Res 52:1786—1790
63. Selye H (1946) The general adaptation syndrome and the disease of adaptation. J Clin Endocrinol 6:117—230
64. Silver MA, Pick R, Brilla CG, Jalil JE, Janicki JS, Weber KT (1990) Reactive and reparative fibrosis in the hypertrophied rat left ventricle: two experimental models of myocardial fibrosis. Cardiovasc Res 24:741—747
65. Tan LB, Jalil JE, Pick R, Janicki JS, Weber KT (1991) Cardiac myocyte necrosis induced by angiotensin II. Circ Res 69:1185—1195
66. Turto H (1977) Collagen metabolism in experimental cardiac hypertrophy in the rat and effect of digitoxin treatment. Cardiovasc Res 11:358—366

67. Weber KT (1989) Cardiac interstitium in health and disease: the fibrillar collagen network. J Am Coll Cardiol 13:1637—1652
68. Weber KT, Brilla CG (1991) Pathological hypertrophy and cardiac interstitium: fibrosis and renin-angiotensin-aldosterone system. Circulation 83:1849—1865
69. Weber KT, Brilla CG, Janicki JS (1990) Structural remodeling of myocardial collagen in systemic hypertension: functional consequences and potential therapy. Heart Failure 6:129—137
70. Weber KT, Brilla CG, Janicki JS (1991) Cell biology of myocardial remodeling: contribution of nonmyocyte cells. J Vasc Med Biol 3:44—49
71. Weber KT, Janicki JS, Shroff SG, Pick R, Abrahams C, Chen RM, Bashey RI (1988) Collagen compartment remodeling in the pressure overloaded left ventricle. J Appl Cardiol 3:37—46
72. Wiener J, Giacomelli F (1973) The cellular pathology of experimental hypertension. VII. Structure and permeability of the mesenteric vasculature in angiotensin-induced hypertension. Am J Pathol 72:221—240
73. Yamada H, Fabris B, Allen AM, Jackson B, Johnston CI, Mendelsohn FAO (1991) Localization of angiotensin converting enzyme in the rat heart. Circ Res 68:141—149
74. Zhou G, Brilla CG, Weber KT (1992) Angiotensin II-mediated stimulation of collagen synthesis in cultured cardiac fibroblasts [Abstract]. FASEB J 6:A1914

Author's address:
Karl T. Weber, MD
Division of Cardiology
University of Missouri-Columbia
Rm. MA432 Medical Science Building
Columbia, MO 65212, U.S.A.

Ventricular remodeling after myocardial infarction. Experimental and clinical studies

G. Ertl, P. Gaudron, K. Hu

Medizinische Klinik, Universität Würzburg

Summary: Changes of ischemic myocardium following coronary occlusion, including active and passive functions, and adaptive changes of non-ischemic surviving myocardium have been summarized under the term "left ventricular remodeling" post myocardial infarction. An increase in left ventricular volume may be a consequence, and associated with an adverse prognosis. Although left ventricular dilatation may increase stroke volume and, thus, be compensatory at first, in about one-fifth of patients it ultimately results in progressive dysfunction and heart failure. Major determinants of this process are time, infarct size, infarct location, global left ventricular function assessed 4 days after infarction by radionuclide ejection fraction and right heart catheter (stroke volume), and morphology of the infarct-associated coronary artery.

The surviving myocardium hypertrophies and may also dilate structurally. Depression of left ventricular ejection fraction chronically after the infarct is due to deterioration of wall motion of chamber segments initially classified normal by radionuclide analysis. Biochemical changes may also occur, including reduction of phosphocreatine, prolongation of time to peak Ca_i^{2+}, and changes in myosin isoforms. Systemic or local humoral factors may be involved in these changes, however, clear evidence is still lacking. Perfusion of surviving myocardium may be altered under various conditions due to morphologic and functional changes of coronary vasculature. Successful prevention of heart failure and death by angiotensin converting enzyme inhibitors in asymptomatic patients with left ventricular dysfunction post-myocardial infarction has supported the pathophysiologic concepts of remodeling.

Key words: Myocardial infarction; left ventricular dysfunction; remodeling

After acute occlusion of a coronary artery, both ischemic and residual non-ischemic myocardium undergo changes (Fig. 1). Ischemic myocardium rapidly loses function, and systolic contraction reverses to systolic expansion, as observed and first reported by Tennant and Wiggers. If coronary occlusion persists, myocardial necrosis develops and progresses like a "wave front" from subendocardial to subepicardial layers, thus ultimately forming a transmural myocardial infarction (36). Necrotic myocardial tissue is substituted by fibrous tissue during days and weeks post-coronary occlusion. Infarcted tissue may either form a solid scar or expand during healing (5). "Infarct expansion" contributes to left ventricular dilatation post myocardial infarction. Increased function of non-ischemic myocardium has been observed early after coronary occlusion. Left ventricular ejection fraction will deteriorate and, thus, end-systolic left ventricular volume will increase when augmented function of non-ischemic myocardium will not outweigh the loss of contractile myocardium. When venous return to the left ventricle from the pulmonary vascular bed remains the same, end-diastolic volume will increase along with an increase in end-diastolic filling pressure. This increase in myocardial fiber length has been defined as "distension" of discretion of structural dilatation of the heart, which may result in normalization of end-diastolic pressure. Elevated filling pressure and augmented volume

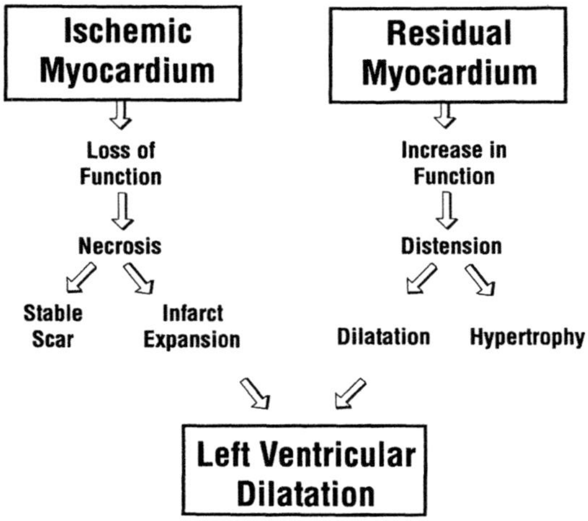

Fig. 1. Schematic diagram of acute and chronic changes in ischemic/infarcted and non-ischemic/overloaded myocardium post-myocardial infarction. The processes which may ultimately result in left ventricular dilatation are summarized under the term "left ventricular remodeling" post-myocardial infarction.

will result in increased left ventricular diastolic wall stress, probably a major stimulus for excentric myocardial hypertrophy and, thus, structural dilatation. These processes have been summarized under the term "remodeling of the left ventricle" post-myocardial infarction.

This review summarizes global and regional changes of the heart during remodeling, their determinants and consequences for global cardiac performance and the residual surviving myocardium.

Left ventricular volume

The pathologist Linzbach described left ventricular dilatation in various cardiac diseases and defined the pathophysiologic importance. His concept was that structural dilatation (*plastische Gefügedilatation*) is the morphologic substrate of heart failure, and he suggested an important role of cardiac deposition of connective tissue for left ventricular dysfunction (26).

Left ventricular dilatation and prognosis

The prognostic importance of cardiac size post-myocardial infarction was also reported as early as 1966 by Waris and colleagues on the basis of chest roentgenograms (44). Serial changes of "left heart size" have been observed by Kostuk and associates, and progressive dilatation correlated closely with an adverse prognosis (22). Chest roentgenograms proved to be relatively insensitive to changes of left ventricular volume. White and his group used contrast angiography and defined end-systolic volume being of higher ($X^2 = 82.9$) predictive value for survival than end-diastolic volume ($X^2 = 59.0$) or ejection fraction ($X^2 = 46.6$) determined 1 to 2 months post-myocardial infarction (47).

Compensatory and non-compensatory dilatation

The high prognostic impact of left ventricular enlargement post-myocardial infarction suggests a potential pathophysiologic role of dilatation. In fact, for geometric reasons, an increase in cardiac volume may compensate for reduced ejection fraction (14). This compensatory effect of dilatation could, however, be outweighed by an increase in systolic wall stress which increases according to Laplace (14). A prospective study was, therefore, undertaken by Gaudron et al. to clarify compensatory and non-compensatory aspects of left ventricular dilatation (10). Serial measurements of left ventricular volume by gated SPECT (single photon emission computed tomography) were performed in patients 4 days, 4 weeks, and 6 months after a first myocardial infarction. Cardiac output was measured by Swan-Ganz catheter, left ventricular ejection fraction by conventional radionuclide ventriculography. Patients were classified as having had large or small myocardial infarctions according to plasma creatine kinase activity. Bicycle exercise tests at identical work load were performed 4 weeks and 6 months after infarction. No differences were found between patient groups (large vs. small) or among various time points of heart rate, arterial, right atrial, pulmonary artery, or wedge pressure, pulmonary vascular, or systemic vascular resistance at rest. Figure 2 shows that ejection fraction was

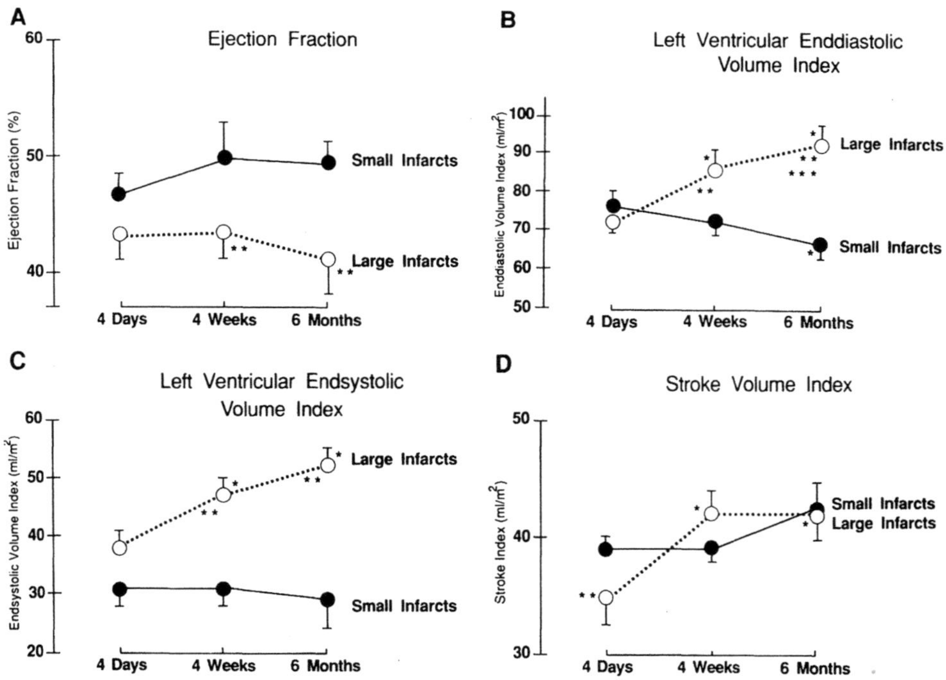

Fig. 2. Time-course of left ventricular ejection fraction (A), end-diastolic (B), end-systolic (C), and stroke volume index (D) in patients with small (●--●) and large (○--○) infarctions. Four weeks and 6 months after large infarction, ejection fraction was depressed, end-diastolic and end-systolic volume were increased. Stroke volume in patients with large infarctions was depressed at 4 days, restored to normal at 4 weeks, and remained constant until 6 months. In patients with small infarctions, ejection fraction was maintained and end-diastolic volume, in contrast to patients with large infarctions, had decreased at 6 months. Values are mean ± SEM. $p < 0.05$ as compared with values at 4 days (*) and 4 weeks (***), and in patients with small infarctions (**). (From Gaudron et al., Am Heart J 1992, with permission.)

depressed in patients with large infarcts with a tendency to deterioration 6 months after infarction. Left ventricular end-diastolic and end-systolic volumes progressively increased in these patients. Stroke volume was subnormal 4 days but normalized 4 weeks after infarction and remained stable thereafter in patients with large infarcts. Figure 3 shows exercise hemodynamics in these patients. Stroke volume index rose during exercise 4 weeks but not 6 months after infarction, and pulmonary capillary wedge pressure rose more at 6 months than at 4 weeks after infarction. It was concluded that left ventricular dilatation was compensatory and normalized stroke volume during 4 weeks after the infarction, while thereafter it was accompanied by deterioration of exercise hemodynamics. Compensatory and non-compensatory dilatation occurred only in patients classified as having large infarcts.

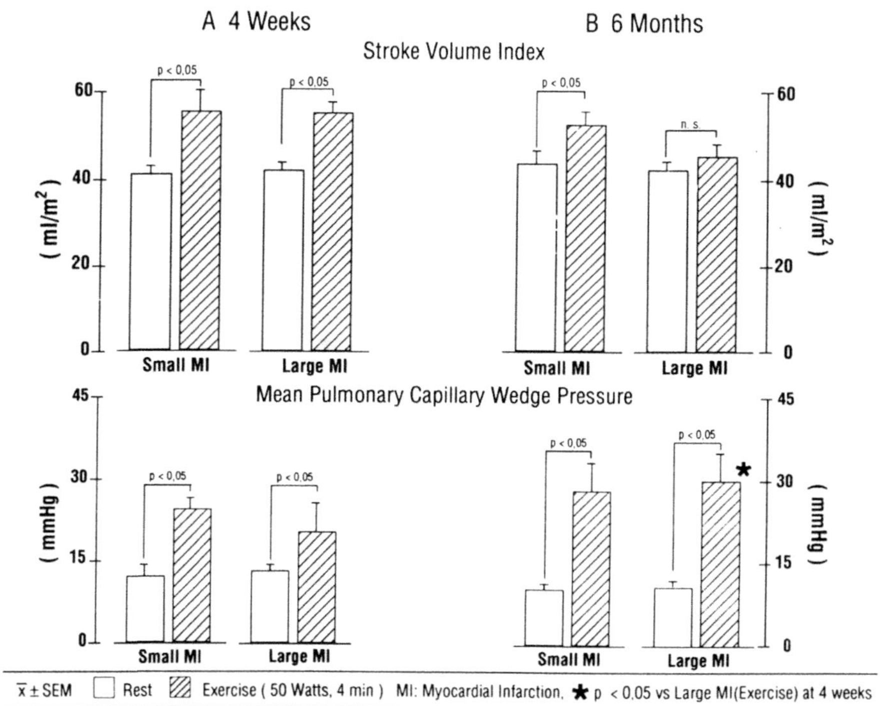

Fig. 3. Stroke volume index and mean pulmonary capillary wedge pressure at rest (open bars) and during steady-state, supine, bicycle exercise at 50 W (hatched bars) 4 weeks (A) and 6 months (B) after small or large infarction. At 6 months capability to augment stroke volume during exercise was preserved in the group with small infarctions but was lost in the group with large infarctions. Values are mean ±SEM. (From Gaudron et al., Am Heart J 1992, with permission.)

Progressive dilatation

A follow up study of Gaudron et al. which will be published in near future, observed patients with progressive dilatation for 3 years (11). This study proved that progressive dilatation was accompanied by progressive left ventricular dysfunction as indicated by deterioration of ejection fraction, cardiac and stroke volume index and an increase in wedge pressure at rest and during exercise. After 3 years, patients shifted to higher classes in the New York Heart Association (NYHA) classification, indicating manifestation of hemodynamic deterioration in clinical symptoms. Thus, initially compensatory dilatation may ultimately result in heart failure.

Determinants of left ventricular dilatation

Determinants or risk factors for left ventricular dilatation post-myocardial infarction have not been so well defined. Hort, a collaborator of Linzbach, found a relation of survival to left ventricular volume after an experimental myocardial infarction in rats, and of left ventricular volume to *infarct size* (18). Pfeffer and coworkers showed in rats that infarct size and time after myocardial infarction were major determinants of left ventricular volume, volume to mass ratio and, thus, wall stress (34). These data supported the concept of progressive dilatation and progressive wall stress forming a vicious circle. Gaudron and associates confirmed in patients the impact of infarct size on left ventricular dilatation (9). Figure 4 shows that between 4 and 28 days after a first myocardial infarction, left ventricular end-diastolic volume index measured by gated SPECT tended to decrease in patients with small myocardial infarctions. In contrast, volume tended to increase in patients with moderate infarct size and increased significantly more in patients with infarcts estimated to be large by CK-analysis (9). This and a follow-up study showed a prevalence of anterior myocardial infarctions in the group defined having large infarct sizes (9, 11). *Infarct location* appears to have an independent impact for the probability of a patient to develop left ventricular dilatation (11). However, progressive dilatation occurred in patients with large inferior and anterior infarcts.

It may be anticipated that *coronary artery morphology*, extension and progression of coronary heart disease, and, especially, recurrent myocardial infarction may have an impact on left ventricular dysfunction and dilatation. General discussion of prognosis of coronary heart disease would be complex and beyond the scope of this review. Relevance of perfusion of the infarct-associated artery has, however, recently

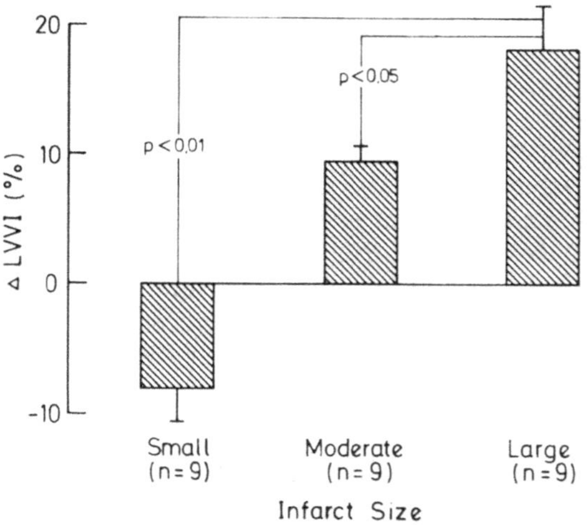

Fig. 4. Changes of left ventricular end-diastolic volume index (LVVI) measured by gated single photon emission computed tomography (SPECT) in patients with a first myocardial infarction (MI) between 4 and 28 days. Patients with an infarction classified as small, showed a reduction of LVVI, while patients with moderate and large infarcts showed an increase (9).

been stressed. Since *perfusion of the infarct-related artery* may be diagnosed early after myocardial infarction, therapeutic interventions could be established at that time. Jeremy and his group have shown that all patients with a completely occluded infarct-related artery and no collaterals developed a more than 20% increase in left ventricular end-diastolic volume between 48 hours and 1 month post-myocardial infarction. Volume remained stable in patients with some perfusion of their infarct (20). Importance of collateral circulation for prevention of left ventricular aneurysm (16) and left ventricular dilatation (48) was supported by further retrospective studies. The rate of left ventricular dilatation depended, not only on the presence or absence of total coronary occlusion (2) or collaterals, but the severity of residual coronary stenosis was also important (25). Thus, it must be questioned whether recanalization or dilatation of a severe stenosis of the infarct-related coronary artery might be indicated to prevent left ventricular dilatation post-myocardial infarction. Controlled prospective studies are requested to address this clinically important question and to clarify at which time after myocardial infarction such an intervention had to be performed.

Late reperfusion which did not improve systolic left ventricular function, had favorable effects on cavity dilatation in one (41) but not in another (45) study. In the GISSI trial, for comparable extents of infarct size, end-systolic volume was smaller in patients who received streptokinase than in those without thrombolytic therapy (29). This finding was confirmed in other studies (24, 43). Thus, reduction of mortality by thrombolytic therapy may in part be due to beneficial effects on left ventricular remodeling.

In conclusion, various determinants contribute to left ventricular dilatation post-myocardial infarction, including infarct size and, thus, extent of left ventricular regional dysfunction. Depression of regional function is resembled by depression of global ejection fraction and stroke volume. Most recently, left ventricular *ejection fraction* and *stroke volume* index measured 4 days after infarction, angiographically determined *infarct size* 4 weeks after infarction, *infarct location* (anterior/inferior) and grade of perfusion ("TIMI grade") of infarct-associated artery were identified as independent predictors of left ventricular dilatation progressive during 3 years after myocardial infarction (11). Thus, a score was developed based on these variables which correctly predicted progressive left ventricular dilatation associated with progressive left ventricular dysfunction and clinical manifestation of heart failure in 89% of patients (11).

Surviving myocardium

As discussed above, there is good evidence that geometrical changes of the heart, especially a vicious circle of dilatation and overload of surviving myocardium, are prominent pathophysiologic factors which participate in development of heart failure. The pathophysiology of the heart post-myocardial infarction is, however, complex due to inhomogeneity of the insult and compensatory processes (Fig. 1). Studies of this pathophysiology are, therefore, difficult and mostly inconclusive.

Morphology and mechanics

The mechanical situation of surviving myocardium is characterized by increased diastolic wall stress due to elevated end-diastolic pressure and/or volume. Animal experiments have shown that excentric (dilatation) and concentric hypertrophy occur in dependence of myocardial infarct size (1). Large infarcts invariably result in a progressive increase in volume-to-mass ratio which may be used as an estimate of wall stress (34). Left ventricular dilatation was proved to be structural in rats with larger infarcts by analysis of pressure/volume curves obtained from in situ arrested hearts (34). Complete diastolic pressure volume curves are difficult to obtain in patients. Figure 5 presents data on pulmonary capillary wedge pressure and left ventricular volume from the study of Gaudron et al. discussed above (10). The graph shows that the increase in left ventricular volume in patients with large infarcts occurs independently of major changes of wedge pressure used as an estimate of left ventricular filling pressure. Thus, this study supports the animal data which have shown that dilatation is structural during weeks to months post-myocardial infarction.

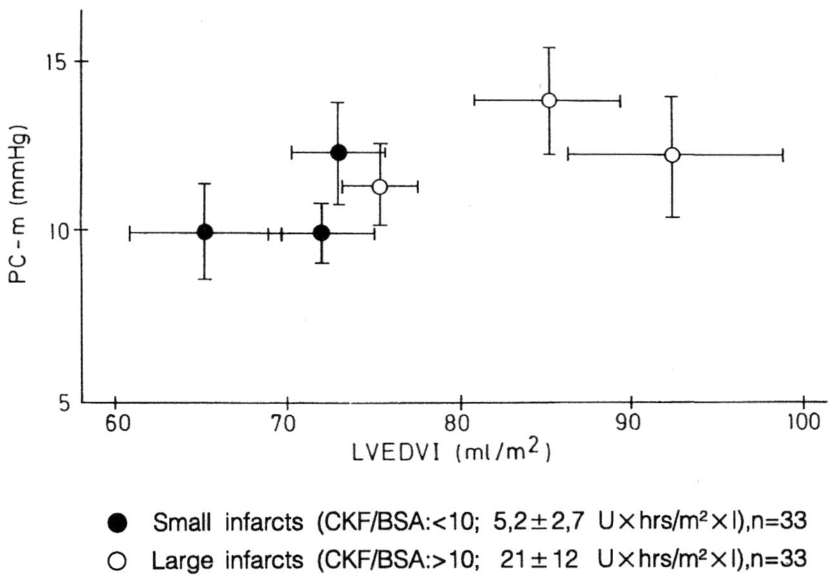

Fig. 5. Relation of mean pulmonary capillary wedge pressure (PC-m) on y-axis to left ventricular end-diastolic volume index (LVEDVI) on x-axis in patients with small (filled circles) and large (open circles) myocardial infarctions, respectively. Measurements were obtained 4 days, 4 weeks, and 6 months after infarction. No significant differences were found of PC-m between the two groups and among various time points. The increase of LVEDVI occurred in patients with large infarcts independent of PC-m, suggesting "structural" dilatation of the ventricle.

Clinical studies suggested that an increase in left ventricular volume during 2 weeks after infarction was mainly due to dilatation of the infarcted segment, i.e. "infarct expansion" (5). The same group, however, reported segmental dilatation of the posterior wall in patients with dilatation of the anterior wall 3 weeks after anterior myocardial infarction (6). Thus, the surviving myocardium dilated as well. Hypertrophy was also detected by echocardiography of non-infarcted myocardium in patients 9 months after myocardial infarction (13). Contractility was reduced, and stiffness increased of non-infarcted papillary muscle from rats 6 weeks after coronary artery ligation (27). The fall of global left ventricular ejection fraction in patients during 3 years after myocardial infarction was due to reduced wall motion of segments classified "normal" by gated SPECT (11). Infarct segments maintained stable, albeit depressed, wall motion. These data suggest that progressive left ventricular dysfunction post-myocardial infarction is associated with progressive dysfunction of surviving myocardium. It remains unclear, however, whether in patients failure of surviving myocardium represents failure of the cardiac myocyte or geometric disadvantage of the dilated heart.

Myocardial metabolism

Morphologic changes of the cardiac myocytes, geometric changes of the left ventricle, and hemodynamic changes due to loss of contractile myocardium most likely result in changes of cardiac energy demand. While some alterations, like reduced stroke work or arterial pressure, would suggest a reduced energy demand, others, like increased wall stress, would go along with enhanced energy demand. Recent studies from our laboratory have shown that for a lower developed pressure and rate-pressure product, rat hearts isolated 8 weeks after a myocardial infarction need the same amount of oxygen as control hearts (40). Thus, the efficiency of these ventricles appears to be reduced. Energy reserve estimated by the myocardial phosphocreatine/ATP ratio measured by 31-P-NMR spectroscopy was less in hearts post-myocardial infarction than in control hearts (33). Time-to-peak tension and time-to-peak Ca_i^{2+} was prolonged, the inotropic response to isoproterenol blunted despite of a large increase in amplitude of Ca_i^{2+} transient in non-infarcted papillary muscle from rat hearts 6 weeks after a myocardial infarction (28). Thus, a defect in excitation-contraction coupling might be involved in failure of chronically overloaded surviving myocardium. This defect was partially normalized by chronic treatment with the angiotensin converting enzyme inhibitor captopril (28). Finally, the isomyosin pattern is changed in surviving myocardium. The V3 form is increased, the V1 form lost (32). An increase in V3 and reduction of V1 would result in *higher* efficiency of surviving myocardium. It has been doubted, however, that V1 to V3 myosin isoenzyme shifts could be of physiological significance on the basis of studies on human myocardium obtained from transplant recipients in end-stage heart failure (31). Thus, biochemical and molecular analysis of surviving myocardium is at its beginning and the results are still highly controversial.

Arrhythmias

The high prognostic impact of an enlarged heart is mostly interpreted from a hemodynamic point of view. Detailed analysis of cardiac deaths which were best predicted by an enlarged end-systolic volume in the study of White et al. shows, however, that 70% of these patients died suddenly (Table 1), whereas only 8% died in heart failure (47). It remains unclear from the publication whether a larger fraction of patients were in heart failure before they died suddenly. These data suggest that mechanisms other than end-stage heart failure may be involved in excess mortality of patients with dilated hearts. Patients with enlarged hearts post-myocardial

Table 1. Mortality 15 months to 13 years after myocardial infarction (adapted from White et al., 1987).

	n	%
Patients	605	100
Deaths	120	20
Cardiac deaths	101	17
— sudden	71	70
— reinfarction	17	17
— heart failure	8	8
cardiac surgery	5	5

infarction had a three times higher incidence of ventricular arrhythmias than patients with normal heart size (7). Experimental studies documented stretch-activated arrhythmias (8) and enhanced vulnerability to ventricular fibrillation of hypertrophied hearts (23, 39). On the other hand, most recent large multicenter trial showed that drugs which reduce left ventricular enlargement and mortality post-myocardial infarction, also prevent *reinfarction* (35, 38). Thus, the exact mechanism of death in patients with left ventricular dilatation remains unclear.

Myocardial perfusion

Anversa et al. have shown, in post-myocardial infarction rats that concentric and excentric hypertrophy of residual myocardium is not accompanied by proportional vascularization. Thus, a relative rarefication occurred of microvessels in this myocardium (1). Coronary flow to hearts isolated from rats 8 weeks after a myocardial infarction was similar to that of control hearts (15). The coronary constrictor effects of angiotensin I and II were unchanged (own data, unpublished) while the dose-response curve for leukotriene D4 was shifted to the left in the infarcted vs. control hearts (15). Thus, coronary vasculature of these hearts appeared to be more sensitive to this eikosanoid. The coronary constrictor effect of N^6-monomethyl-L-arginine (L-NMMA) is attenuated in rats post-myocardial infarction (3). Thus, basal relaxing tone of the endothelial derived relaxing factor NO appears to be impaired. Finally, maximal coronary flow achievable by carbochrome was significantly less in surviving myocardium post-myocardial infarction than in control hearts (21). Thus, complex morphological and functional disturbances of the coronary circulation are present in this model.

Humoral influences

Humoral factors might influence remodeling of the heart post-myocardial infarction in various ways. Loading conditions may be altered by changes of systemic vascular resistance (afterload) or venous return (preload). Hormone systems may act as vasoconstrictors (angiotensin II) or retain sodium (aldosterone). In addition, circulating or local hormones may affect repair processes of infarcted tissue or adaptive processes of surviving myocardium (46). Plasma atrial natriuretic peptide (ANP) may be increased in rats and patients after myocardial infarction in dependence of infarct size (12, 30, 42) and expression of ANP messenger RNA is induced in atrial (30) and ventricular myocardium (4). In the rat model, plasma renin activity, angiotensin II and ANP, but not aldosterone were increased (19). Cardiac angiotensin converting enzyme messenger RNA and angiotensin converting enzyme activity are increased in this model (17). The pathophysiologic relevance of these findings remains to be determined.

Therapeutic implication

Prevention of deleterious consequences of left ventricular remodeling has been the goal of large clinical trials recently published (35, 37, 38). It is beyond the scope of this review to discuss these trials in great detail. The SAVE (Survival and Left Ventricular Enlargement) study, which showed that mortality and clinical manifestation of heart failure could be prevented by treatment with an ACE-inhibitor of patients with severe left ventricular dysfunction after a myocardial infarction, supported the pathophysiologic concepts discussed in this review. Whether the ACE-inhibitor acts by simple mechanical unloading or by a specific effect on surviving myocardium remains to be clarified.

References

1. Anversa P, Beghi C, Kikkawa Y, Olivetti G (1986) Myocardial infarction in rats. Infarct size, myocyte hypertrophy, and capillary growth. Circ Res 58:26—37
2. Cigarroa RG, Lange RA, Hillis LD (1989) Prognosis after acute myocardial infarction in patients with and without residual anterograde coronary blood flow. Am J Cardiol 64:155—160
3. Drexler H, Hablawetz BS, Lu W, Riede U, Christes A (1992) Effects of inhibition of nitric oxide formation of regional blood flow in experimental myocardial infarction. Circulation 86:255—262
4. Drexler H, Hanze J, Finckh M, Lu W, Just H, Lang RE (1989) Atrial natriuretic peptide in a rat model of cardiac failure. Circulation 79:620—633
5. Eaton LW, Weiss JL, Bulkley BH, Garrison JB, Weisfeldt ML (1979) Regional cardiac dilatation after acute myocardial infarction. N Engl J Med 300:57—62
6. Erlenbacher JA, Weiss JL, Eaton LW, Kallman C, Weisfeldt ML, Bulkley BH (1982) Late effects of acute infarct dilation on heart size: A two-dimensional echocardiagraphic study. Am J Cardiol 49:1120—1126
7. Ertl G, Just H, Lang K (1976) Herzrhythmusstörungen in der chronischen Phase des Myokardinfarktes. Dtsch Med Wschr 101:845—849
8. Franz MR, Cima R, Wang D, Profitt D, Kurz R (1992) Electrophysiological effects of myocardial stretch and mechanical determinants of stretch-activated arrhythmias. Circulation 86:968—978
9. Gaudron P, Eilles C, Ertl G, Kochsiek K (1990) Early remodelling of the left ventricle in patients with myocardial infarction. Eur Heart J 11:(Suppl B), 139—146

10. Gaudron P, Eilles C, Ertl G, Kochsiek K (1992) Compensatory and noncompensatory left ventricular dilatation after myocardial infarction: Time course and hemodynamic consequences at rest and during exercise. Am Heart J 123:377—385
11. Gaudron P, Eilles C, Kugler I, Ertl G (1993) Progressive left ventricular dysfunction and remodelling following myocardial infarction: Potential mechanisms and early predictors. Circulation 87:755—763
12. Gaudron PJ, Eilles Ch, Neuser D, Ertl G, Kochsiek K (1988) Plasma ANP in patients with acute myocardial infarction: time course, relation to infarct size, central hemodynamics and left ventricular volume. Circulation 78(Suppl II):II—63
13. Ginzton LE, Conant R, Rodrigues DM, Laks MM (1989) Functional significance of hypertrophy of the noninfarcted myocardium after myocardial infarction in humans. Circulation 80:816-822
14. Gülch RW, Jacob R (1988) Geometric and muscle physiological determinants of cardiac stroke volume as evaluated on the basis of model calculation. Basic Res Cardiol 83:476—485
15. Han H, Neubauer S, Gaudron P, Hu K, Ertl G (1992) Effects of Leukotriene D4 and its specific antagonist L-660,711 in isolated rat heart after myocardial infarction. J Moll Cell Cardiol 24(Suppl V):51
16. Hirai T, Fujita M, Nakajima H, Asanoi H, Yamanishi K, Ohno A, Sasayama S (1989) Importance of collateral circulation for prevention of left ventricular aneurysm formation in acute myocardial infarction. Circulation 79:791—796
17. Hirsch AT, Talsness CE, Schunkert H, Paul M, Dzau VJ (1991) Tissue-specific activation of cardiac angiotensin converting enzyme in experimental heart failure. Circulation Research 69:475—482
18. Hort W (1965) Ventrikeldilatation und Muskelfaserdehnung als früheste morphologische Befunde beim Herzinfarkt. Virchows Arch Path Anat 339:71—82
19. Hu K, Gaudron P, Bahner U, Palkovits M, Ertl G (1991) Atrial natriuretic factor (ANF) in brain areas of rats post myocardial infarction (MI). Eur Heart J 12(Suppl):702
20. Jeremy RW, Hackworthy RA, Bautovich G, Hutton BF, Harris PJ (1987) Infarct artery perfusion and changes in left ventricular volume in the month after acute myocardial infarction. J Am Coll Cardiol 9:989—995
21. Karam R, Healy BP, Wicker P (1990) Coronary reserve is depressed in postmyocardial infarction reactive cardiac hypertrophy. Circulation 81:238—246
22. Kostuk WJ, Kazamias TM, Gander MP, Simon AL, Ross J (1973) Left ventricular size after acute myocardial infarction. Serial changes and their prognostic significance. Circulation 47:1174—1179
23. Kowey PR, Friehling TD, Sewter J, Wu Y, Sokil A, Paul J, Nocella J (1991) Electrophysiological effects of left ventricular hypertrophy. Effect of calcium and potassium channel blockade. Circulation 83:2067—2076
24. Lavie CJ, O'Keefe JH, Chesebro JH, Clements IP, Gibbons RJ (1990) Prevention of late ventricular dilatation after acute myocardial infarction by successful thrombolytic reperfusion. Am J Cardiol 66:31—36
25. Leung W-H, Lau C-P (1992) Effects of severity of the residual stenosis of the infarct related coronary artery on left ventricular dilation and function after acute myocardial infarction. J Am Coll Cardiol 20:307—313
26. Linzbach AJ, Linzbach M (1951) Die Herzdilatation. Klin Wochenschr 29:621—630
27. Litwin SE, Litwin CM, Raya TE, Warner AL, Goldman S (1991) Contractility and stiffness of noninfarcted myocardium after coronary ligation in rats. Effects of chronic angiotensin converting enzyme inhibition. Circulation 83:1028—1037
28. Litwin SE, Morgan JP (1992) Captopril enhances intracellular calcium handling and β-adrenergic responsiveness of myocardium from rats with postinfarction failure. Circulation Research 71:797—807
29. Marino P, Zanolla L, Zardini P (1989) on behalf of the Gruppo Italiano per lo Studio della Streptochinasi nell Infarto Miocardico (GISSI): Effect of streptokinase on left ven-

tricular modeling and function after myocardial infarction: The GISSI (Gruppo Italiano per lo Studio della Streptochinasi nell Infarto Miocardico) trial. J Am Coll Cardiol 14:1149—1158
30. Mendez RE, Pfeffer JM, Ortola FV, Bloch KD, Anderson S, Seidman JG, Brenner BM (1987) Atrial natriuretic peptide transcription, storage, and release in rats with myocardial infarction. Am J Physiol 253:H1449—H1455
31. Mercadier JJ, Bouveret P, Gorza L, Schiaffino S, Clark WA, Zak R, Swynghedauw B, Schwartz K (1983) Myosin isoenzymes in normal and hypertrophied human ventricular myocardium. Circ Res 53:52—62
32. Mercadier JJ, Lomprè AM, Wisnewsky C, Samuel JL, Bercovici J, Swynghedauw B, Schwartz K (1981) Myosin isoenzymic changes in several models of rat cardiac hypertrophy. Circ Res 49:525—532
33. Neubauer S, Horn M, Gaudron P, Hu K, Laser M, Voll J, Tian R, Ingwall J, Ertl G (1991) Susceptibility of chronically infarcted rat heart to hypoxia and reoxygenation. A 31P-NMR study. Circulation 84(Suppl II):275
34. Pfeffer JM, Pfeffer MA, Fletcher PJ, Braunwald E (1991) Progressive ventricular remodeling in rat with myocardial infarction. Am J Physiol 260:H1406—H1414
35. Pfeffer MA, Braunwald E, Moye LA, Basta L, Brown EJ, Cuddy TE, Davis BR, Geltmann EM, Goldman S, Flaker GC, Klein M, Lamas GA, Packer M, Rouleau J, Rouleau JL, Rutherford J, Wertheimer JH, Hawkins CM (1992) on Behalf of the SAVE Investigators: Effect of captopril on mortality and morbidity in patients with left ventricular dysfunction after myocardial infarction. N Engl J Med 327:669—677
36. Reimer KA, Lowe JE, Rasmussen MM, Jennings RB (1977) The Wavefront phenomenon of ischemic cell death. 1. Myocardial infarct size vs duration of coronary occlusion in dogs. Circulation 56:786—794
37. Swedberg K, Held P, Kjekshus J, Rasmussen K, Ryden L, Wedel H (1992) on Behalf of the CONSENSUS II Study Group: Effects of the early administration of enalapril on mortality in patients with acute myocardial infarction. N Engl J Med 327: 678—684
38. The SOLVD Investigators: Effect of enalapril on mortality and the development of heart failure in asymptomatic patients with reduced left ventricular ejection fractions. N Engl J Med 327:685—691
39. Thollon C, Kreher P, Charlon V, Rossi A (1989) Hypertrophy induced alteration of action potential and effects of the inhibition of angiotensin converting enzyme by perindopril in infarcted rat hearts. Cardiovasc Res 23:224—230
40. Tian R, Gaudron P, Hu K, Han H, Neubauer S, Ertl G (1991) Pressure-Volume Relation and Oxygen Consumption in Isolated Rat Hearts with Chronic Myocardial Infarction. Eur Heart J 12(Suppl):133
41. Topol EJ, Califf RM, Vandormael M, Grines CL, George BS, Sanz ML, Wall T, O'Brien M, Schwaiger M, Aguirre FV, Young S, Popma JJ, Sigmon KN, Lee KL, Ellis SG (1992) A randomized trial of late reperfusion therapy for acute myocardial infarction. Circulation 85:2090—2099
42. Tsunoda K, Hodsman GP, Sumithran E, Johnston CI (1986) Atrial natriuretic peptide in chronic heart failure in the rat: A correlation with ventricular dysfunction. Circ Res 59:256—261
43. Villari B, Piscione F, Bonaduce D, Golino P, Lanzillo T, Condorelli M, Chiariello M (1990) Usefulness of late coronary thrombolysis (recombinant tissue-type plasminogen activator) in preserving left ventricular function in acute myocardial infarction. Am J Cardiol 66:1281—1286
44. Waris EK, Siitonen L, Himanka E (1966) Heart size and prognosis in myocardial infarction. Am Heart J 71:187—195
45. Warren SE, Royal HD, Markis JE, Grossman W, McKay RG (1988) Time course of left ventricular dilatation after myocardial infarction: Influence of infarct-related artery and success of coronary thrombolysis. J Am Coll Cardiol 11:12—19

46. Weber KT, Janicki JS (1989) Angiotensin and the remodelling of the myocardium. Br J clin Pharmac 28:141S—150S
47. White HD, Norris RM, Brown MA, Brandt PWT, Whitlock RML, Wild CJ (1987) Left ventricular end-systolic volume as the major determinant of survival after recovery from myocardial infarction. Circulation 76:44—51
48. Wolf R, Nötges A, Sinn R, Lichtlen PR (1991) Einfluß koronarer Kollateralgefäße auf den Verlauf der linksventrikulären Dilatation nach Myokardinfarkt. Z Kardiol 8:614—621

Authors' address:
Prof. Dr. G. Ertl
Medizinische Klinik der Universität Würzburg
Josef-Schneider-Straße 2
D-8700 Würzburg

"Cardioprotection" by ACE-inhibitors in acute myocardial ischemia and infarction?

K. Przyklenk and R. A. Kloner

Heart Institute, Hospital of the Good Samaritan and
University of Southern California, Los Angeles, CA., USA

Summary: Coronary artery occlusion results in the acute activation of the renin-angiotensin system and production of angiotensin II, a potent vasoconstrictor and positive inotropic agent. This has raised the possibility that angiotensin converting enzyme (ACE) inhibitors might be "cardioprotective" (that is, might attenuate myocardial injury, dysfunction and necrosis) in the setting of acute ischemia and infarction. Captopril, enalapril and ramipril have, in fact, been reported to acutely limit myocardial injury and necrosis in models of permanent coronary artery occlusion. The mechanisms responsible for this cardioprotection are complex, but include favorable alterations in myocardial oxygen supply/demand, and, in some instances, inhibition of bradykinin metabolism and/or increased prostaglandin synthesis. Other studies, however, have failed to document a reduction in infarct size with ACE inhibitor treatment. Results obtained in models of coronary occlusion/reperfusion have also been mixed. In models of brief transient ischemia not associated with necrosis, captopril and zofenopril have consistently been found to attenuate postischemic contractile dysfunction of the viable but "stunned" myocardium during the early hours following relief of ischemia. In contrast, there is no consensus on the effects of enalapril on the stunned myocardium: both positive and negative results have been obtained. Similar disparity has been reported in models of more prolonged ischemia/reperfusion resulting in subendocardial necrosis: some studies have reported myocardial salvage, while others have provided disturbing evidence of apparent exacerbation of myocardial necrosis with captopril and enalapril therapy. Thus, after a decade of investigative effort, the question of whether ACE inhibitors are "cardioprotective" in the setting of acute myocardial ischemia and infarction remains unresolved. Nonetheless, clinical protocols are in progress to assess the effects of early ACE inhibitor treatment in patients with acute myocardial infarction.

Key words: Coronary artery occlusion; coronary artery reperfusion; myocardial infarct size; creatine kinase; myocardial contractile function

Considerable evidence indicates that activation of the renin-angiotensin system (RAS) and the resultant release of angiotensin II plays an important role in the pathophysiology of various cardiovascular disease states, including hypertension, congestive heart failure, and cardiac hypertrophy (13, 18). It is therefore not surprising that angiotensin converting enzyme (or ACE) inhibitors such as captopril and enalapril have become a front-line form of therapy in the management of these disorders (17, 18).

ACE inhibitor therapy has also been shown to be of benefit when administered during the weeks-months following myocardial infarction (MI). Specifically, captopril attenuates infarct expansion and left-ventricular dilitation in both animals models (19, 40) and in patients (41). In addition, captopril and enalapril improve long-term survival following experimental infarction (42, 55).

These aforementioned studies have focused on the role of ACE inhibitor therapy in the chronic healing phase postMI. However, both experimental (15, 16) and clinical reports (33) have revealed that *coronary artery occlusion results in an acute activation of the RAS*. These data have lead to speculation that activation of the RAS may exacerbate myocardial ischemic injury (16, 21), and, if this is the case, have raised the possibility that ACE inhibitors might be "cardioprotective" (that is, might attenuate myocardial injury, dysfunction and necrosis) in the setting of *acute* ischemia and infarction (18, 25, 29, 30, 35, 45, 49). What are the properties of these agents that might render them cardioprotective if administered during the early minutes-hours after the onset of ischemia? Focusing on results obtained from in vivo models of acute ischemia and infarction, what is the experimental evidence that ACE inhibitors preserve myocyte viability, limit infarct size, or maintain myocardial contractile function? Do ACE inhibitors have a role in the clinical management of acute MI? These are the questions we address in the current review.

The promise: why should ACE inhibitors be cardioprotective?

Angiotensin II is a potent vasoconstrictor and positive inotropic agent (21, 29) generated by both the endocrine and local (i.e., cardiac) paracrine/autocrine components of the RAS (29, 30, 39). ACE inhibitors, although a structurally diverse class of compounds, all, by definition, blunt the conversion of angiotensin I to angiotensin II. It is therefore not surprising that the benefits of ACE inhibitor therapy in hypertension and heart failure have largely been attributed to the profound and well documented hemodynamic consequences (including reductions in afterload and preload, reductions in coronary vascular resistance, and increases in coronary blood flow) associated with the blunting of angiotensin II formation. These hemodynamic alterations, if initiated during acute ischemia, would clearly have a favorable effect on the precarious imbalance between myocardial oxygen supply and demand, and represent the primary mechanism by which ACE inhibitors might limit myocardial injury and dysfunction in ischemia and infarction.

In addition to reducing myocardial oxygen demand and increasing oxygen supply, ACE inhibitors have been reported to exert direct and potentially protective effects on the heart, including inhibition of bradykinin metabolism, increased prostaglandin synthesis, and inhibition of catecholamine release (7, 22, 32, 50, 51, 58). However, in contrast to the common hemodynamic consequences achieved by the blunting of angiotensin II formation, many of these latter effects appear to depend upon the specific molecular structure of each agent. Similarly, it has been suggested that ACE inhibitors which contain a sulfhydryl (SH) group (i.e., captopril and zofenopril) may be cardioprotective by virtue of the proposed antioxidant or oxygen radical scavenging properties of the SH moiety (1, 26, 61, 62). While oxygen radicals produced during myocardial ischemia have been shown to contribute to myocardial necrosis in models of permanent coronary occlusion (44), production of free radicals is greatly accelerated upon restoration of blood flow to previously ischemic tissue (4). One might therefore predict that SH-containing ACE inhibitors could be of particular benefit in models of coronary occlusion followed by reperfusion: this controversial topic of ACE inhibitor therapy for "reperfusion injury" has been reviewed in detail in this volume by Bolli (3). In any case, it is these various diverse mechanisms — including favorable alterations in myocardial oxygen supply/demand; inhibition of bradykinin metabolism; enhanced prostaglandin synthesis; inhibition of catechol-mine release; and scavenging of oxygen free radicals — which form the basis for the promise that ACE inhibitors might limit injury and dysfunction in instance of acute myocardial ischemia and infarction.

The reality: evidence from experimental models

Models of permanent coronary artery occlusion (Table 1)

The first evidence that ACE inhibitors might be cardioprotective in the setting of acute coronary artery occlusion was provided one decade ago by Ertl and colleagues (16). Using the anesthetized open-chest canine model, captopril or saline were continuously infused from 30 min to 6 h after the onset of ischemia. Infarct size assessed at 6 h postocclusion averaged 57% of the occluded coronary artery bed in captopril-treated dogs, which was significantly smaller than the value of 75% obtained in the saline-treated controls (Fig. 1A). This reduction in infarct size was most probably due to the increase in collateral perfusion to the ischemic zone and reductions in afterload and preload associated with captopril treatment (16).

This initial observation was quickly followed by reports of cardioprotection with other ACE inhibitors. Using left-ventricular creatine kinase (CK) activity as an indirect index of myocyte viability, Hock et al. (21) reported that enalaprilat, ad-

Table 1. ACE inhibitors in models of permanent coronary artery occlusion.

Author/Reference	Model	Agent	Index	"Cardio-protection"?
Ertl et al. (16)	Anesthetized dog: 6 h CO	Captopril: during CO	Infarct size	Yes
Liang et al. (28)	Conscious dog: 24 h CO	Teprotide + captopril: during CO	Infarct size; segment shortening	No; No
Lefer et al. (27)	Anesthetized cat: 5 h CO	Enalapril: during CO	ST-segment elevation; CK activity	Yes; Yes
Daniell et al. (8)	Conscious dog: 24 h CO	Captopril: during CO	Infarct size	No
Hock et al. (21)	Rat: 48 h CO	Enalaprilat: during CO	CK activity	Yes
Martorana et al. (31)	Anesthetized dog: 6 h CO	Ramiprilat: before CO	Infarct size	Yes

CO = coronary occlusion

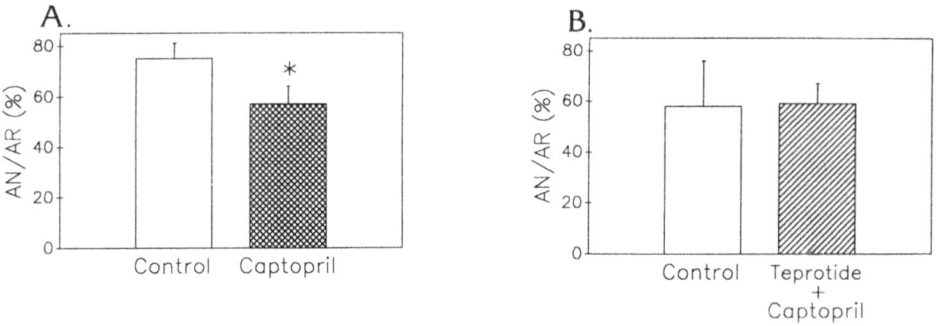

* $p < 0.05$ vs. controls

AN = area of necrosis; AR = area of occluded myocardium at risk infarction

Fig. 1. ACE inhibitors in models of permanent coronary artery occlusion. **A)** Treatment with captopril (0.25 mg/kg bolus + 0.25 mg/kg/hour), begun 30 min after the onset of ischemia, significantly reduced infarct size assessed 6 h following coronary occlusion in the anesthetized canine model. (Adapted from Ertl et al. (16.) **B)** In contrast, teprotide (25 μg/kg/min) + oral captopril (3 × 10 mg/kg), begun 40 min after the onset of ischemia, did not limit infarct size assesed 24 h following occlusion in conscious dogs. (Adapted from Liang et al. (28).)

ministered at 2 min and 24 h after coronary artery ligation is rats, significantly blunted tissue CK depletion and reduced ischemic damage to the heart. Using these data, the authors estimated that approximately 28% of the LV remained viable following 48 h of occlusion in control rats, as compared with 45% of the myocardium in rats treated with enalaprilat (21). Infusion of enalapril, initiated 30 min after the onset of ischemia, similarly attenuated tissue CK depletion, blunted the increase in plasma CK levels, and reversed ST-segment elevation in cats subjected to 5 h of coronary artery occlusion (27). This apparent salvage of ischemic myocardium in the feline model was attributed primarily to a favorable reduction in myocardial oxygen demand with enalapril treatment (27).

More recently, profound reduction in myocardial injury has been reported with low-dose intracoronary infusion of ramiprilat: infarct size measured at 6 h following coronary occlusion in the canine model averaged 25% of the myocardium at risk in the ramiprilat-treated group vs. 53% of the risk region in control dogs (31). In this instance, the protective effects of ACE inhibitor treatment were not a consequence of hemodynamic alterations. However, as co-administration of the bradykinin antagonist HOE 140 abolished the reduction in infarct size achieved with ramiprilat, the authors concluded that the benefits of ramiprilat in this model were due in large part to inhibition of bradykinin metabolism (31).

In contrast, two studies have failed to document a cardioprotective effect of ACE inhibitor therapy following permanent coronary occlusion (8, 28). For example, Liang and colleagues (28) compared the effects of teprotide + captopril or placebo, initiated 40 min after the onset of ischemia, in conscious dogs subjected to 24 h of coronary artery occlusion. The adequacy of ACE inhibition was verified in this study by assessing the pressor response to angiotensin I challenge: control dogs exhibited an increase in mean aortic pressure on the order of 20 mm Hg in response to angiotensin I injection, while treated dogs showed no net pressor response.

Although teprotide + captopril resulted in modest vasodilation and attenuated the increase in peripheral vascular resistance associated with coronary occlusion, these agents did not limit myocardial necrosis: infarct size averaged approximately 60% of the occluded bed in both control and treated groups (Fig. 1B). Moreover, teprotide + captopril did not preserve contractile function of the ischemic myocardium: the ischemic region remained essentially akinetic in both groups following treatment (28). A similar failure of captopril to limit infarct size following 24 h of coronary occlusion in conscious dogs has also been reported by Daniell et al. (8).

How can these disparate observations be explained? As the answer does not appear to lie with the dose and treatment regimens, it is tempting to speculate that the discrepancy may be a consequence of the two most glaring differences among the protocols: assessment of cardioprotection at 6 h postocclusion in anesthetized animals vs. 24 h postocclusion in conscious dogs. There is evidence that barbiturate anesthesia per se stimulates renin release, and that the vasodilator effects of ACE inhibitors are potentiated by anesthesia (28, 36). In addition, there is evidence that some pharmacologic agents (i.e., superoxide dismutase + catalase; deferoxamine; iloprost) delay, *but do not prevent* mycoardial necrosis; reduction in infarct size with these agents was observed acutely at 6 h after the onset of ischemia, but was no longer evident at 24—48 h following occlusion (44, 48, 54). A systematic comparison of the effects of ACE inhibitors at 6 h vs. 1 day postocclusion in conscious vs. anesthetized animals would obviously be required to resolve this question.

Models of coronary occlusion/reperfusion

With the advent of thrombolysis, angioplasty, and other forms of reperfusion therapy as the treatment of choice for acute myocardial infarction, it is not suprising that more recent studies involving ACE inhibition have focused on the effects of these agents in models of ischemia/reperfusion. ACE inhibitors have been evaluated both in experimental models of brief transient ischemia not associated with myocardial necrosis (i.e. simulating angina) and in models of more prolonged (1—2 h) coronary artery occlusion followed by reflow (simulating timely reperfusion for the treatment of acute MI).

Brief transient occlusion: ACE inhibitors and the "stunned" myocardium (Table 2)

While a brief (i.e., $\leqslant$15 min) episode of transient coronary artery occlusion does not result in myocardial necrosis in the canine model, the contractile function of the viable but previously ischemic tissue remains profoundly depressed or "stunned" for hours to days following restoration of blood flow (5). Do ACE inhibitors provide cardioprotection — that is, attenuate postischemic dysfunction — in the setting of brief transient ischemia?

Our first indication that ACE inhibitors might improve contractile function of the stunned myocardium was obtained in 1987 (43): we observed that high doses of enalapril, adminstered 45 min after a brief, 15 min ischemic insult, increased segment shortening to 50—60% of normal baseline values in enalapril-treated dogs, as compared with values averaging 20% of baseline in control animals. This improvement in function may have been due at least in part to the significant reduction in

Table 2. ACE inhibitors in models of brief occlusion/reperfusion (i.e., models of "stunned" myocardium).

Author/Reference	Model	Agent	Index	"Cardio-protection"?
Przyklenk et al. (43)	Dog: 15 min CO + 3.25 h reflow	Enalapril: after reflow	Segment shortening	Yes
Westlin et al. (62)	Dog: 15 min CO + 3 h reflow	Captopril: before CO	Segment shortening	Yes
Westlin et al. (62)	Dog: 15 min CO + 3 h reflow	Captopril: at reflow	Segment shortening	Yes
Westlin et al. (62)	Dog: 15 min CO + 3 h reflow	Enalaprilat: before CO	Segment shortening	No*
Przyklenk et al. (47)	Dog: 15 min CO + 3 h reflow	Zofenopril: at reflow	Segment shortening	Yes
Przyklenk et al. (46)	Dog: 15 min CO + 3 h reflow	Zofenopril: at reflow	Segment shortening	Yes
Przyklenk et al. (46)	Dog: 15 min CO + 3 h reflow	Enalaprilat: at reflow	Segment shortening	Yes
Bittar et al. (2)	Dog: 15 min CO + 3 h reflow	Captopril: before CO	Segment shortening	Yes

CO = coronary occlusion * contractile dysfunction was exacerbated with enalaprilat treatment.

mean arterial pressure and, hence, afterload, associated with enalapril treatment (43).

This issue was further addressed by Westlin and Mullane (62), who reported that captopril, administered either before occlusion or at the time of reperfusion, significantly enhanced postischemic contractile function of canine myocardium stunned by 15 min of coronary occlusion: segment shortening during the initial 3 h of reperfusion averaged 50—60% of normal baseline values in captopril-treated dogs vs. 10% of baseline in the control group (Fig. 2A).

Evidence from our laboratory (46, 47) and others (2) further confirmed the observation that SH-containing ACE inhibitors improve contractile function of the stunned myocardium. Using the same canine model, we observed that zofenopril given at the time of reperfusion restored segment shortening to 50—75% of baseline, as compared with values of 0—20% observed in control animals (46, 47, Fig. 2B). Similarly, Bittar et al. (2) reported that captopril administered before coronary occlusion attenuated postischemic dysfunction. Treatment with captopril did, in the

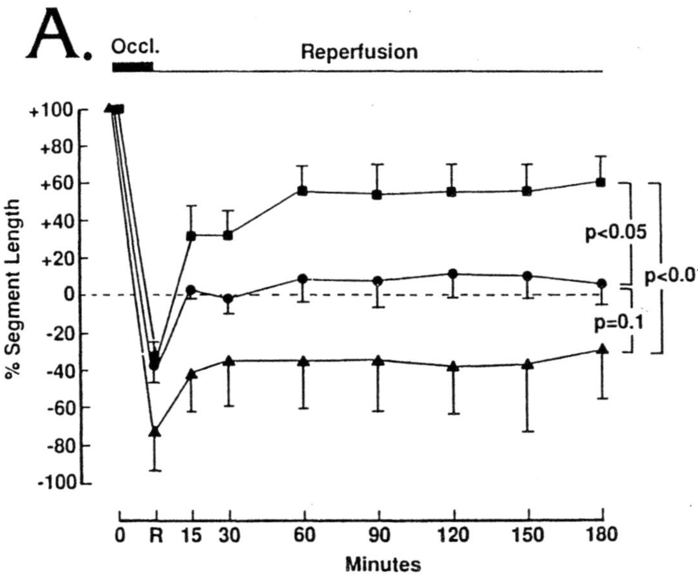

Fig. 2. ACE inhibitors in models of brief occlusion/reperfusion not resulting in myocardial necrosis (models of "stunned" myocardium). **A)** Captopril (5 mg/kg), given 15 min before ischemia, significantly enhanced the recovery of % segment length (an index of regional contractile function) following a brief 15-min episode of coronary occlusion in the canine model. However, pretreatment with enalaprilat (mean dose of 1.6 mg/kg) exacerbated contractile dysfunction both during occlusion and following reperfusion. Squares = captopril-treated group; triangles = enalaprilat-treated group; circles = controls. (Reprinted with permission of the American Heart Association from Westlin and Mullane (62).)

study of Bittar et al., result in a significant reduction in rate-pressure product (2). However, in both our protocol (46) and that of Westlin and Mullane (62), the improvement in function with zofenopril and captopril could not be attributed to alterations in systemic hemodynamic parameters alone (46, 62) or to increases in myocardial blood flow (46).

In contrast to the consistent reports of cardioprotection obtained with captopril and zofenopril in this model, the effects of enalapril on the stunned myocardium are controversial. In our hands, enalapril administered following reflow (43) or enalaprilat given at the time of reperfusion (46) attenuated postischemic contractile dysfunction to the same extent as that achieved with zofenopril. Interesting, however, the mechanisms of action of enalaprilat and zofenopril appear to differ. The beneficial effects of enalaprilat were essentially reversed by infusion of indomethacin, suggesting that the improved function achieved with this agent was due at least in part to a prostaglandin-mediated mechanism. In contrast, the improved function associated with zofenopril treatment appeared to be independent of prostaglandin metabolism, and may have been a consequence of the purported antioxidant properties of the SH group (46); Fig. 2B). However, in marked contrast to our observations, Westlin and Mullane observed that enalaprilat administered prior to

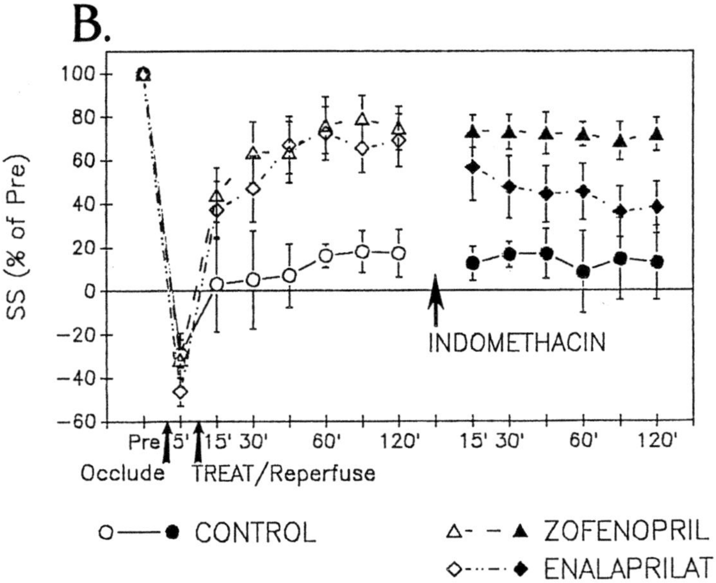

Fig. 2. B) In contrast, both zofenopril (5 mg/kg) and enalaprilat (1.5 mg/kg), given at the time of reperfusion, significantly attenuated postischemic dysfunction following 15 min of brief transient ischemia in the canine model. However, the mechanisms of action of the two agents appeared to differ: infusion of indomethacin essentially reversed the improvement in contractile function achieved with enalaprilat, but had no effect in dogs that had been treated with zofenopril. That is, enalaprilat — but not zofenopril — improved contractile function of stunned myocardium by a prostaglandin-mediated mechanism. (Reprinted with permission from Przyklenk and Kloner (46).) SS = segment shortening, expressed as a % of preocclusion (Pre) values.

coronary occlusion failed to improve segment shortening of the stunned myocardium: in fact, contractile dysfunction was *exacerbated* in enalaprilat-treated dogs, both during occlusion and following reperfusion, when compared with controls (62; Fig. 2A). This discrepancy may be due to differences between the two protocols in terms of the choice of anesthetic agents and the timing of enalaprilat treatment. In addition, as Westlin and Mullane (62) did not assess collateral blood flow during coronary artery occlusion, it is possible that enalaprilat-treated dogs were more severely ischemic than the control group. However, a definitive explanation for the improved function with enalaprilat treatment in our study and exacerbated dysfunction observed by Westlin and Mullane is lacking.

Prolonged occlusion/reperfusion: ACE inhibitors in models of subendocardial infarction (Table 3)

Early evidence that ACE inhibitors might preserve myocyte viability following transient ischemia was provided by Hock et al. (21): enalaprilat given 2 min after the onset of ischemia blunted tissue CK depletion in rats subjected to 10 min of coronary occlusion (sufficient to cause some myocardial necrosis in this model) and 48 h

Table 3. ACE inhibitors in models of sustained occlusion/reperfusion (i.e., models of subendocardial necrosis).

Author/Reference	Model	Agent	Index	"Cardio-protection"?
Hock et al. (21)	Rat: 10 min CO + 48 h reflow	Enalaprilat: during CO	CK activity	Yes
de Graeff et al. (10)	Pig: 1 h CO + 2 h reflow	Captopril: before CO (low dose and high dose)	CK activity	Yes (high dose only)
de Graeff et al. (9)	Pig: 1 h CO + 2 weeks reflow	Captopril: during CO	CK activity	Yes
Brown et al. (6)	Dog: 3 h CO + 3 h reflow	Enalapril: before reflow	Infarct size	No*
Tio et al. (56)	Pig: 45 min CO + 2 weeks reflow	Zofenopril: before CO	CK activity	No
Noda et al. (38)	Dog: 90 min CO + 3 h reflow	Captopril: during CO	Infarct size	Yes
Tobe et al. (57)	Pig: 45 min CO + 2 weeks reflow	Perindoprilat: during CO	CK activity; Infarct size	No; No
Hartman et al. (20)	Rabbit: 30 min CO + 2 h reflow	Ramiprilat: during CO	Infarct size	Yes
de Lorgeril et al. (11)	Dog: 2 h CO + 6 h reflow	Captopril: during CO	Infarct size	Yes in subgroup with low collateral flow; No* in subgroup with high collateral flow

CO = coronary occlusion   * Infarct size was increased with ACE inhibitor treatment

of reperfusion. Using these data to estimate myocardial salvage, the authors calculated that 65% of the myocardium remained viable in the control group, whereas 85% was viable in enalaprilat-treated rats (21).

This issue was subsequently pursued in a more rigorous manner in a series of experiments by de Graeff, van Gilst, and colleagues. In the first of these studies (10), anesthetized closed-chest pigs received either low-dose captopril, high-dose captopril or saline, and then underwent 1 h of coronary occlusion and 2 h of reperfusion.

Plasma CK concentration following reflow — an indirect index of myocardial injury — tended to be attenuated in the low-dose captopril group, and was significantly reduced in pigs treated with high-dose captopril when compared with controls (Fig. 3A). In addition, high-dose captopril treatment also blunted the ischemia-induced efflux of inosine (a catabolite of adenosine triphosphate (ATP)) and noradrenaline into the coronary sinus (10). These three pieces of evidence lead the authors to conclude that captopril reduced myocardial injury in a dose-dependent manner is this porcine model, perhaps due to an increase in collateral blood flow to the ischemic myocardium, inhibition of the sympathetic nervous system, and/or scavenging of oxygen radicals (10). Similar results were reported from these investigators with administration of a captopril bolus during coronary occlusion: CK release following 1 h of transient coronary occlusion was again blunted in captopril-treated pigs when compared with controls (9).

Direct evidence of myocardial salvage — in this case, with ramiprilat — has recently been reported in the rabbit model (20). Infarct size following 30 min of occlusion and 2 h of reperfusion averaged 41% of the myocardium at risk in control rabbits, but was reduced to 20% of the risk region in rabbits treated with ramiprilat prior to reperfusion. This protective effect of ramiprilat was not due to hemodynamic alterations, but was completely reversed by coadministration of the bradykinin antagonist HOE 140 (20). Thus, as in the studies of Martorana et al. in the canine model of permanent coronary occlusion (31), the reduction in infarct size with ramiprilat following ischemia/reperfusion was due in part to preservation of endogeneous bradykinin. Similar results have also been reported with captopril in nephrectomized dogs (38): captopril reduced infarct size produced by 90 min of transient coronary occlusion, but, interestingly, this was *not* accompanied by a reduction in angiotensin II release from the ischemic myocardium. This lead the authors to conclude that the cardioprotective effects of captropril are are not dependent upon the blunting of cardiac angiotensin II production (38), and to speculate that the reduction in infarct size may have been due to inhibition of bradykinin metabolism (32, 38).

However, as was the case with the other experimental models, not all studies of ACE inhibitors have yielded positive results. For example, zofenopril treatment, begun 2 days prior to a 45-min ischemic insult in the porcine model, attenuated the efflux of adrenaline, noradrenaline, and ATP catabolites into the coronary sinus, and reduced the inducibility of ventricular tachycardia assessed by programmed electrical stimulation at 2 weeks following reflow (56). There was a modest reduction in plasma CK release in zofenopril-treated pigs, but this trend toward myocardial salvage did not attain statistical significance (56). Perindoprilat, initiated 30 min after the onset of occlusion in this same porcine model, did not blunt catecholamine or purine release into the coronary sinus, did not attenuate plasma CK concentrations, and did not reduce infarct size measured at 2 weeks following reflow (57, 60). Moreover, perindoprilat treatment had no effect on electrocardiographic stability assessed at 2 weeks post reperfusion (57). Interestingly, however, the authors noted that, for all animals in the study — *irrespective of treatment group* — survival postinfarction correlated inversely with plasma renin activity measured before coronary occlusion. That is, mortality was significantly greater in pigs with high renin levels at baseline (60). In addition, concentrations of prostaglandin E_2 in the coronary sinus measured during coronary occlusion were higher in survivors vs. non-

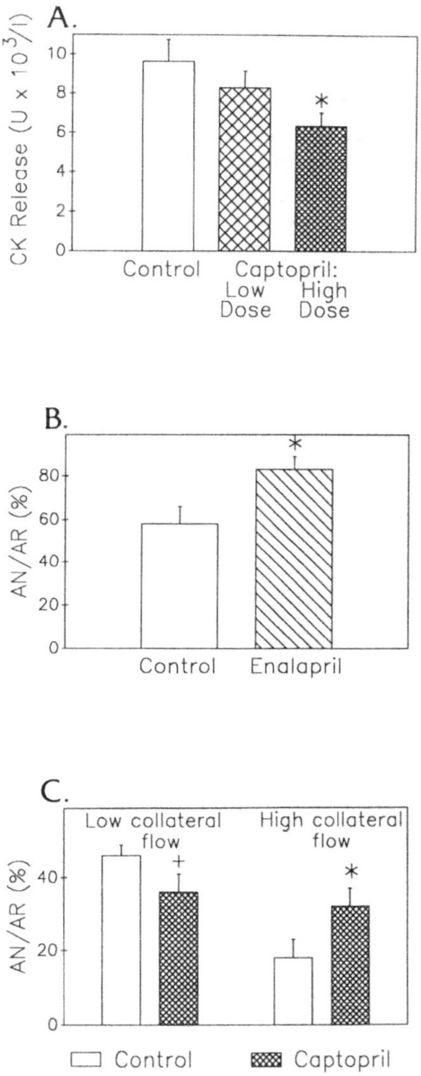

Fig. 3. ACE inhibitors in models of sustained occlusion/reperfusion resulting in subendocardial necrosis.

A) In a porcine model of 1 h of coronary occlusion and 2 h of reperfusion, pretreatment with captopril attenuated creatine kinase (CK) release in a dose-dependent manner: plasma CK levels following 2 h of reflow tended to be blunted in pigs that received low-dose captopril (0.6 mg/kg bolus + 0.0025 mg/kg/min), and were significantly attenuated in pigs treated with high-dose captopril (6 mg/kg bolus + 0.025 mg/kg/min). (Adapted from de Graeff et al. (10).)
* $p < 0.05$ vs. controls

B) In contrast, enalapril given before reperfusion failed to limit infarct size in dogs subjected to 3 h of coronary occlusion and 3 h of reflow. In fact, infarct size was significantly larger in enalapril-treated dogs when compared with controls. (Adapted from Brown et al. (6).) AN = area of necrosis; AR = area of occluded myocardium at risk of infarction.
* $p < 0.05$ vs. controls

C) Captopril treatment (5 mg/kg bolus + 0.25 mg/kg/h), begun 1 h after the onset of ischemia, had no overall effect on infarct size in dogs that underwent 2 h of coronary occlusion and 6 h of reperfusion. However, post-hoc analysis revealed that captopril tended to reduce infarct size in the subgroup of dogs that were severely ischemic during coronary occlusion (i.e., dogs in which collateral blood flow averaged approximately 10% of nonischemic values), and increased infarct size in dogs with high collateral blood flow (a mean of approximately 40% of nonischemic values) during occlusion. (Adapted from de Lorgeril et al. (11).) AN = area of necrosis; AR = area of occluded myocardium at risk of infarction. + $p = 0.09$ and * $p < 0.05$ vs. corresponding controls.

survivors (60). Thus, although perindoprilat was not cardioprotective in this model, these data support the hypothesis that activation of the RAS — and the relationship between the RAS and prostaglandin metabolism — plays an important and deleterious role in the setting of coronary occlusion/reperfusion. Finally, a preliminary report by Brown and colleagues (6) indicated that enalapril given before reperfusion failed to reduce infarct size in dogs subjected to 3 h of coronary occlusion and 3 h of reperfusion. In fact, infarct size was greater in enalapril-treated dogs when compared with controls, averaging 83% and 58% of the myocardium at risk, respectively (Fig. 3B). No reason was offered, however, for this apparent exacerbation of myocardial necrosis with enalapril (6).

An intriguing explanation for these disparate results — that could potentially be extrapolated to models of permanent occlusion as well as occlusion/reperfusion — was recently provided by de Lorgeril and colleagues (11). Treatment with captopril begun 1 h after the onset of ischemia had no overall effect on infarct size in anesthetized open-chest dogs submitted to 2 h of coronary occlusion and 6 h of reperfusion. However, post-hoc analysis revealed that captopril tended to reduced infarct size in the subgroup of dogs that was severely ischemic during coronary occlusion, and *increased* infarct size in the subgroup of animals with high collateral blood flow during ischemia (Fig. 3C). Moreover, the worsening of myocardial injury in the high-flow subgroup was attributed to coronary vasodilation and a subsequent decrease in collateral perfusion to the ischemic tissue (i.e., an apparent situation of "coronary steal") following captopril treatment (11). These results raise the possibility that ACE inhibitors might be cardioprotective in models characterized by low native collateral perfusion (i.e., the rat, rabbit, and pig), and, in the canine model of highly variable collateral flow, in subgroups of animals with a paucity of native collateral vessels. The results further suggest that ACE inhibitors might have no benefit — and might, in fact, be deleterious — in models or subgroups with extensive collateral perfusion. Verification of this hypothesis awaits further prospective evaluation.

The first efforts: early ACE inhibitor treatment in patients with acute myocardial infarction

Despite the decidedly mixed results that have been obtained in the experimental laboratory, clinical protocols are in progess to assess the effects of early ACE inhibitor treatment in patients with acute MI (12, 14, 23, 24, 37, 52, 59). Initial studies using intravenous captopril in the early hours postinfarction were complicated by profound hypotension (14, 23). More recent data, however, indicate that oral captopril is better tolerated (12, 24), and that intravenous enalapril can be safely given to patients if carefully titrated (53). Early captopril treatment has been shown to improve global ejection fraction in patients with Q-wave infarction, with no apparent difference between patients who did or did not undergo thrombolysis (52). In studies in which captopril was given as adjuvant therapy with thrombolytic agents, ACE inhibitor treatment was associated with significant reductions in the incidence of early and late arrhythmias (12, 24) and lower catecholamine levels following reperfusion (24). Adjuvant therapy with captopril has also been reported to attenuate early left-ventricular dilatation and enlargement (in good agreement with experimental results from the canine model (34)), but failed to improve ejection fraction during the initial 7 days following treatment (37). Thus, even in these first protocols, the effects of early ACE inhibitor therapy following acute MI are not entirely positive.

Did ACE inhibitor therapy actually *salvage* ischemic myocardium in these clinical studies? Accurate and definitive assessment of infarct size is obviously beyond the scope of these protocols. However, di Pasquale and colleagues have reported that plasma CK concentrations were lower in 25 patients who received captopril 15 min before thrombolysis when compared with 23 controls who received thrombolysis alone (12). This interesting, but indirect and preliminary evidence of apparent infarct size reduction with ACE inhibitor therapy obviously demands confirmation in larger randomized trials.

Conclusion

Do ACE inhibitors provide "cardioprotection" in in vivo models of acute myocardial ischemia and infarction? There is evidence that captopril, enalapril, and ramipril can acutely limit myocardial injury in models of permanent coronary artery occlusion. The mechanisms responsible for this cardioprotection are complex, but appear to involve favorable alterations in myocardial oxygen supply/demand, and, in some instances, inhibition of bradykinin metabolism and/or increased prostaglandin synthesis. However, there is some indication that this acute reduction in infarct size may represent a delay, rather than prevention of myocardial cell death. Results obtained in models of coronary occlusion/reperfusion have also been mixed. In models of brief transient ischemia not associated with necrosis, captopril and zofenopril have consistently been found to attenuate postischemic contractile dysfunction of the viable but "stunned" myocardium during the early hours following relief of ischemia. In contrast, there is no consensus on the effects of enalapril on the stunned myocardium: both positive and negative results have been obtained. Similar disparity has been reported in models of more prolonged ischemia/reperfusion resulting in subendocardial necrosis: some studies have reported myocardial salvage, while others have provided disturbing evidence of apparent exacerbation of myocardial necrosis with captopril and enalapril therapy. Thus, after a full decade of investigative effort, the question of whether ACE inhibitors are "cardioprotective" in the setting of acute myocardial ischemia and infarction remains unresolved. Nonetheless, clinical protocols are in progress to assess the effects of early ACE inhibitor treatment in patients with acute myocardial infarction.

References

1. Bagchi D, Prasad R, Das DK (1989) Direct scavenging of free radicals by captopril, an angiotensin converting enzyme inhibitor. Biochem Biophys Res Comm 158:52—57
2. Bittar N, Zheng HN, Nwosu EA (1991) Captopril is more effective than dipyridamole or labetolol in attenuating myocardial stunning in the dog. Proceedings of the Second International Symposium on ACE Inhibition, London UK, p P—179 (abstract)
3. Bolli R (1992) Attenuation of reperfusion injury by ACE inhibitiors? Basic Res Cardiol: in press
4. Bolli R, Patel BS, Jeroudi MO, Lai EK, McCoy PB (1988) Demonstration of free radical generation in "stunned" myocardium of intact dogs with the use of the spin trap alpha phenyl N-Tert-Butyl Nitrone. J Clin Invest 82:476—485
5. Braunwald E, Kloner RA (1982) The stunned myocardium: prolonged postischemic ventricular dysfunction. Circulation 66:1146—1149
6. Brown EJ Jr, Swinford RD, Shatkin BJ, Honig SC, Cohn PF (1988) Massive reperfusion injury: paradoxical effect of combined angiotensin-converting enzyme inhibition plus myocardial reperfusion. J Am Coll Cardiol 11:50A (abstract)
7. Cushman DW, Ondetti MA (1980) Inhibitors of angiotensin-converting enzyme. Prog Med Chem 17:41—104
8. Daniell HB, Carson RR, Ballard KD, Thomas GR, Privitera PJ (1984) Effects of captopril on limiting infarct size in conscious dogs. J Cardiovasc Pharmacol 6:1043—1047
9. de Graeff PA, de Langen CDJ, van Gilst WH, Bel K, Scholtens E, Kingma JH, Wesseling H (1988) Protective effects of captopril against ischemia/reperfusion-induced arrhythmias in vitro and vivo. Am J Med 84 (Suppl 3A):67—74

10. de Graeff PA, van Gilst WH, de Langen CDJ, Kingma JH, Wesseling H (1987) Concentration-dependent protection by captopril against myocardial damage during ischemia and reperfusion in a closed chest pig model. J Cardiovasc Pharmacol 9 (Suppl 2):S37—S42
11. de Lorgeril M, Ovize M, Delaye J, Renaud S (1992) Importance of the flow perfusion deficit in the response to captopril in experimental myocardial infarction. J Cardiovasc Pharmacol 19:324—329
12. di Pasquale P, Barone G, Paterna S, Cannizaro S, Giubilato A (1990) Efficacy of captopril before thrombolysis in acute myocardial infarction: preliminary findings. Drugs Exp Clin Res 15:581—589
13. Dzau VJ (1988) Tissue renin-angiotensin system: physiologic and pharmacologic implications. Circulation 77 (Suppl I):I1—13
14. Ertl G (1988) Converting enzyme inhibitors and ischemic heart disease. Eur Heart J 9:716—727
15. Ertl G, Alexander RW, Kloner RA (1983) Interactions between coronary occlusion and the renin-angiotensin system in the dog. Basic Res Cardiol 78:518—533
16. Ertl G, Kloner RA, Alexander RW, Braunwald E (1982) Limitation of experimental infarct size by an angiotensin-converting enzyme inhibitor. Circulation 65:40—48
17. Gavras H (1990) Angiotensin converting enzyme inhibition and its impact on cardiovascular disease. Circulation 81:381—388
18. Gavras H, Gavras I (1991) Cardioprotective potential of angiotensin converting enzyme inhibitors. J Hypertension 9:385—392
19. Gay RG (1990) Early and late effects of captopril treatment after large myocardial infarction in rats. J Am Coll Cardiol 16:967—977
20. Hartman JC, Wall TM, Hullinger TG (1992) Role of bradykinin in reduction of myocardial infarct size by ramiprilat. J Mol Cell Cardiol 24 (Suppl III):S.11 (abstract)
21. Hock CE, Ribeiro GT, Lefer AM (1985) Preservation of ischemic myocardium by a new converting enzyme inhibitor, enalaprilic acid, in acute myocardial infarction. Am Heart J 109:222—228
22. Johnston CI, Clappison BH, Anderson WP, Yasuzjima M (1982) Effect of angiotensin-converting enzyme inhibition on circulating and local kinin levels. Am J Cardiol 49:1401—1404
23. Kingma JH, van Gilst WH, de Graeff PA, Louwerenburg HW, Six AJ, Wesseling H (1989) Captopril during thrombolysis in acute myocardial infarction: feasibility, tolerance and beneficial neurohumoral effects. In: MacGregor GA, Sever PS (eds) Current Advances in ACE Inhibition; Churchill Livingstone, Edinburgh, pp 291—295
24. Kingma JH, van Gilst WH, Peels CH, Jaarsma W, Verheught FW (1990) Converting enzyme inhibition during thrombolytic therapy in acute myocardial infarction. Circulation 82 (Suppl III):III—666 (abstract)
25. Kloner RA, Przyklenk K (1992) Cardioprotection with angiotensin converting enzyme inhibitors: redefined for the 1990's. Clin Cardiol: in press
26. Kukreja RC, Kontos HA, Hess ML (1990) Captopril and enalaprilat do not scavenge the superoxide anion. Am J Cardiol 65:241—271
27. Lefer AM, Peck RC (1984) Cardioprotective effects of enalapril in acute myocardial ischemia. Pharmacology 29:61—69
28. Liang CS, Gavras H, Black J, Sherman LG, Hood WB (1982) Renin-angiotensin system inhibition in acute myocardial infarction in dogs: effects on systemic hemodynamics, myocardial blood flow, segmental myocardial function and infarct size. Circulation 66:1249—1255
29. Linder C, Heusch G (1990) ACE inhibitor for the treatment of myocardial ischemia? Cardiovasc Drugs Therapy 4:1375—1384
30. Lindpaintner K, Ganten D (1991) Tissue renin-angiotensin systems and their modulation: the heart as a paradigm for new aspects of converting enzyme inhibition. Cardiology 79 (Suppl 1):32—44

31. Martorana PA, Kettenbach B, Breipohl G, Linz W, Scholkens BA (1990). Reduction of infarct size by local angiotensin-converting enzyme inhibition is abolished by a bradykinin antagonist. Eur J Pharmacol 182:395—396
32. Martorana PA, Linz W, Scholkens BA (1991) Does bradykinin play a role in the cardiac antiischemic effect of the ACE inhibitor? Basic Res Cardiol 86:293—296
33. McAlpine HM, Cobbe SM (1988) Neuroendocrine changes in acute myocardial infarction. Am J Med 84 (Suppl 3A):61-74
34. Mehta PM, Alker KJ, Kloner RA (1988) Functional infarct expansion, left ventricular dilation and isovolumic relaxation time after coronary occlusion: a two-dimensional echocardiographic study. J Am Coll Cardiol 11:630—636
35. Mehta PM, Przyklenk K, Kloner RA (1990) Cardioprotective effects of captopril in myocardial ischemia. ischemia/reperfusion and infarction. Eur Heart J 11 (Suppl B):94—99
36. Murphy VS, Waldron TL, Goldberg ME (1978) Inhibition of angiotensin-converting enzyme by SQ 14,225 in anesthetized dogs: hemodynamics and renal vascular effects. Proc Soc Exp Biol Med 157:121—129
37. Nabel EG, Topol EJ, Galeana A, Ellis SG, Bates ER, Werns SW, Walton JA, Muller DW, Schwaiger M, Pitt B (1991) A randomized placebo-controlled trial of combined early intravenous captopril and recombinant tissue-type plasminogen activator therapy in acute myocardial infarction. J Am Coll Cardiol 17:467—473
38. Noda K, Sagaguri M, Ideishi M, Ikeda M, Arakawa K (1990) Cardioprotection by ACE inhibitor in ischemic heart is independent of the local angiotensin II formation. J Hypertension 8 (Suppl 3):106
39. Paul M, Bachman J, Ganten D (1992) The tissue renin-angiotensin systems in cardiovascular disease. Trends Cardiovasc Med 2:94—99
40. Pfeffer JM, Pfeffer MA, Braunwald E (1985) Influence of chronic captopril therapy in the infarcted left ventricle in the rat. Circ Res 57:84—95
41. Pfeffer MA, Lamas GA, Vaughan DE, Parisi AF, Braunwald E (1988) Effect of captopril on progressive ventricular dilation after anterior myocardial infarction. N Engl J Med 319:80—86
42. Pfeffer MA, Pfeffer JM, Steinberg C, Finn P (1985) Survival after an experimental myocardial infarction: beneficial effects of long-term therapy with captopril. Circulation 72:406—412
43. Przyklenk K, Kloner RA (1987) Acute effects of hydralazine and enalapril on contractile function of postischemic stunned myocardium. Am J Cardiol 60:934—936
44. Przyklenk K, Kloner RA (1987) Effect of oxygen-derived free radical scavengers on infarct size following six hours of permanent coronary artery occlusion: salvage or delay of myocyte necrosis? Basic Res Cardiol 82:146—158
45. Przyklenk K, Kloner RA (1989) Relationships between structure and effects of ACE inhibitors: comparative effects in myocardial ischemic/reperfusion injury. Br J Clin Pharmacol 28:167S—175S
46. Przyklenk K, Kloner RA (1991) Angiotensin converting enzyme inhibitors improve contractile function of stunned myocardium by different mechanisms of action. Am Heart J 121:1319—1330
47. Przyklenk K, Whittaker P, Kloner RA (1989) Zofenopril, a newly developed sulfhydryl-containing converting enzyme inhibitor, enhances contractile function of stunned myocardium. In: MacGregor GA, Severs PS (eds) Current Advances in ACE Inhibition; Churchill Livingstone, Edinburgh, pp 279—282
48. Reddy BR, Wynne J, Kloner RA, Przyklenk K (1991) Pretreatment with the iron chelator deferoxamine fails to provide sustained protection against myocardial ischemia-reperfusion injury. Cardiovasc Res 25:711—718
49. Scholkens BA, Linz W (1990) Cardioprotective effects of ACE inhibitors: experimental proof and clinical perspectives. Clin Physiol Biochem 8 (Suppl 1):33—43
50. Schwartz SL, Williams GH (1982) Angiotensin-converting enzyme inhibition and prostaglandins. Am J Cardiol 49:1405—1409

51. Schwartz SL, Williams GH, Hollenberg NK, Levine TB, Dluhy RC, Moore TJ (1980) Captopril-induced changes in prostaglandin production. J Clin Invest 65:1257—1264
52. Sharpe N, Smith H, Murphy J, Greaves S, Hart H, Gamble G (1991) Early prevention of left ventricular dysfunction after myocardial infarction with angiotensin-converting-enzyme inhibition. Lancet 337:872—876
53. Sigurdsson A, Held P, Andersson G, Swedberg K (1991) Enalaprit in acute myocardial infarction: tolerability and effects on the renin-angiotensin system. Int J Cardiol 33:114—124
54. Simpson PJ, Mickelson J, Fantone JC, Gallagher KP, Lucchesi BR (1987) Sustained myocardial protection by iloprost with prolonged infusion in a canine model of temporary regional ischemia. Fed Proc 46:1144 (abstract)
55. Sweet CS, Ludden CT, Stabilito II, Emmert SE, Hey JF (1988) Beneficial effects of milrinone and enalapril on long-term survival of rats with healed myocardial infarction. Eur J Pharmacol 147:29—38
56. Tio RA, de Langen CDJ, de Graeff PA, van Gilst WH, Bel KJ, Wolters GTP, Mook PH, van Wijngaarden J, Wesseling H (1990) The effects of oral pretreatment with zofenopril, an angiotensin-converting enzyme inhibitor, on early reperfusion and subsequent electrophysiologic stability in the pig. Cardiovasc Drugs Therapy 4:695—704
57. Tobe TJM, de Langen CDJ, Weersink EGL, van Wijngaarden J, Bel KJ, de Graeff PA, van Gilst WH, Wesseling H (1992) The angiotensin converting enzyme inhibitor perindopril improves survival after experimental myocardial infarction in pigs. J Cardiovasc Pharmacol 19:732—740
58. van Gilst, de Graeff PA, Wesseling H, de Langen CDJ (1986) Reduction of reperfusion arrhythmias in the ischemic isolated rat heart by angiotensin converting enzyme inhibitors: a comparison of captopril, enalapril, and HOE 498. J Cardiovasc Pharmacol 8:722—728
59. van Gilst WH, Kingma JH for the CATS Investigators Group (1991) Early intervention with angiotensin-converting enzyme inhibitors during thrombolytic therapy in acute myocardial infarction: rationale and design of captopril and thrombolysis study. Am J Cardiol 68:111D—115D.
60. van Wijngaarden J, Tobe TJM, Weersink EGL, Bel KJ, de Graeff PA, de Langen CDJ, van Gilst WH, Wesseling H (1992) Effects of early angiotensin-converting enzyme inhibition in a pig model of myocardial ischemia and reperfusion. J Cardiovasc Pharmacol 19:408—416
61. Weglicki WB, Mak IT, Simic MG (1990) Mechanisms of cardiovascular drugs as antioxidants. J Mol Cell Cardiol 22:1199—1208
62. Westlin W, Mullane K (1988) Does captopril attenuate reperfusion-induced myocardial dysfunction by scavenging free radicals? Circulation 77 (Suppl I):130—139

Authors' address:
Karin Przyklenk, PhD.
Heart Institute/Research
Hospital of the Good Samaritan
616 South Witmer Street
Los Angeles, CA. 90017 USA.

Effect of angiotensin-converting enzyme inhibitors on myocardial ischemia/reperfusion injury: an overview

M. E. Zughaib, J.-Z. Sun, R. Bolli

Experimental Animal Laboratory, Section of Cardiology,
Department of Medicine, Baylor College of Medicine, Houston, TX

Summary: There are multiple mechanisms whereby ACE inhibitors could be beneficial during myocardial ischemia and reperfusion, including: i) reduced formation of angiotensin II, ii) decreased metabolism of bradykinin, iii) antioxidant activity, and iv) possibly other unknown mechanisms. Reduced formation of angiotensin II should be beneficial because this peptide exerts several actions that are potentially detrimental to the ischemic/reperfused myocardium, including vasoconstriction, increased release of norepinephrine, stimulation of phospholipase C and/or A2, and increased afterload with an attendant increase in oxygen demands. Reduced metabolism of bradykinin could be beneficial by increasing myocardial glucose uptake, by causing vasodilation, and by stimulating production of endothelium-derived relaxing factor and prostacyclin. Although earlier studies suggested that sulfhydryl-containing ACE inhibitors scavenge superoxide anions, recent data have shown that these drugs scavenge hydroxyl radical and hypochlorous acid with no effect on superoxide anion. Studies in isolated hearts have demonstrated that ACE inhibitors attenuate the metabolic, arrhythmic, and contractile dearangements associated with ischemia and reperfusion, and have suggested that such beneficial effects are mediated by potentiation of bradykinin and/or increased synthesis of prostacyclin. Studies in models of myocardial stunning after brief (15-min) ischemia in vivo (anesthetized dogs) suggest that ACE inhibitors enhance the recovery of contractile function after a single brief ischemic episode. No data are available regarding the effect of these drugs on myocardial stunning after a prolonged, partly reversible episode, after multiple consecutive brief ischemic episodes, and after global ischemia. The mechanism for the salutary effects of ACE inhibitors on stunning remains a mystery. It may involve an antioxidant action (in the case of thiol-containing molecules) or potentiation of prostaglandins (in the case of non-thiol-containing molecules). What is clear is that the enhanced recovery of function effected by these drugs is not due to hemodynamic effects, inhibition of the converting enzyme per se, or an "antiischemic" action (since the drugs were effective when given at the time of reperfusion). The effects of ACE inhibitors on myocardial infarct size remain controversial.

Further studies will be necessary to conclusively establish whether ACE inhibitors can protect against the detrimental effects of myocardial ischemia and reperfusion. Nevertheless, the evidence provided thus far is encouraging and warrants an in-depth assessment of the role of these drugs in attenuating myocardial ischemia/reperfusion injury.

Key words: Reperfusion injury; postischemic myocardial dysfunction; reperfusion arrhythmias; angiotensin-converting enzyme inhibitors; captopril; enalapril; zofenopril

1. The concept of myocardial reperfusion injury

Coronary reperfusion by means of thrombolytic therapy, percutaneous transluminal angioplasty, or bypass surgery is rapidly emerging as the fundamental strategy in the management of acute ischemic syndromes. In addition, it is now recognized that spontaneous reperfusion after coronary spasm or thrombosis is a common occur-

Supported in part by NIH Grants HL-43151 and SCOR Grant HL-42267.

rence in patients with coronary artery disease. The explosive growth of interventional recanalization, coupled with the recent appreciation of the role of spontaneous reperfusion in the natural history of coronary artery disease, has provided the impetus to investigate the consequences of restoring blood flow to the ischemic myocardium. Experimental studies have demonstrated that although early reperfusion limits or even prevents necrosis, restoration of blood flow is associated with a constellation of characteristic structural and functional derangements (5, 33), which are collectively referred to as "reperfusion injury" (7). Among these, three may have particular clinical importance: i) ventricular arrhythmias (reperfusion arrhythmias), ii) transient mechanical dysfunction or myocardial "stunning", and iii) cell death.

Reperfusion arrhythmias develop within seconds after restoration of flow to acutely ischemic myocardium in experimental animals, and are frequently malignant (e.g., ventricular fibrillation). Their clinical significance continues to be debated, but it is possible that they occur in patients after spontaneous relief of coronary spasm or early lysis of thrombus, particularly when thrombolytic therapies are administered outside of the hospital. *Myocardial stunning* is the prolonged contractile dysfunction that occurs despite the absence of irreversible injury. Considerable evidence indicates that it is caused in part by a component of injury specifically associated with reperfusion (6). This phenomenon has been well characterized in animal models, and there is mounting evidence that it occurs in patients with coronary artery disease in a variety of situations in which the heart is exposed to transient ischemia followed by reperfusion, such as unstable angina, acute myocardial infarction with coronary recanalization, open-heart surgery, and cardioplegia (8). In these situations, the development of myocardial stunning may contribute significantly to morbidity and mortality (8). *Cell death* is obviously the most serious consequence of ischemia and reperfusion, and has been postulated to be produced by both of these conditions. However, while ischemia *per se* can undoubtedly cause death of myocardial cells, there is little conclusive evidence that reperfusion in itself can cause *lethal* injury (i.e., that it can kill myocytes that up until the time of reperfusion had only sustained reversible ischemic injury and thus were potentially salvageable) (1). Regardless of this, however, reduction of infarct size after ischemia/reperfusion remains an important therapeutic goal. In view of the uncertainty regarding the relative contributions of ischemia and reperfusion to myocardial injury, in this essay we will use the term "ischemia/reperfusion injury".

Although numerous mechanisms have been proposed for the adverse sequelae of myocardial ischemia and reperfusion, the two most plausible are the generation of cytotoxic oxygen-derived free radicals and a perturbation of calcium homeostasis (in particular, a transient calcium overload in the early phase of reperfusion followed by a relative calcium deficiency due to excitation-contraction uncoupling) (7). It is important to stress that these two mechanisms are not mutually exclusive and, in fact, may represent two facets of the same phenomenon (6). At present, there is considerable evidence that both oxyradical-mediated injury and impaired calcium homeostatis play an important role in the pathogenesis of reperfusion arrhythmias and myocardial stunning (6). In contrast, the role of these derangements in cell death remains highly controversial (7).

Although oxidative stress and altered calcium fluxes appear to be the two major mechanisms responsible for ischemia/reperfusion injury, other derangements are likely to be involved as well. It must be kept in mind that ischemia and reperfusion trigger a complex cascade of events. Furthermore, both the generation of reactive oxygen metabolites and the disturbance of calcium homeostatis can be modulated by many mediators and by several physiological and pathological processes.

In recent years, considerable evidence has accumulated which suggests a significant role of the cardiac renin-angiotensin system (RAS) in myocardial ischemia/reperfusion injury and a beneficial influence of angiotensin-converting enzyme (ACE) inhibitors in this setting. The purpose of this article is to review the evidence for a pathogenetic contribution of the cardiac RAS to the sequelae of myocardial ischemia and reperfusion and for a cardioprotective effect of therapy with ACE inhibitors. Particular emphasis will be placed on the possible mechanisms of action of these drugs, which is currently the subject of considerable controversy and intense investigation. Because the effect of ACE inhibitors on infarct size is discussed in detail by Przyklenk et al. in an accompanying article, this review will primarily examine the ability of these drugs to influence postischemic recovery of function.

2. The myocardial RAS

ACE inhibitors have been used clinically for years as one of the mainstays of therapy for hypertension and congestive heart failure. Their beneficial effects in these disorders were initially attributed to extracardiac actions, i.e., the reduced formation of angiotensin II in the lungs from the angiotensin I released by the kidneys. However, the existence of a local myocardial production of angiotensin II was suspected because plasma renin activity often did not correlate with the efficacy of ACE inhibitors (37). Local RAS have now been demonstrated in various tissues, including the adrenal gland, the brain, the blood vessels (predominantly in the luminal plasma membrane of the endothelial cells but also in the vascular wall itself (54)), and the heart (reviewed in (14)). The presence of a cardiac RAS is supported by the following lines of evidence:

i) Renin and angiotensinogen mRNA are expressed in rat hearts (28), suggesting that the corresponding proteins are synthesized in mammalian hearts (34).

ii) Sodium depletion can increase cardiac renin activity in dogs (31).

iii) Myocardial angiotensin II production has been demonstrated in nephrectomized rats in the face of absent *plasma* angiotensin II (64).

iv) A cardiac ACE has been identified using an iodine-labeled enalapril analogue as a marker (43).

v) The administration of angiotensin I to isolated hearts (34) or to intact nephrectomized rabbits (27) results in the recovery of angiotensin II in the coronary sinus effluent; this myocardial production of Ang II can be abolished by ACE inhibitors (27, 34).

vi) Membrane-bound angiotensin II receptors have been demonstrated in cardiac myocytes (3). The stimulation of these receptors activates the membrane-bound phosphoinositidase (phospholipase C) which catalyzes the hydrolysis of phosphatidylinositol biphosphate to diacylglycerol (which activates Ca^{++}-sensitive protein kinase C) and inositol triphosphate (which increases intracellular $[Ca^{++}]$ by different mechanisms). The end-result of the activation of this *phosphatidylinositol signaling pathway* (described both in animals (3) and in humans (60)) is the regula-

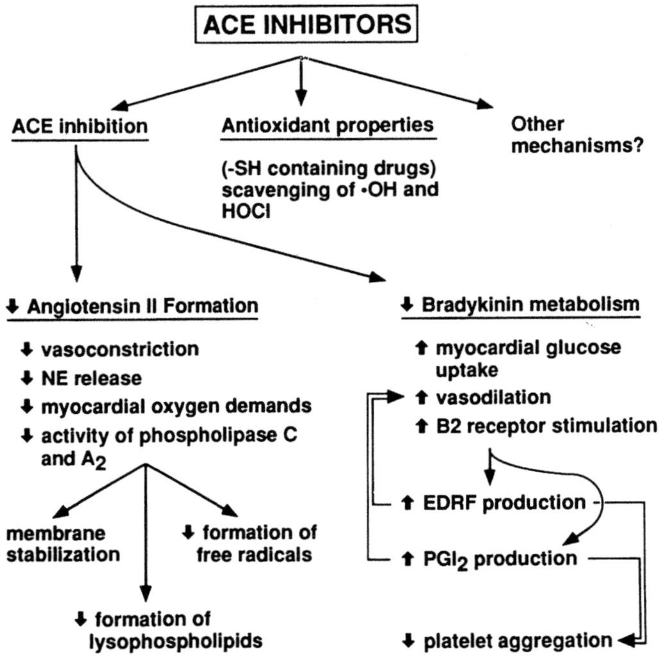

Fig. 1. Schematic diagram showing the potential mechanisms whereby ACE inhibitors may exert a protective effect in acute myocardial ischemia and reperfusion. For details see text. NE, norepinephrine; EDRF, endothelium-derived relaxing factor

tion of cytosolic Ca^{++} (9). Interestingly, these angiotensin II receptors have also been found in adrenergic nerve fibers in both healthy and diseased hearts (60), suggesting another important possible site of action of ACE inhibitors besides the myocytes themselves (e.g., for suppression of arrhythmias — see below).

3. Cardioprotective potential of ACE inhibitors

ACE inhibitors can be beneficial during myocardial ischemia and reperfusion by various mechanisms including: i) reduced formation of angiotensin II, ii) decreased metabolism of bradykinin, iii) antioxidant activity, and iv) possibly other unknown mechanisms (Fig. 1).

i) *Reduced formation of angiotensin II:* Angiotensin II exerts several actions which could be detrimental to the ischemic/reperfused myocardium. First, it is a potent vasoconstrictor and therefore could conceivably exacerbate ischemia (26). Second, it facilitates the activity of the cardiac sympathetic nervous system, leading to increased release of norepinephrine (26). This results in an indirect positive inotropic effect as well as in an increased propensity to arrhythmias (37). Third, as mentioned above, it stimulates phospholipase C and/or A2 (48). The consequent increase in degradation of membrane phospholipids may result in membrane destabilization and impaired function of subcellular organelles, in accumulation of toxic byproducts such as lysophospholipids, and in generation of free radicals through peroxidation of polyunsaturated fatty acids (48). Fourth, it may increase myocardial oxygen demands by increasing cardiac afterload. Finally, it exerts a direct positive inotropic action in vitro (15) in supraphysiologic concentrations (35). This property is usually not observed in vivo because the concentration of angiotensin II is lower and also possibly because a positive inotropic effect is overridden by the concomitant increase in afterload (1). Angiotensin II may also have a potential role in the regulation of cellular metabolism, as suggested by the finding of binding sites for angiotensin II on mitochondria (57), but little is known regarding this issue.

In view of these considerations, the reduced formation of angiotensin II would be expected to be beneficial during myocardial ischemia and reperfusion through a variety of mechanisms, including reduced oxygen demands, increased oxygen supply, preservation of membrane integrity, and reduced adrenergic stimulation.

ii) *Decreased metabolism of bradykinin:* In addition to producing angiotensin II, the converting enzyme is also the major enzyme responsible for the catabolism of bradykinin. Accordingly, ACE inhibitors prevent the degradation of bradykinin, a potent vasodilator. In this regard, it has recently been appreciated that bradykinin is released in the myocardium in response to experimental and clinical ischemia or infarction (29, 30), leading to the hypothesis that it may have cardioprotective properties (29). In endothelial cells bradykinin stimulates the B_2 receptors, resulting in increased production of endothelium-derived relaxing factor (EDRF) and prostacyclin (PGI_2) (42). Both EDRF and PGI_2 are potent vasodilators and platelet aggregation inhibitors. Indeed, the ACE inhibitor ramiprilat produces increases in PGI_2 and EDRF in endothelial cells (39). In addition, bradykinin increases myocardial glucose uptake (52). Taken together, these considerations support the concept that the anti-ischemic effect of ACE inhibitors is due in part to potentiation of bradykinin. This concept is corroborated by recent data indicating that blockade of bradykinin receptors with a bradykinin B_2 receptor antagonist abolished the cardioprotective effect of ramiprilat (38, 39, 55, 63).

iii) *Possible antioxidant activity:* The superoxide ($O_2^{\cdot-}$)-scavenging properties of sulfhydryl-containing ACE inhibitors (captopril, zofenopril and SQ 14,534) were reported by Westlin and Mullane (62) using data from three different in vitro systems: a) the superoxide-dependent autooxidation of epinephrine to adrenochrome c; b) the purine xanthine oxidase reaction (which generates $O_2^{\cdot-}$); and c) the activation of canine neutrophils activated with phorbol myristate acetate, which also generates $O_2^{\cdot-}$ (62). These observations were concordant with those of Bagchi et al. (2), who reported (using other assays) that captopril was an extremely potent free radical scavenger, with quenching abilities as potent as SOD against superoxide, or dimethylthiourea against $OH^{\cdot}$, and better than allopurinol against HOCl. Both Westlin and Mullane (62) and Bagchi et al. ascribed the free radical scavenging properties of ACE inhibitors to the —SH moiety.

However, the above findings were challenged by Kukreja et al. (36), who clearly demonstrated, using several superoxide-generating systems that captopril has no direct $O_2^{\cdot-}$-scavenging properties. These authors also demonstrated that captopril reduces cytochrome c directly and ascribed the results of Westlin and Mullane (62) to this unrecognized effect of the drug on the assay of superoxide used. Using a method initially described by Misra and Fridovich (45), Chopra et al. (10, 11) reported that the sulfhydryl-containing ACE inhibitors captopril, epicaptopril, and zofenopril were potent free radical scavengers at 4×10^{-5} M, but they scavenged "general" radicals, such as alkyl ($R^{\cdot}$) and alkoxyl ($ROO^{\cdot}$), and not superoxide (10, 11). In addition, Becker et al. demonstrated that captopril suppressed the chemiluminescence reaction elicited from luminol in the presence of $OH^{\cdot}$ (4). Engelman et al. (20) reported that captopril is a weak $O_2^{\cdot-}$ scavenger, but behaves as a potent scavenger of $OH^{\cdot}$ and HOCl.

In summary, the antioxidant properties of ACE inhibitors remain to be elucidated. It appears that these drugs do not scavenge $O_2^{\cdot-}$. However, because of the presence of a reduced thiol group, which acts as an electron acceptor, it seems plausible that SH-containing ACE inhibitors may scavenge $OH^{\cdot}$ and HOCl (most drugs that contain an —SH group are good $OH^{\cdot}$ scavengers (46)). The important question is: do ACE inhibitors in pharmacologic doses achieve cellular concentrations sufficiently high for the $OH^{\cdot}$ scavenging properties to become relevant? This question remains unanswered.

4. Effects of ACE inhibitors on myocardial ischemia/reperfusion injury

The properties of ACE inhibitors discussed above provide a sound rationale for testing the effects of these drugs in myocardial ischemia/reperfusion injury. A large number of studies have addressed this issue and the results can be summarized as follows. In the experimental setting, ACE inhibitors have been suggested to increase collateral flow (22), decrease the propensity for reperfusion arrhythmias (19, 40, 41, 61, 62), attenuate myocardial stunning (50, 51, 62), and decrease infarct size (13, 16, 21, 22, 32, 44). In the clinical setting, ACE inhibitors have assumed a prominent role in the treatment of the long-term adverse effects of myocardial ischemia and reperfusion. It is now well established that ACE inhibitors improve survival in congestive heart failure (12, 59), and in LV dysfunction after myocardial infarction (58). They also decrease ventricular remodeling (49) and infarct expansion, and promote regression of LV hypertrophy (17, 47). *However, there are, as yet, no data suggesting a beneficial effect of ACE inhibitors in acute myocardial ischemia and reperfusion in humans.*

As mentioned earlier, the effect of ACE inhibitors on infarct size will not be discussed in this article. We will focus on ischemia/reperfusion injury in vitro and myocardial stunning.

1) *Effect of ACE inhibitors on myocardial ischemia/reperfusion in vitro*

Using isolated perfused rat hearts, Linz et al. reported that ramiprilat (the deesterified active form of the ACE inhibitor ramipril) exerted beneficial effects when added to the perfusate at 10 µg/ml in the setting of regional (LAD) 15-min ischemia followed by 30 min of reflow (40). In addition to a decreased incidence of ventricular fibrillation, treated hearts exhibited less release of cardiac enzymes, higher levels of glycogen, ATP, and creatine phosphate, and higher left-ventricular pressure, Pp/dt_{max} and coronary flows compared with controls (40). The salutary effects of ACE inhibitors in this model were confirmed by other investigators using ramipril (53, 61) and captopril (61).

However, Van Gilst et al. (61), in their model of 15 min of regional ischemia followed by 30 min of reperfusion in isolated rat hearts, observed that the cardioprotective effects of captopril (80 μg/ml) and HOE 498 (ramiprilat, 15 μg/ml) could not be reproduced with enalapril 68 μg/ml), despite the fact that equipotent (ACE inhibiting) doses of the three drugs were used (61). Whereas captopril and ramiprilat maintained the pressure-rate product (a measure of mechanical function), decreased purine and norepinephrine overflow at reperfusion and limited the occurrence of VF, no such effects were demonstrated with enalapril (61). The reason for this discrepancy is unclear, but may be due to the infusion of the substance in its inactive (prodrug) rather than its active (enalaprilat) form.

Besides prevention of angiotensin II formation, there could be other mechanism(s) for the protection effected by ACE inhibitors in these in vitro experiments. One such mechanism could be the prevention of bradykinin metabolism. In this regard, Schoelkens et al. (53) found that ramiprilat or bradykinin were equally cardioprotective, and that the beneficial effects of ramiprilat were completely abolished by the infusion of a bradykinin antagonist. Another mechanism could be prostaglandin-related. Prostaglandins have been suggested as possible mediators of the actions of ACE inhibitors (56) and captopril indirectly stimulates PGI_2 synthesis in vascular tissue through bradykinin (18) (see above). An important role of prostaglandins was demonstrated in the Van Gilst study (61), in which the infusion of indomethacin abolished all the cardioprotective effects of captopril and ramiprilat (see above).

Taken together, these in vitro studies clearly demonstrate that ACE inhibitors can prevent the occurrence of deleterious metabolic, arrhythmic, and contractile abnormalities, and that these effects are produced by a wide array of structurally diverse substances. Since in isolated hearts there is no systemic production of angiotensin II, these beneficial effects must reflect either inhibition of a myocardial RAS or other mechanisms.

However, the aforementioned in vitro studies must be interpreted with caution, since the concentration of ACE inhibitors used in several of them was substantially higher than that needed for in vitro inhibition of the converting enzyme. Moreover, a distinction between an anti-ischemic vs. an anti-reperfusion injury effect could not be made because the drugs were often infused throughout the experimental protocols (encompassing both ischemia and reperfusion). Finally, these artificial models have limited physiologic relevance and the results need to be confirmed in intact animal models before any meaningful conclusions can be drawn.

2) *Effect of ACE inhibitors on myocardial stunning in intact animals*

Westlin and Mullane reported that captopril and SQ 14,534 (a captopril stereoisomer), but not enalaprilat, were scavengers of superoxide radicals in vitro and were protective in an open-chest dog model of 15-min ischemia and 3 h reperfusion in vivo (62). The authors found that administration of captopril before ischemia resulted in a significant improvement in the recovery of myocardial segment shortening after reperfusion. In contrast, an equihypotensive dose of enalaprilat (an ACE inhibitor that lacks a —SH moiety) failed to improve recovery of function (62). Dogs given captopril immediately before restoring coronary blood flow showed a return of function similar to that observed in animals treated with the drug before occlusion. SQ 14,534, the isomer of captopril, which is 100-fold less potent as an ACE inhibitor but equipotent in scavenging superoxide anion, also improved reperfusion-induced cardiac dysfunction when administered at reperfusion (62). The authors concluded that captopril alleviates myocardial stunning by a mechanism independent of ACE inhibition. Such a mechanism may involve an antioxidant property conferred by the —SH moiety, which is shared by captopril and its isomer, but not by enalaprilat. Furthermore, they concluded that the beneficial effects of captopril on myocardial stunning are due (at least in large part) to the prevention of a component of injury related to reperfusion (e.g., oxyradical-mediated damage) (62).

The effect of ACE inhibitors on myocardial stunning was further explored by Przyklenk and Kloner in the same canine model (15-min coronary occlusion followed by 3 h of reperfusion) (51). These authors compared the effects of zofenopril (an ACE inhibitor with an —SH moiety), SQ 14,534 (an —SH-containing stereoisomer of captopril which, as mentioned above, has essentially no ACE inhibitory properties), and enalaprilat (an ACE inhibitor without an —SH moiety). All groups of animals were similar with respect to hemodynamic variables and coronary collateral flow. All treated groups exhibited a significantly greater recovery of contractile function compared to controls (51). Since the ACE inhibitors were given *at the time of reperfusion,* this study (51) further supports the notion that these drugs alleviate a component of injury that occurs *after* restoration of flow. In contrast to the study of function similar to that observed in animals treated with the drug before occlusion. SQ 14,534, the isomer of captopril, which is 100-fold less potent as an ACE inhibitor but equipotent in scavenging superoxide anion, also improved reperfusion-induced cardiac dysfunction when administered at reperfusion (62). The authors concluded that captopril alleviates myocardial stunning by a mechanism independent of ACE inhibition. Such a mechanism may involve an antioxidant property conferred by the —SH moiety, which is shared by captopril and its isomer, but not by enalaprilat. Furthermore, they concluded that the beneficial effects of captopril on myocardial stunning are due (at least in large part) to the prevention of a component of injury related to reperfusion (e.g., oxyradical-mediated damage) (62).

The effect of ACE inhibitors on myocardial stunning was further explored by Przyklenk and Kloner in the same canine model (15-min coronary occlusion followed by 3 h of reperfusion) (51). These authors compared the effects of zofenopril (an ACE inhibitor with an —SH moiety), SQ 14,534 (an —SH-containing stereoisomer of captopril which, as mentioned above, has essentially no ACE inhibitory properties), and enalaprilat (an ACE inhibitor without an —SH moiety). All groups of animals were similar with respect to hemodynamic variables and coronary collateral flow. All treated groups exhibited a significantly greater recovery of contractile function compared to controls (51). Since the ACE inhibitors were given *at the time of reperfusion,* this study (51) further supports the notion that these drugs alleviate a component of injury that occurs *after* restoration of flow. In contrast to the study by Westlin and Mullane (62), in this study enalaprilat was found to attenuate postischemic dysfunction, a discrepancy that the authors ascribed to methodological differences (anesthesia protocol, timing of treatment, and the presence of collateral flow measurements) between the two studies. In addition, Przyklenk and Kloner found that indomethacin, given 2 h after reperfusion, largely reversed the beneficial effects of enalaprilat, suggesting that enalaprilat attenuates postischemic dysfunction at least in part by a prostaglandin-mediated mechanism. In contrast, indomethacin had no effect on the improved recovery of function associated with zofenopril, suggesting that this drug exerts its protective effects by a mechanism independent of prostaglandin synthesis (51). In this regard, it is known that ACE inhibitors can enhance the synthesis of prostaglandins (especially PGI_2) indirectly through the inhibition of bradykinin metabolism (18). Moreover, recent evidence has implicated the cyclooxygenase pathway in the pathogenesis of myocardial stunning (23—25).

In another study (50), Przyklenk and Kloner demonstrated that enalapril given 45 min *after* reperfusion attenuated myocardial postischemic dysfunction in open-chest dogs subjected to a 15-min occlusion. However, these results are difficult to interpret because enalapril reduced mean arterial pressure by approximately 20% and because stunned myocardium is known to have an exquisite sensitivity to decrease in afterload. The authors attributed the improved functional recovery effected by enalapril to increased blood flow to the previously ischemic region (50).

In summary, the available evidence suggests that ACE inhibitors can attenuate myocardial stunning after a brief, reversible ischemic episode. No data are available regarding the effect of these drugs on myocardial stunning after a prolonged, partly reversible ischemic episode, after multiple consecutive brief ischemic episodes, and after global ischemia (that is, cardioplegia). The mechanism for the salutary effects of ACE inhibitors on stunning remains a mystery. It may involve an antioxidant action (in the case of SH-containing molecules such as captopril, SQ 14,534, and zofenopril) or potentiation of prostaglandin actions (in the case of non-SH-containing compounds such as enalaprilat). *However, it must be emphasized that there is, as yet, no direct evidence that ACE inhibitors prevent free radical reactions or increase prostanoid synthesis in in vivo models of stunned myocardium.* What is clear is that the enhanced recovery of function effected by these drugs is *not* due to i) favorable hemodynamic effects, ii) inhibition of the converting enzyme *per se* (i.e., reduced synthesis of angiotensin II or increased half-life of bradykinin), or iii) an "anti-ischemic" action (i.e., an improved balance between oxygen supply and demand during ischemia). Further work will be needed to elucidate this issue, but the ability of ACE inhibitors to alleviate stunning when given at the time of reperfusion makes them attractive for clinical use.

5. Concluding remarks and future direction

We are only at the beginning of the process of assessing the benefits of ACE inhibitors in acute myocardial ischemia and reperfusion. The hypothesis that these drugs could be useful in this setting is very recent, the data supporting it are still scanty, and the evidence is far from being conclusive. Nevertheless, the available studies warrant an in-depth, thorough assessment of the utility of ACE inhibitors in attenuating myocardial stunning and in limiting infarct size, and, indeed, raise enthusiasm regarding the potential benefits that can be accrued with this form of therapy. The fact that ACE inhibitors have shown cardioprotective actions when given *at the time of reperfusion,* and the fact that they are generally well tolerated by patients, suggest that these agents may have an important clinical role as an adjunctive maneuver to alleviate the detrimental effects of ischemia and reperfusion of the heart. If this is the case, this would be one more item in a long series of clinical disorders that have been proven to be favorably affected by ACE inhibitor therapy.

However, before we conclude that the these drugs are a panacea, additional studies need to be done in the experimental as well as clinical settings. In the experimental setting, the beneficial effects of ACE inhibitors against myocardial stunning and in limiting infarct size need to be demonstrated in *conscious* animal models, i.e., in physiological animal preparations. Further insights must be gained into the mechanism of action of these compounds; in particular, it is necessary to demonstrate that they can exert antioxidant effects and/or enhance prostacyclin in in vivo models of myocardial ischemia and reperfusion. If the latter effect is proven, the next logical question that needs to be addressed is: how does prostacyclin protect against myocardial stunning or infarction? The issue of whether the presence of a reduced thiol group augments the cardioprotective potential of an ACE inhibitor must be settled by conducting careful, dose-ranging studies comparing SH-containing and non-SH-containing drugs in the same setting. It is also important to elucidate whether ACE inhibitors inhibit stunning only after a brief, reversible ischemic insult or also in other situations, for example, after a prolonged, partly irreversible ischemic insult (myocardial infarction) or in the setting of global cardiac ischemia (i.e., cardioplegia). At this point, the mechanism of action of ACE inhibitors in acute myocardial ischemia is so enigmatic that it seems plausible that it involves some as yet unrecognized effect on the myocardium.

ACE inhibitors are already a mainstay in our therapeutic armamentarium and already represent one of the major advances in cardiology in the last two decades. It will be fascinating to follow the progress of our knowledge in the next few years and to determine whether these drugs can exert beneficial effects in acute myocardial ischemia and reperfusion comparable to those already shown in many other situations.

References

1. Ahmed SS, Levinson GE, Weisse AB, Regan TJ (1975) The effect of angiotensin on myocardial contractility. J Clin Pharmacol 15:276—285
2. Bagchi D, Prasad R, Das DK (1989) Direct scavenging of free radicals by captopril, an angiotensin converting enzyme inhibitor. Bioch Biophys Res Com 158(1):52—57
3. Baker KM, Companile CP, Trachte GJ, Peach MJ (1984) Identification and characterization of the rabbit angiotensin II myocardial receptor. Circ Res 54:286—293
4. Becker BF, Reinholz N, Leipert B, Raschke P, Gerlach E (1991) Are the radical scavenging properties of ace inhibitors with sulfhydryl groups in therapeutically effective concentrations of quantitative significance? Klin Wochenschr 69(Suppl 24):6—9
5. Becker LC, Ambrosio G (1987) Myocardial consequences of reperfusion. Prog Cardiovasc Dis 30:23—44
6. Bolli R (1990) Mechanism of myocardial "stunning". Circulation 82(3):723—738
7. Bolli R (1991) Oxygen-derived free radicals and myocardial reperfusion injury: an overview. Cardiovasc Drugs Ther 5:249—268
8. Bolli R, Hartley CJ, Rabinovitz RS (1991) Clinical relevance of myocardial "stunning". Cardiovasc Drugs Ther 5:877—890
9. Cecil's Textbook of Medicine (1992) Wyngaarden JB, Smith LH, Bennett JC (eds) W. B. Saunders Company, pp 1197—1198
10. Chopra M, McMurray J, Stewart J, Dargie HJ, Smith WE (1990) Free radical scavenging: a potentially beneficial action of thiol-containing angiotensin converting enzyme inhibitors. Biochem Soc Trans 18:1184—1185
11. Chopra M, Scott N, McMurray J, McLay J, Bridges A, Smith WE, Belch JJF (1989) Captopril: a free radical scavenger. Br J Clin Pharmacol 27:396—399

12. CONSENSUS Trial Study Group (1987) Effects of enalapril on mortality in severe congestive heart failure. N Engl J Med 316:1429—1435
13. de Graeff PA, van Gilst WH, Bel K, de Langen CDJ, Kingma JH, Wesseling H (1987) Concentration-dependent protection by captopril against myocardial damage during ischemia and reperfusion in a closed chest pig model. J Cardiovasc Pharmacol 9(Suppl 2):S37—S42
14. Deboben A, Inagami T, Ganten D (1983) Tissue renin. In: Genest J, Kuchel O, Hamet P, Cantin M (eds) Hypertension — physiopathology and treatment. New York: McGraw-Hill Book Company:194—209
15. Dempsey PJ, McCallum ZT, Kent KM, Cooper T (1971) Direct myocardial effects of angiotensin II. Am J Physiol 220:477—481
16. DiPasquale P, Barone G, Paterna S, Cannizaro S, Giubilato A (1990) Efficacy of captopril before thrombolysis in acute myocardial infarction: preliminary findings. Drugs Exp Clin Res 16(11):581—589
17. Dunn FG, Oigman W, Ventura HO, Messerli FH, Kovrin I, Fohlich ED (1984) Enalapril improves systemic and renal hemodynamics and allows regression of left ventricular mass in essential hypertension. Am J Cardiol 53:105—108
18. Dusing R, Scherag R, Landsberg G, Glanzer K, Kramer HJ (1983) The converting enzyme inhibitor captopril stimulates prostacyclin synthesis by isolated rat aorta. Eur J Pharmacol 91:501—504
19. Elfellah MS, Ogilivie RI (1985) Effect of vasodilator drugs on coronary occlusion and reperfusion arrhythmias in anesthetized dogs. J Cardiovasc Pharmacol 7:826—832
20. Engelman RM, Rousou JA, Iyengar J, Das DK (1991) Captopril, an ACE inhibitor, for optimizing reperfusion after acute myocardial infarction. Ann Thorac Surg 52:918—926
21. Ertl G, Gaudron P, Kochsiek K (1990) Influence of angiotensin-converting enzyme inhibition on cardiac function in myocardial infarction. Am J Cardiol 65:70G-73G
22. Ertl G, Kloner RA, Alexander RW, Braunwald E (1982) Limitation of infarct size by an angiotensin-converting enzyme inhibitor. Circulation 1:40—48
23. Farber NE, Gross GJ (1989) Prostaglandin E_1 attenuates postischemic contractile dysfunction after brief coronary occlusion and reperfusion. Am Heart J 18:17
24. Farber NE, Gross GJ (1990) Prostaglandin redirection by thromboxane synthetase inhibition: attenuation of myocardial stunning in canine heart. Circulation 81:369
25. Farber NE, Pieper GM, Thomas JP, Gross GJ (1988) Beneficial effects of iloprost in the stunned canine myocardium. Circ Res 62:204
26. Fowler NO, Holmes JC (1964) Coronary and myocardial actions of angiotensin. Circ Res 14:191—201
27. Ganten D, Balz W, Hense H, Jung W, Rohde A, Bayer C (1985) Angiotensin (ANG) peptides in tissue of rabbits: characterization and regulation after nephrectomy and converting enzyme inhibitor (CEI) treatment. Naunyn-Schmiedbergs Arch Pharmacol 329(Suppl):R63
28. Ganten D, Ludwig G, Hennhoefer C (1986) Genetic control of renin in the tissues of different strains of mice [Abstract]. Nauyn Schmiedebergs Arch Pharmacol 332: R—59
29. Hashimoto K, Hamamoto H, Honda Y, Hirose M, Furakawa S, Kimura E (1978) Changes in components of kinin system and hemodynamics in acute myocardial infarction. Am Heart J 95:619—626
30. Hashimoto K, Hirose M, Furukawa S, Hayakawa H, Kimura E (1977) Changes in hemodynamics and bradykinin concentration in coronary sinus blood in experimental coronary occlusion. Jap Heart J 18:679—689
31. Hadyuk K, Boucher R, Genest J (1970) Renin activity and content in various tissues in dogs under different pathophysiological states. Proc Soc Exp Biol Med 134:252—255
32. Hock CE, Ribeiro LGT, Lefer AM (1985) Preservation of ischemic myocardium by a new converting enzyme inhibitor, enalaprilic acid, in acute myocardial infarction. Am Heart J 109:222—228

33. Jennings RB, Reimer KA (1983) Factors involved in salvaging ischemic myocardium. Effects of reperfusion of arterial blood. Circulation 68(Suppl):I25—I36
34. Jin M, Wilhelm MJ, Lang RE, Unger T, Lindpainter K, Ganten D (1988) Endogeneous tissue renin-angiotensin systems: from molecular biology to therapy. Am J Med 84(Suppl 3A):28—36
34b. Klein J, Colin P, Scherer E, Levy M, Koren G (1990) Simple measurement of captopril in plasma by high-performance liquid chromatography with ultraviolet detection. Ther Drug Monit 12(1):105—110
35. Koch-Weser J (1965) Nature of inotropic action of angiotensin. Circ Res 16:230—237
36. Kukreja RC, Kontos HA, Hess ML (1990) Captopril and enalaprilat do not scavenge the superoxide anion. Am J Cardiol 65:24I—27I
37. Lindpainter K, Jin M, Wilhelm MJ, Suzuki F, Linz W, Schoelkens BA, Ganten D (1988) Intracardiac generation of angiotensin and its physiologic role. Circulation 77(Suppl I):I—18—23
38. Linz W, Martorana PA, Grotsch H, Bei-Yin Q, Scholkens BA (1990) Antagonizing bradykinin obliterates the cardioprotective effects of bradykinin and angiotensin-converting enzyme (ACE) inhibitors in ischemic hearts. Drugs Dev Res 19:393—408
39. Linz W, Martorana PA, Scholkens BA (1990) Local inhibition of bradykinin degradation in ischemic hearts. J Cardiovasc Pharmacol 15(Suppl 6):99—109
40. Linz W, Scholkens BA, Han YF (1986) Beneficial effects of the converting enzyme inhibitor, ramipril, in ischemic rat hearts. J Cardiovasc Pharmacol 8(Suppl 10): S91—S99
41. Linz W, Scholkens BA, Manwen J, Wilhelm M, Ganten D (1986) The heart as a target for converting enzyme inhibitors: studies in ischemic isolated working rat hearts. J Hypert 4(Suppl 6):S477—S479
42. Martorana PA, Linz W, Scholkens BA (1991) Does bradykinin play a role in the cardiac antiischemic effect of ACE inhibitors? Basic Res Cardiol 86:293—296
43. Mebazzaa A, Chevalier B, Mercadier JJ, Echter E, Rappaport L, Swynghedauw B (1989) A review of the renin-angiotensin system in the normal heart. J Cardiovasc Pharmacol 14(Suppl 4):S16—20
44. Mehta PM, Przyklenk K, Kloner RA (1990) Cardioprotective effects of captopril in myocardial ischaemia, ischaemia/reperfusion and infarction. Eur Heart J 11(Suppl B):94—99
45. Misra HP, Fridovich I (1977) Superoxide dismutase: a photochemical augmentation assay. Arch Biochem Biophys 187:303—307
46. Myers ML, Bolli R, Lekich RF, Hartley CJ, Roberts R (1986) N-2-mercaptopropionylglycine improves recovery of myocardial function after reversible regional ischemia. J Am Coll Cardiol 8:1161
47. Nakashima Y, Fouad FM, Tarazi RC (1984) Regression of left ventricular hypertrophy from systemic hypertension by enalapril. Am J Cardiol 53:1044—1049
48. Peach MJ (1981) Molecular actions of angiotensin. Biochem Pharmacol 30: 2745—2751
49. Pfeffer JM, Pfeffer MA (1988) Angiotensin converting enzyme inhibition and ventricular remodeling in heart failure. Am J Med 84(Suppl 3A):37—44
50. Przyklenk K, Kloner RA (1987) Acute effects of hydralazine and enalapril on contractile function of postischemic "stunned" myocardium. Am J Cardiol 60:934—936
51. Przyklenk K, Kloner RA (1991) Angiotensin converting enzyme inhibitors improve contractile function of stunned myocardium by different mechanism of action. Am Heart J 121:1319—1330
52. Rosen P, Eckel J, Reinauer H (1983) Influence of bradykinin on glucose uptake and metabolism studied in isolated cardiac myocytes and isolated perfused rat hearts. Hoppe Seylers Z Physiol Chem 364:431—438
53. Scholkens BA, Linz W (1991) Ace inhibition: mechanisms of cardioprotection in acute myocardial ischemia. Klin Wochenschr 69(Suppl 24):1—5

54. Scholkens BA, Linz W, Han Y-F (1987) Heart and vascular wall as targets for tissue converting enzyme inhibition. Clin Exp Hypertens 9(2—3):427—433
55. Scholkens BA, Linz W, Konig W (1988) Effects of the angiotensin converting enzyme inhibitor, ramipril in isolated rat heart are abolished by a bradykinin antagonist. J Hypertension 6(Suppl 4):25—28
56. Schwartz SL, Williams GH, Hollenberg NK, Levine L, Dluhy RG, Moore FJ (1980) Captopril-induced changes in prostaglandin production. J Clin Invest 65:1257
57. Sweet CS (1990) Issues surrounding a local cardiac renin system and the beneficial actions of angiotensin-converting enzyme inhibitors in ischemic myocardium. Am J Cardiol 65:11I—13I
58. The SAVE Trial: Data presented at the 41st Annual Scientific Sessions of the American College of Cardiology — Dallas, April 1992
59. The SOLVD Investigators (1991) Effect of enalapril on survival in patients with reduced left ventricular ejection fractions and congestive heart failure. N Engl J Med 325:293—302
60. Urata H, Healy B, Stewart RW, Pumpus FM, Husain A (1989) Angiotensin II receptors in normal and failing human hearts. J Clin Endocrinol Metab 69:54—66
61. van Gilst WH, de Graeff PA, Wesseling H, de Langen CDJ (1986) Reduction of reperfusion arrhythmias in the ischemic isolated rat heart by angiotensin converting enzyme inhibitors: a comparsion of captopril, enalapril and HOE 498. J Cardiovasc Pharmacol 8:722—728
62. Westlin W, Mullane K (1988) Does captopril attenuate reperfusion-induced myocardial dysfunction by scavenging free radicals? Circulation 77(Suppl I)I—30—39
63. Wiemer G, Becker RHA (1991) Die Ramiprilat-stimulierte cGMP und PGI2-Bildung in Endothel-zellen ist Bradykinin-vermittelt. Kardiol 80(Suppl 3):120
64. Wilhelm MJ, Lindpainter K, Jin M, Zimmerman F, Bayer C, Ganten D (1987) The intrinsic cardiac renin-angiotensin system: capability for independent local regulation. Hochdruck 8:18

Author's address:
Roberto Bolli, M.D.
Section of Cardiology
Baylor College of Medicine
6535 Fannin, MS F-905
Houston, TX 77030

Angiotensin-converting enzyme inhibitor in a human model of restenosis

G. R. Heyndrickx and the MERCATOR ("Multicenter European Research Trial with Cilazapril after Angioplasty to Prevent Transluminal Coronary Obstruction and Restenosis") study group

Introduction

Percutaneous transluminal coronary angioplasty (PTCA) was introduced by Andreas Gruentzig in 1977, as an alternative treatment for coronary artery bypass grafting (CABG) to restore coronary blood flow in patients with obstructive coronary artery disease (15). Increased experience and advances in technology have resulted in a high primary success rate (over 90%) and a low complication rate (death, non-fatal myocardial infarction; 4—5%) (9). However, the late restenosis rate (17% to 40%) still limits the long-term benefit of the procedure (21, 23, 47, 52).

The cause of restenosis is unclear, but factors such as platelet aggregation, formation of mural thrombi, intimal proliferation of smooth muscle cells, elastic recoil, and active vasoconstriction at the site of PTCA injury have all been implicated (14, 24, 26, 41, 43, 50, 53). A decade of intensive clinical and pharmacological research has not succeeded in altering the restenosis rate (5, 48). Various treatments such as intravenous administration of heparin, antiplatelet therapy (aspirin, dipyridamole, ticlopidine, prostacyclin, ciprostene, thromboxane A2 receptor blocker), anticoagulants (coumadin), calcium channel blockers (nifedipine, diltiazem, verapamil) and other agents such as corticosteroids and colchicine, have failed to reduce the restenosis rate (18, 47). Fish oil and cholesterol-lowering agents have shown promises, although the published results are conflicting (18, 42).

Balloon angioplasty extensively damages the medial smooth muscle cells as well as the endothelial lining of the coronary vessel wall (11). Recent data have shown that mitogens from platelets are not wholly responsible for initiating the proliferative response in balloon catheter-injured arteries, since smooth muscle cell proliferation occurred in the absence of platelets (12). The smooth muscle cell proliferation was correlated with the severity of trauma inflicted by the denuding technique to the arterial wall, which would suggest a role for endogenous factors possibly released from damaged endothelial and smooth muscle cells (24, 25). The basic fibroblastic growth factor (b-FGF) is one of the main culprit factors as it is released from disrupted cultured vascular cells and is a growth factor for smooth muscle cells in vitro and in vivo (12, 20). Platelet derived growth factor may regulate the migration of the smooth muscle cells from the media into the intima (16, 28). In this process, angiotensin II might act as a co-mitogen and stimulate increased proliferation of smooth muscle cells which have been activated to enter the cell cycle and have migrated to the subintima (28). Based on the hypothesis that a local angiotensin system may regulate the vascular response to endothelial injury, Powell et al. (34) examined the effects of various doses of the angiotensin converting enzyme inhibitor cilazapril on neointimal proliferation in the rat carotid artery. Administration of a

The study was sponsored by F. Hoffmann-La Roche Ltd., Basel, Switzerland.

high dose resulted in a 80% reduction in neointima formation in this balloon-artery injury model.

The present multicenter, randomized, double-blind, placebo-controlled trial was designed to test in man whether ACE inhibition can prevent late restenosis after PTCA.

Methods

Study population

After informed consent a total of 735 patients scheduled for PTCA with an angiographically proven functionally significant narrowing in one or more major coronary arteries, either symptomatic or asymptomatic were randomly assigned to cilazapril or placebo. Only 693 patients with a successful PTCA (defined as a visually assessed diameter stenosis of less than 50% post-PTCA) who met all in and exclusion criteria as stated in the protocol, continued the trial and formed the study population. Forty-two patients were excluded for the following reasons: 1) PTCA procedure not performed, 2) PTCA procedure unsuccessful, 3) PTCA procedure complicated by myocardial infarction, 4) Baseline film could not be quantitatively analyzed, 5) Exclusion criterion overlooked at the time of screening.

Trial medication was given for the first time in the evening after successful PTCA and consisted of either capsules of cilazapril (first evening 2.5 mg, then 5 mg bid) or matching placebo for 6 months. In addition, all patients received 75 to 125 mg aspirin bid started before coronary PTCA until follow-up angiography (2, 44).

Follow-up evaluation

Patients returned to the outpatient clinic after 1, 2, 4, and 6 months for an interview, a cardiac examination, ECG, laboratory tests and a capsule count. Follow-up angiography was performed at the 6-month visit after the trial medication was discontinued. If symptoms recurred within 6 months, coronary angiography was carried out earlier. If no definite restenosis was present and the follow-up time was less than 3 months, the patient was asked to undergo another coronary angiogram at 6 months.

One to 4 days prior to follow-up angiography, but after discontinuation of the trial medication, a symptom-limited exercise test was performed on a bicycle ergometer according to a standard protocol. The test was performed in a sitting position, starting with a workload of 20 watts which was increased by 20 watts every minute. Exercise was continued until anginal symptoms, or a drop in systolic blood pressure, or severe arrhythmia, or a ST-depression of more than 1 mm occurred, or the patient stopped because of fatigue. A 12-lead ECG was recorded during exercise and recovery. ST-changes were measured 80 ms after the J-point.

PTCA procedure and angiographic analysis

PTCA was performed using standard procedures. Choice of balloon type, inflation duration and pressure were left to the operator.

Three coronary angiograms were obtained in each patient, one just before PTCA, one immediately after PTCA and one at follow-up, in such a way that they were suitable for quantitative analysis by the Coronary Angiography Analysis System

(CAAS) which has been validated and described in detail (13, 38, 39). All angiographic analyses including qualitative assessment of certain lesion characteristics (1, 10, 27) were performed at a core laboratory which was blinded as regards treatment allocation and did not have access to clinical data.

End-points

The primary end-point of this study was the within-patient change in minimal lumen diameter as determined by quantitative angiography immediately post-PTCA and at follow-up. In case the clinical condition required re-PTCA, the angiogram made prior to re-PTCA was used to obtain follow-up values, irrespective of the timing of re-PTCA (hours, days or weeks).

For each dilated segment the minimal lumen diameter was taken as the mean value from multiple matched projections. Within-patient change was defined as the follow-up minus the post-PTCA value. In case more than one segment was dilated (multi-vessel or multi-site procedures), the mean change over all lesions dilated was taken as end-point.

Secondary end-points were restenosis rates, exercise test results and clinical events. These were: death (irrespective of cause), NYHA III/IV due to congestive heart failure, non-fatal myocardial infarction (symptoms, ECG-changes and CK enzymes above twice the upper limit of normal), coronary revascularization (CABG, repeat PTCA, stent implantation or atherectomy at the same site or other site) and recurrent angina requiring initiation or increase in medical therapy, or none of the above. Only those revascularizations that were done before the 6-month time window (6 months ± 3 weeks) were counted as a clinical event.

Statistical methods and analysis

Since restenosis should be viewed as a continuous process, it was measured by the mean overall change in absolute minimal luminal diameter and not by applying arbitrarily selected cut-off criteria of "50% diameter stenosis at follow-up" or "$\geqslant$0.72 mm change in minimal diameter between post-PTCA and follow-up". With the assumption of a change of —0.40 ± 0.50 mm in mean minimal lumen diameter between postangioplasty and follow-up angiogram in the control group and —0.25 ± 0.50 mm (i.e., a 37.5% difference) in the active drug group (two-sided test with an alpha error of 0.05 and a power of 0.90), the minimal sample size was estimated to be 233 patients in each group.

To test the hypothesis that the mean change in minimal lumen diameter is equal in the two treatment groups, an analysis of variance was done with treatment and center as main factors and treatment times center as interaction term. As the change in minimal luminal diameter after PTCA follows a near Gaussian distribution, parametric tests were allowed to be used (40). The treatment effect was defined as the difference in mean change in minimal lumen diameter between the two treatment groups. In addition, 95% confidence intervals of the treatment effect were obtained from the analysis of variance.

Comparison of the clinical outcome was done for the intention-to-treat population. Each patient was assigned at the time of follow-up to the most serious applicable event on the scale described above. For comparison of the clinical outcome between the two treatment groups, standard non-parametric statistical methods were used.

Results

Baseline characteristics and clinical follow-up

Selected demographic and clinical characteristics of the two study groups were evenly distributed except for patients with pain at rest and patients currently smoking, who were more frequently encountered in the control group.

Clinical follow-up was obtained for all 693 patients. During the course of the study, five patients died (control 2, cilazapril 3). The cause of death was in four cases cardiovascular and in one case of other origin. The occurrence of non-fatal myocardial infarction, bypass surgery, atherectomy, stent implantation or recurrent angina was not significantly different (adjusted chi square test) between the two groups. Table 1 shows the number of events on a per-patient basis, with only the most serious event listed.

Table 1. Ranking per patient based on most serious clinical event during 6-month follow-up.

	Control N = 352 Pts	Cilazapril N = 341 Pts
Death	2 (<1%)	3 (<1%)
NYHA III/IV	0	0
Non-fatal myocardial infarction	8 (2.3%)	5 (1.4%)
Coronary revascularization	51 (14.5%)	53 (15.5%)
Angina recurrence	67 (19.0%)	68 (19.9%)
No event	224 (63.6%)	212 (62.2%)

NYHA = New York Heart Association classification for congestive heart failure was used; Pts = Patients.

Angiographic efficacy analysis

Table 2 summarizes the quantitative angiographic findings in the per-protocol population. On per-protocol basis, the loss at follow-up in minimal lumen diameter was —0.29 ± 0.49 mm in the control group and —0.27 ± 0.51 mm in the cilazapril treated group (treatment effect, 0.023 mm; 95% Cl: —0.06 to 0.11 mm). Figure 1 represents a cumulative frequency curve of the minimal lumen diameter observed in both groups prior to PTCA, after PTCA and at 6-month follow-up.

Discussion

I. Rationale for ACE inhibition after PTCA

Over the past decade, it has been repeatedly demonstrated that treatment of chronic hypertensive rats with ACE inhibitors reduces the medial hypertrophy of muscular arteries (31, 32, 33). Therefore, it has been postulated that the local renin-angiotensin system may participate in regulating the vascular response to arterial injury. This

Table 2. Quantitative analysis in the per-protocol population.

	Control N = 309 Pts	Cilazapril N = 286 Pts
Obstruction diameter (mm)		
pre-angioplasty	0.98 ± 0.35	1.05 ± 0.35
post-angioplasty	1.77 ± 0.34	1.80 ± 0.36
follow-up	1.48 ± 0.54	1.54 ± 0.54
Reference diameter (mm)		
pre-angioplasty	2.61 ± 0.54	2.66 ± 0.51
post-angioplasty	2.67 ± 0.48	2.72 ± 0.49
follow-up	2.68 ± 0.56	2.74 ± 0.52
Difference in obstruction diameter (mm)		
post — pre-angioplysty	0.79 ± 0.42	0.75 ± 0.37
follow-up — post-angioplasty	—0.29 ± 0.49	—0.27 ± 0.51
Percentage stenosis (%)		
pre-angioplasty	61.4 ± 13.4	60.1 ± 12.3
post-angioplasty	32.9 ± 9.0	33.0 ± 10.0
follow-up	44.2 ± 18.0	43.5 ± 17.2
Difference in percentage stenosis (%)		
post — pre-angioplasty	—28.5 ± 15.3	—27.1 ± 13.7
follow-up — post-angioplasty	11.3 ± 18.2	10.5 ± 18.0

Plus — minus values are means ± sd; Pts = Patients.

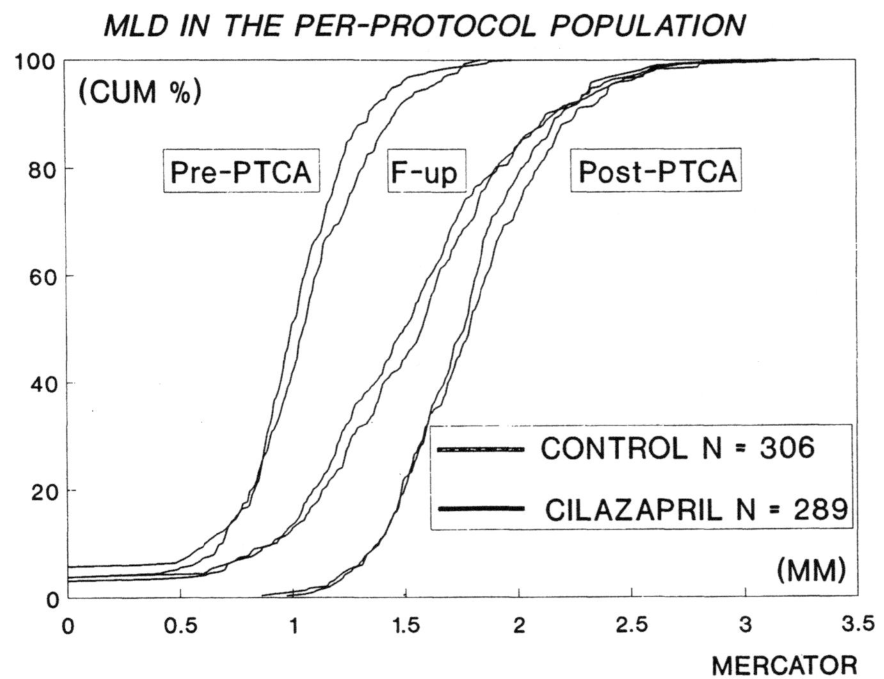

Fig. 1. Cumulative distribution curve of the minimal lumen diameter (MDL) pre-PTCA, post-PTCA and at 6-month follow-up in both treatment groups. (From Serruys PW et al. Circulation 1991; 84:1568—1580. Reproduced with permission).

hypothesis has prompted the investigation of the role of angiotensin II after injury. For this purpose, the effect of the long-acting ACE inhibitor cilazapril on the proliferative response to arterial injury was examined by Powell et al. (34) in an animal model. This inhibitor was selected because at a dose of 10 mg/kg/day, it lowered blood pressure over a 24-h period and reduced the medial hypertrophy of hypertensive rats. Using the same dose of cilazapril, neointima formation was decreased by 80% and lumen integrity was preserved in normotensive rats in which the left carotid artery was subjected to endothelial denudation and injury by balloon catheterization (26).

More recently, several groups have studied the effects of angiotensin II on smooth muscle cell proliferation in vitro as well as the influence of ACE inhibition on smooth muscle cell proliferation. Angiotensin II induced expression of several growth factor genes, such as genes encoding platelet-derived growth factor (PDGF), transforming growth factor-β (TGF-β) and thrombospondin (TS) (29, 35, 36, 46). These results demonstrate that, in cultured cells, angiotensin II induces mRNAs to encode several important growth factor genes and thus induces cell proliferation. Cilazapril or its active metabolite did not have a direct effect by itself, but the antiproliferative effect was mediated through angiotensin II. Consequently, the inhibition of angiotensin II production may prevent the proliferative response that occurs after PTCA in man.

II. Trial design: quantitative angiography as primary end-point

The (re-)appearance of angina as a sole criterion of restenosis underestimates the angiographic rate of restenosis. The poor value of recurrent anginal symptoms as a marker of restenosis is confirmed by the low predictive value of symptoms found in many studies (15). Similarly, the usefulness of ergometry to detect restenosis after PTCA has been questioned since several studies have found that the presence of exercise test induced angina or ST-segment depression/elevation or both are not highly predictive for restenosis if the test is performed early or late after PTCA (15). A drug tested for its ability to prevent restenosis may be shown to be beneficial following PTCA by reducing angina during exercise-test and yet have no effect on intimal hyperplasia following balloon induced injury. In the present study, fewer patients in the cilazapril-treated group experienced anginal pain during the exercise test; this symptomatic beneficial effect was not corroborated by either an increase in workload or in double product nor by STT-changes. It must be emphasized that this difference in behavior between the two groups remains unexplained and had no bearing on the general outcome of the trial.

In contradistinction, the prognostic value of the change in sequential coronary angiogram has been largely underestimated as a surrogate endpoint for clinical atherosclerotic events. In the phase II of pharmacological investigation, the main emphasis should be put on the physiopathological mechanism of prevention of restenosis in the post-injury model and the improvement in clinical outcome should be viewed as a secondary benefit dependent on the anatomical status.

III. Lack of effect on angiographic restenosis

Several explanations (which are not mutually exclusive) may account for the apparent failure of cilazapril to decrease the rate of coronary restenosis.

A. Dose related

The dose selected for this trial was based on pharmacokinetic data in healthy volunteers, demonstrating that a single dose of 5 mg cilazapril reduced the plasma ACE activity to virtually unmeasurable levels (4, 30). Pharmacokinetic data from hypertensive patients demonstrate that after a single dose of 5 mg cilazapril the plasma angiotensin II concentration starts to return to baseline in 8 to 10 h, although a sustained blood pressure reduction is achieved. Therefore, the dosage of 5 mg bid was chosen.

After the trial was designed, it has been shown that inhibition of neointima formation is a dose-dependent phenomenon and the dose required for inhibition of neointimal formation appears to be somewhat higher than for lowering blood pressure (35). In the rat model, this dose relationship for the anti-proliferative effect of cilazapril is different from the dose relationship for the anti-hypertensive effect. Thus, a possible explanation for the lack of effect in MERCATOR is that the dose used was too low, as the dose used in the rat model was 70 times higher (10 mg/kg/day). The ongoing American-Canadian sister trial to MERCATOR, MARCATOR, which is similar in design but randomizes between 1, 5, and 10 mg of cilazapril bid will give us the unique opportunity to further investigate this relationship in humans. If the anti-hypertensive effect in the 10 mg bid subset of patients does not materially differ from that in the two other arms of the trial (1 and 5 mg bid), while a direct antiproliferative effect is observed, then further investigation of the role of the renin-angiotensin system in tissue proliferation after vascular injury seems warranted.

B. Time-related

As in animal experiments, no major difference in inhibition of neointimal proliferation has been observed whether the drug was given 1 h prior to or within 2 days after the wall injury, it was assumed that ACE inhibition by cilazapril could be started immediately after PTCA (34).

In experimental studies the strongest inhibition of neointima formation was obtained when treatment was started 6 days before injury. It could be that a period of drug impregnation prior to injury might be required to obtain an inhibitory effect, although a significant, but slightly attenuated effect was observed when started 2 days after injury.

C. Species-related

Powell et al. compared the effects of high doses of cilazapril (10 mg/kg/day) and captopril (100 mg/kg/day) on neointimal proliferation in the rat carotid artery model (35). Both agents were highly effective and, in addition, concomitant heparin therapy appeared to exert a synergistic antiproliferative effect. Similarly, in the atherosclerotic rabbit iliac model, cilazapril (5 mg/kg/day) reduced the incidence of restenosis following balloon injury (3). In contrast, Lam et al. found no benefit of high-dose cilazapril (20 mg/kg bid) in the porcine carotid artery injury model (22). Churchill et al. and Huber et al. could not demonstrate any significant benefit of captopril or enalapril in preventing restenosis in the swine model (7, 19). Despite the fact that all species show an effect on blood pressure, the post-injury proliferation in baboons and pigs was not clearly affected by cilazapril at the doses used, whereas rats, guinea pigs and rabbits did respond (17). Rakugi et al. have shown that vascular injury results in the induction of ACE in proliferating cells in the neointima and support the role of the local renin-angiotensin system in restenosis (37). Although quite attractive, the close parallel between the muscular response to experimental arterial injury and the development of restenosis in humans after therapeutic angioplasty remains a working hypothesis. The response of atherosclerotic human arteries may be modulated by cellular and molecular influences that are not exactly similar to those acting in non-diseased non-human arteries.

D. Alternative pathways of angiotensin II production

Enzymes other than angiotensin converting enzyme are known for their ability to metabolize angiotensin I to angiotensin II (chymase, tonin and cathepsin). It could well be that these alternative pathways resulted in sufficient level of angiotensin II to activate or to stimulate the restenosis process. As no actual measurement was done of angiotensin I or II, it is difficult to say if these alternative pathways were active. However, we found a significant decrease in blood pressure immediately after the first drug intake, in patients randomized to cilazapril as compared to patients taking placebo. This effect was maintained during the whole 6-month follow-up period. Thus, clinically there was an effect of cilazapril by reducing blood pressure presumably by lowering the level of angiotensin II. The use of an angiotensin II receptor blocker might be worth exploring (6), as in this case all angiotensin II, irrespective of the metabolic pathway that is used, is blocked.

E. Possible mitogenic effect of angiotensin I

Another explanation for failure of cilazapril to reduce restenosis is that, as a logical consequence by the use of ACE-inhibitors, the concentration of angiotensin I is increased, which has been shown to be mitogenetic for arterial muscle cells (36). This unavoidable side-effect of ACE-inhibitors may, perhaps only in some species annihilate their favorable actions exerted through A II suppression.

IV. Relevance of mechanism of action

The most recent theory on restenosis put forward by Clowes indicates that the b-FGF released after disruption and cell necrosis of the endothelium and media is the factor which initiates the proliferation and duplication of the smooth muscle cells (24). These subsequently activated smooth muscle cells tend to migrate in the subintima of the vessel where they are attracted by the PDGF, stemming from the aggregated platelets. It is in this location and stage that angiotensin II is acting upon them as a comitogen. This complex interaction may be the predominant biological scenario in certain species, such as rat and rabbit, but may be inoperative in other species such as the baboon and the guinea pig.

Recently, Forrester et al. hypothesized that restenosis is a manifestation of the general wound-healing process expressed specifically in vascular tissue (14). They list five different groups of growth factors PDGF, FGF, EGF (Epidermal Growth Factor), IGF (Insulin-like growth factor), and TGF (Transforming growth factor), each with a specific role and with possible many interactions. It is, of course, possible that angiotensin II has only a minor role in this complex process and therefore ACE inhibition did not result in less angiographic restenosis.

In contrast, Schwartz et al. hypothesizes that mural thrombus is the most important factor in the restenosis process. It is seen in all treated animals after injury, after 3 days it is covered by endothelium and, later on, smooth muscle cells start to grow downward towards the media, suggesting that neointimal cells are not likely derived from arterial media at the immediate injury site (45).

Conclusion

Long-term angiotensin converting enzyme inhibition with cilazapril in a dose of 5 mg bid does not prevent restenosis and does not favorably influence the overall clinical outcome following PTCA in patients. The final report on the Mercator trial has been recently published (51). The results of the MARCATOR trial have to be awaited before determining whether a higher dose of cilazapril has any effect on angiographic restenosis.

APPENDIX I

Steering Committee, writing group and authors of the manuscript

Patrick W Serruys, MD (Chairman), Wolfgang Rutsch, MD, Nicolas Danchin, MD, William Wijns, MD, Hakan Emanuelsson, MD, François Chappuis, MD, Walter RM Hermans, MD.

MERCATOR Study Group

Participating Clinics and Investigators

The following institutions and investigators participated in MERCATOR. The number of patients enrolled at each center are given in parenthesis. Log-keeping centers are identified with an asterisk*⁾.
The London Chest Hospital, London, England (21)⁾:* R. Balcon, MD, Principal Investigator; J. Timmins, MD, D. C. Springings, MD, S. J. D. Brecker, MD, S. W. Davies, MD.
Hôpital TIMONE, Marseille, France (14)⁾:* J. L. Bonnet, MD, Principal Investigator; F. d'Houdain, MD.
University Hospital Leiden, Leiden, The Netherlands (41)⁾:* B. Buis, MD, Principal Investigator; A. L. M. Bakx, MD, M. I. Sedney, MD.
Ospidale Nuguarda CA'Granda, Milan, Italy (12)⁾:* L. Campolo, MD. Principal Investigator; G. B. Danzi, MD, A. M. de Biase, MD.

Hôpital Cantonal, Geneva, Switzerland (20): F. Chappuis, MD, Principal Investigator; W. Rutishauser, MD, P. Urban, MD, B. Meier, MD.
CHU Brabois, Vandoeuvre, France (40)⁾:* N. Danchin, MD, Principal Investigator; Y. Juillière, MD, V. Voilquin-Thomas, MD.
University of Göteborg, Göteborg, Sweden (44)⁾:* H. Emanuelsson, MD, Principal Investigator; P. Albertsson, MD, K. Selin, MD, L. Ekström, MD.
Medizinische Klinik, München, Germany (32): R. von Essen, MD, Principal Investigator; H. Nebelsieck, MD, A. Uberreiter, MD, K. Igerl, MD.
Onze Lieve Vrouw Ziekenhuis, Aalst, Belgium (44)⁾:* G. R. Heyndrickx, MD, Principal Investigator; P. Nellens, MD, B. de Bruyne, MD, M. Goethals, MD.
Städtisches Krankenhaus Bogenhausen, München, Germany (23)⁾:* T. Ischinger, MD, Principal Investigator; M. Fischer, MD, K. Coppenrath, MD.
Albert-Ludwigs-Universität, Freiburg, Germany (18)⁾:* H. J. Just, MD, Principal Investigator; H. Wollschläger, MD, H. Drexler, MD, G. Elias, MD.
Medizinische Poliklinik, Zürich, Switzerland (20): H. P. Krayenbühl, MD, Principal Investigator; O. Hess, MD, F. W. Amann, MD, R. Schläpfer, MD, M. Büchi, MD.
Universität Erlangen, Erlangen, Germany (28): B. Kunkel, MD, Principal Investigator; T. Fürste, MD.
CHRU — Hôpital Cardiologique, Lille, France (40)⁾:* J. M. Lablanche, MD, Principal Investigator; J. M. Joris, MD, T. Eeman, MD, M. Henry, MD.
Kantonsspital Basel, Basel, Switzerland (24): M. Pfister, MD, Principal Investigator; F. Burkart, MD, W. Kiowski, MD, E. Straumann, MD, R. Schäfers, MD.
Medizinische Hochschule, Hannover, Germany (24)⁾:* W. Rafflenbeul, MD, Principal Investigator; D. Gulba, MD.
Hôpital Trousseau, Tours, France (12)⁾:* P. Raynaud, MD, Principal Investigator; B. Desvaux, MD, L. Quillet, MD.
Freeman Hospital, Newcastle-upon-Tyne, England (12)⁾:* D. S. Reid, FRCP, Principal Investigator; M. Been, MD, T. K. Oliver, DCRR, CHSM.
Herzzentrum Hirslanden, Zürich, Switzerland (8): M. Rothlin, MD, Principal Investigator; R. Tartini, MD, U. Dürst, MD, H. O. Hirzel, MD.
Universitäts Klinikum Virchow, Berlin, Germany (56): W. Rutsch, MD, H. Schmutzler, MD, Principal Investigators; J. Bott, MD.
Universitätsklinik, Kiel, Germany (32): R. Simon, MD, Principal Investigator; M. Höfig, MD, G. Herrmann, MD.
UCL Clinique de Mont-Godinne, Yvoir, Belgium (24)⁾:* E. Schroeder, MD, Principal Investigator; R. Krémer, MD, B. Marchandise, MD, P. Chenu, MD.
Thoraxcenter, Rotterdam, The Netherlands (56)⁾:* P. W. Serruys, MD, Principal Investigator; W. R. M. Hermans, MD, B. J. Rensing, MD.
Walsgrave Hospital, Coventry, England (15)⁾:* M. Fai Shiu, MD, Principal Investigator; J. Escaned, MD, R. Ahmed, MD.
Medizinische Klinik I, Aachen, Germany (40): R. Uebis, MD, Principal Investigator; J. vom Dahl, MD, C. Stellbrink, MD, S. Nase-Hüppmeier, MD.
St. Luc University Hospital, Brussels, Belgium (35)⁾:* W. Wijns, MD, Principal Investigator; J. M. Detry, MD, J. Col, MD, J. Cosyns, MD, C. Hanet, MD, X. Michel, MD, J. Renkin, MD.

Data Coordinating and Analysis

F. Hoffmann-La Roche Ltd., Basel, Switzerland
SOCAR SA, Givrins, Switzerland

Angiographic Core Laboratory

Cardialysis/Thoraxcenter, Rotterdam, The Netherlands: P. W. Serruys, MD, B. J. Rensing, MD, W. R. M. Hermans, MD, J. Pameyer.

Angiographic Assessment Committee

P. W. Serruys, MD (Chairman), W. R. M. Hermans, MD, R. Balcon MD, R. Uebis, MD, J. M. LaBlanche, MD, W. Rafflenbeul, MD.

Study Directors

Th. Widmann, MD, F. Hoffmann-La Roche Ltd., Basel, Switzerland.
P. G. Hugenholtz, MD, Ferme Mont-de-Vaux, Echichens, Switzerland.

References

1. Ambrose JA, Winters SL, Stern A, Eng A, Teichholz LE, Gorlin R, Fuster V (1985) Angiographic morphology and the pathogenesis of unstable angina pectoris. J Am Coll Cardiol 5:609—616
2. Barnathan ES, Schwartz JS, Taylor L, Laskey WK, Kleveland JP, Kussmaul WG, Hirshfeld JW (1987) Aspirin and dipyridamole in the prevention of acute coronary thrombosis complicating coronary angioplasty. Circulation 76:125—134
3. Bilazarian SD, Currier JW, Haudenschild C, Heyman D, Powell J, Ryan TJ, Faxon DP (1991) Angiotensin converting enzyme inhibition reduces restenosis in experimental angioplasty [abstract]. J Am Coll Cardiol 17:2:268A
4. Burnier M, Mooser V, Nussberger J, Waeber B, Brunner HR (1989) Correlation between plasma concentration of cilazapril and hemodynamic and hormonal effects in healthy man. Br J Clin Pharmac 27:189S—197S
5. Califf RM, Ohman EM, Frid DJ, Fortin DF, Mark DB, Hlatky MS, Herndon JE, Bengtson JR (1990) Restenosis: The clinical issues, in Topol EJ (ed): Textbook of Interventional Cardiology. Philadelphia, WB Saunders Co, 63:394
6. Christen Y, Waeber B, Nussberger J, Porchet M, Borland RM, Lee RJ, Shum L, Timmermans PBMWH, Brunner HR (1991) Oral administration of DuP 753, a specific angiotensin II receptor antagonist, to normal male volunteers. Inhibition of pressor response to exogenous angiotensin I and II. Circulation 83:1333—1342
7. Churchill DA, Siegel CO, Dougherety KG, Raizner A, Minor ST (1991) Failure of enalapril to reduce coronary restenosis in a swine model (abstract). Circulation 84:4:II—297
8. Daemen MJAP, Lombardi DM, Bosman FT, Schwartz SM (1991) Angiotensin II induces smooth muscle cell proliferation in the normal and injured rat arterial wall. Circ Res 68:450—456
9. Detre K, Holubkov R, Kelsey S, Cowley M, Kent K, Williams D, Myler R, Faxon D, Holmes D Jr, Bourassa M, Block P, Gosselin A, Bentivoglio L, Leatherman L, Dorros G, King S III, Galichia J, Al-Bassam M, Leon M, Robertson T, Passamani E, Co-Investigators of the NHLBI PTCA Registry (1988) Percutaneous Transluminal Coronary Angioplasty in 1985—1986 and 1977—1981. The National Heart Lung Blood Institute Registry. N Engl J Med 318:265—270

10. Dorros G, Cowley MJ, Simpson J, Bentifoglio LG, Block PC, Bourassa M, Detre K, Gosselin AJ, Gruentzig AR, Kelsey SF, Kent KM, Mock MB, Mullins SM, Myler RK, Passamani ER, Stertzer SH, Williams DO (1983) Percutaneous transluminal coronary angioplasty: Report of complications from the National Heart, Lung, and Blood Institute PTCA Registry. Circulation 67:4:723—730
11. Fingerle J, Au YPT, Clowes AW, Reidy MA (1990) Intimal lesion formation in rat carotid arteries after endothelial denudation in absence of medial injury. Atheriosclerosis 10:1082—1087
12. Fingerle J, Johnson R, Clowes AW, Majesky MW, Reidy MA (1989) Role of platelets in smooth muscle cell proliferation and migration after vascular injury in rat carotid artery. Proc Natl Acad Sci 86:8412—8416
13. Flemming RM, Kirkeeide RL, Smalling RW, Gould KL, Stuart Y (1991) Patterns in visual interpretation of coronary arteriograms as detected by quantitative coronary arteriography. J Am Coll Cardiol 18:945—951
14. Forrester JS, Fishbein M, Helfant R, Fagin J (1991) A paradigm for restenosis based on cell biology: clues for the development of new preventive therapies. J Am Coll Cardiol 17:758—769
15. Gruentzig AR, Senning A, Siegenthaler WE (1979) Nonoperative dilatation of coronary artery stenosis: Percutaneous transluminal coronary angioplasty. N Engl J Med 301:61—68
16. Hammacher A, Hellman U, Johnsson A, Östman A, Gunnarsson K, Westermark, B, Wasteson Ä, Heldin CH (1988) A major part of platelet-derived growth factor purified from human platelets is a heteromer of one A and one B chain. J Biol Chem 263:16493—16498
17. Hanson SR, Powell JS, Dodson T, Lumsden A, Kelly AB, Anderson JS, Clowes AW, Harker LA (1991) Effects of angiotensin-converting enzyme inhibition with cilazapril on intimal hyperplasia in injured arteries and vascular grafts in the baboon. Hypertension 18 (suppl II):70—76
18. Hermans WRM, Rensing BJ, Strauss BH, Serruys PW (1991) Prevention of restenosis after percutaneous transluminal coronary angioplasty (PTCA): The search for a "magic bullet". Am Heart J 122:1:171—187
19. Huber KC, Schwartz RS, Edwards WD, Camrud AR, Murphy JG, Jorgenson M, Holmes DR (1991) Restenosis and angiotensin-converting enzyme inhibition: effects on neointimal proliferation in a porcine coronary injury model (abstract). Circulation 84:4:II—298
20. Jawien A, Lindner V, Bowen-Pope DF, Schwartz SM, Reidy MA, Clowes AW (1990) Platelet derived growth factor (PDGF) stimulates arterial smooth muscle cell proliferation in vivo (abstract). FASEB 4:342
21. Kaltenbach M, Kober G, Scherer D, Vallbracht C (1985) Recurrence rate after successful angioplasty. Eur Heart J 6:276—281
22. Lam JYT, Bourassa MG, Blaine L, Lachapelle C (1990) Can cilazapril reduce the development of atherosclerotic changes in the balloon injured porcine carotid arteries? (abstract). Circulation 82:4:III—429
23. Leimgruber PP, Roubin GS, Hollman J, Cotsonis GA, Meier B, Douglas JS, King III SB, Gruentzig AR (1986) Restenosis after successful angioplasty in patients with single-vessel disease. Circulation 73:710—717
24. Lindner V, Reidy MA (1991) Proliferation of smooth muscle cells after vascular injury is inhibited by an antibody against basic fibroblast growth factor. Proc Natl Acad Sci 88:3739—3743
25. Lindner V, Lappi DA, Baird A, Majack RA, Reidy MA (1991) Role of basic fibroblast growth factor in vascular lesion formation. Circ Res 68:106—113
26. Liu MW, Roubin GS, King SB (1989) Restenosis after coronary angioplasty. Potential biologic determinants and role of intimal hyperplasia. Circulation 79: 1374—1387

27. Mabin TA, Holmes DR Jr, Smith HC, Vlietstra RE, Bove AA, Reeder GS, Chesebro JH, Bresnahan JF, Orszulak TA (1985) Intracoronary thrombus: Role in coronary occlusion complicating percutaneous transluminal coronary angioplasty. J Am Coll Cardiol 5:198—202
28. Majesky MW, Reidy MA, Bowen-Pope DF, Hart CE, Wilcox JN, Schwartz SM (1990) PDGF ligand and receptor gene expression during repair ligand. J Cell Biol 111:2149—2158
29. Naftilan AJ, Pratt RE, Dzau VJ (1989) Induction of platelet derived growth factor A chain and C-myc gene expressions by angiotensin II in culture rat vascular smooth muscle cells. J Clin Invest 83:1419—1424
30. Nussberger J, Brunner DB, Waeber B, Brunner HR (1985) True versus immunoreactive angiotensin II in human plasma. Hypertension 7 (suppl I):1—17
31. Owens GK, Schwartz SM (1983) Vascular smooth muscle cell hypertrophy and hyperploidy in the Goldblatt hypertensive rat. Cir Res 53:491—500
32. Owens GK, Reidy MA (1985) Hyperplastic growth response of vascular smooth muscle cells following induction of acute hypertension in rats by aortic coarctation. Cir Res 57:659—670
33. Owens GK (1987) Influences of blood pressure on development of aortic medial smooth muscle hypertrophy in spontaneously hypertensive rats. Hypertension 9:178—187
34. Powell JS, Clozel JP, Müller RKM, Kuhn H, Hefti F, Hosang M, Baumgartner HR (1989) Inhibitors of angiotensin-converting enzyme prevent myointimal proliferation after vascular injury. Science 245:186—188
35. Powell JS, Muller RKM, Rouge M, Kuhn H, Hefti F, Baumgartner HR (1990) The proliferative response to vascular injury is suppressed by angiotensin-converting enzyme inhibition. J Cardiovasc Pharmacology 16 (suppl 4):S42—S49
36. Powell JS, Rouge M, Muller RK, Baumgartner HR (1991) Cilazapril suppresses myointimal proliferation after vascular injury: effects on growth factor induction and vascular smooth muscle cells. Basic Research in Cardiology 86 (suppl I):65—74
37. Rakugi H, Krieger J, Wang DS, Dzau VJ, Pratt RE (1991) Induction of angiotensin converting enzyme in neointima after balloon injury (abstract). Circulation 84:4:II—113
38. Reiber JHC, Serruys PW, Kooyman CJ, Wijns W, Slager CJ, Gerbrands M, Schuurbiers JCH, den Boer A, Hugenholtz PG (1985) Assessment of short, medium and long term variations in arterial dimensions from computer assisted quantification of coronary cineangiograms. Circulation 71:280—288
39. Reiber JHC, Serruys PW (1990) Quantitative coronary angiography, in Marcus ML, Schelbert HR, Skorton DJ, Wolf GL (ed): Cardiac Imaging: A Companion to Braunwald's Heart Disease. Philadelphia, WB Saunders Co, pp 211—280
40. Rensing BJ, Hermans WRM, Deckers JW, de Feyter PJ, Tijssen JGP, Serruys PW (1992) Luminal narrowing after percutaneous transluminal coronary balloon angioplasty follows a near gaussian distribution. A quantitative angiographic study in 1445 successfully dilated lesions. J Am Coll Cardiol 9:939—945
41. Ross R (1986) The pathogenesis of atherosclerosis. An update. N Engl J Med 314:488—500
42. Sahni R, Maniet AR, Voci G, Banka VS (1991) Prevention of restenosis by lovastatin after successful angioplasty. Am Heart J 121:1600—1608
43. Schwartz SM, Campbell GR, Campbell JH (1986) Replication of smooth muscle cells in vascular disease. Circ Res 58:427—444
44. Schwartz L, Bourassa MG, Lesperance J, Aldridge HE, Kazim F, Salvatori VA, Henderson M, Bonan R, David PR (1988) Aspirin and dipyridamole in the prevention of restenosis after percutaneous transluminal coronary angioplasty. N Engl J Med 318:1714—1719
45. Schwartz RS, Huber KC, Edwards WD, Camrud AR, Jorgenson M, Holmes DR (1991) Coronary restenosis and the importance of mural thrombus: results in a porcine coronary model (abstract). Circulation 84:4:II—71

46. Scott-Burden T, Resink TJ, Hahn AWA, Bühler FR (1990) Induction of thrombospondin expression in vascular smooth muscle cells by angiotensin II. J Cardiovasc Pharm 16 (suppl 7):17—20
47. Serruys PW, Luijten HE, Beatt KJ, Geuskens R, de Feyter PJ, van den Brand M, Reiber JHC, Ten Katen HJ, van Es GA, Hugenholtz PG (1988) Incidence of restenosis after successful coronary angioplasty: a time related phenomenon. A quantitative angiographic study in 342 consecutive patients at 1, 2, 3 and 4 months. Circulation 77:361—371
48. Serruys PW, Rensing BJ, Luijten HE, Hermans WRM, Beatt KJ (1990) Restenosis following coronary angioplasty. In Meier B (ed) Interventional Cardiology. Bern: Hogrefe and Huber Publishers, 79:115
49. Serruys PW, Rutsch W, Heyndrickx GR, Danchin N, Mast G, Wijns W, Rensing BJ, Vos J, Stibbe J (1991) for the CARPORT study group. Prevention of restenosis after percutaneous transluminal coronary angioplasty with thromboxane A2 receptor blockade. A randomized, double blind, placebo controlled trial. Circulation 84:1568—1580
50. Steele PM, Chesebro JH, Stanson AW, Holmes DR Jr, Dewanjee MK, Badimon L, Fuster V (1985) Balloon angioplasty: Natural history of the pathophysiological response to injury in the pig model. Cir Res 57:105—112
51. The Multicenter European Research Trial with Cilazapril after angioplasty to prevent transluminal coronary obstruction and restenosis (Mercator) study Group (1992) Circulation 86:100—110
52. Vandormael MG, Deligonul U, Kern M, Harper M, Presant S, Gibson P, Galan K, Chaitman BR (1987) Multilesion coronary angioplasty: clinical and angiographic follow-up. J Am Coll Cardiol 10:246—252
53. Wilentz JR, Sanborn TA, Haudenschild CC, Valeri CR, Ryan TJ, Faxon DP (1987) Platelet accumulation in experimental angioplasty: time course and relation to vascular injury. Circulation 75:636—642

Authors' address:
G. R. Heyndrickx, MD, PhD, FACC
Cardiovascular Center
Onze Lieve Vrouw Ziekenhuis
Moorselbaan 164
B-9300 Aalst

Pathophysiology of heart failure and the renin-angiotensin-system

J. Holtz

Institut für Pathophysiologie, Martin-Luther-Universität, Halle-Wittenberg, FRG

Summary: For more than a decade, the inhibition of the renin-angiotensin system in heart failure has been regarded as pure vasodilator therapy. Consequently, the role of the renin-angiotensin system has been seen as contributing to hemodynamic overload by vascoconstriction and volume retention. Meanwhile, clinical experience was indicated that important additional aspects of ACE-inhibition in heart failure are attenuation of the enhanced neuroendocrine activity and reversal or prevention of inappropriate trophic reactions of the overloaded myocardium. In overloaded hearts there is enhanced intracardiac formation of angiotensin due to enhanced expression of angiotensinogen and ACE, and due to accumulation of circulating, nephrogenic active renin. In human hearts, a mast-cell-derived chymase, which is not blocked by ACE-inhibition, contributes to intracardiac angiotensin formation. The enhanced intracardiac angiotensin-II formation in overloaded hearts is involved in coronary constriction, impairment of diastolic relaxation, myocyte enlargement and interstitial fibrosis, which aggravate the diastolic impairment. The major problem in overloaded, hypertrophied cardiocytes is the dedifferentiation with instabilization of Ca^{++}-homeostasis due to an altered program of gene expression. Dedifferentiated cardiocytes have a reduced expression of sarcoplasmic reticulum Ca^{++}-ATPase and an enhanced expression of the sarcolemmal Na^{+}/Ca^{++}-exchanger, resulting in an attenuation of active diastole (Ca^{++}-reaccumulation into the sarcoplasmic reticulum), a depressed force-frequency relation, and an enhanced susceptibility for fatal arrhythmias. Furthermore, an enhanced local renin-angiotensin system in distensible coronary and systemic arteries seems to contribute to a reduced releasability of endothelium-derived relaxing factor, probably by reducing bradykinin availability. This modulation of endothelial function appears to contribute to the localization and progression of atheroma development in presence of risks factors for atherosclerosis.

Key words: Cardiac angiotensin formation; myocardial hypertrophy; cardiocyte dedifferentiation; cardiocyte Ca^{++}-homeostais; sarcoplasmic reticulum Ca^{++}-ATPase; endothelial function

Introduction

The ever growing interest in the role of the renin-angiotensin-system in the pathophysiology of congestive heart failure has been fueled, to a major extent, by the dramatic effects of chronic treatment with ACE-inhibitors in this fatal syndrome. Looking back, one receives the impression of some kind of shift in the general view on the question as to which of the several benefical mechanisms of ACE-inhibition might by relevant for its preventive potential in heart failure. Accordingly, our view on the pathophysiologic role of the renin-angiotensin system in congestive heart failure became more and more complex (Fig. 1).

Originally, ACE-inhibition was regarded as acting mainly by systemic vasodilation, similar to other vasodilators. Therefore, the pathophysiologic role of an activated renin-angiotensin system in failure was seen in its direct constrictor effects, contributing to the vicious cycle of enhanced hemodynamic overload due to compensatory pressoric activation, this overload being enhanced by the renal and adrenal effects of the activated RAS with the resultant retention of salt and volume.

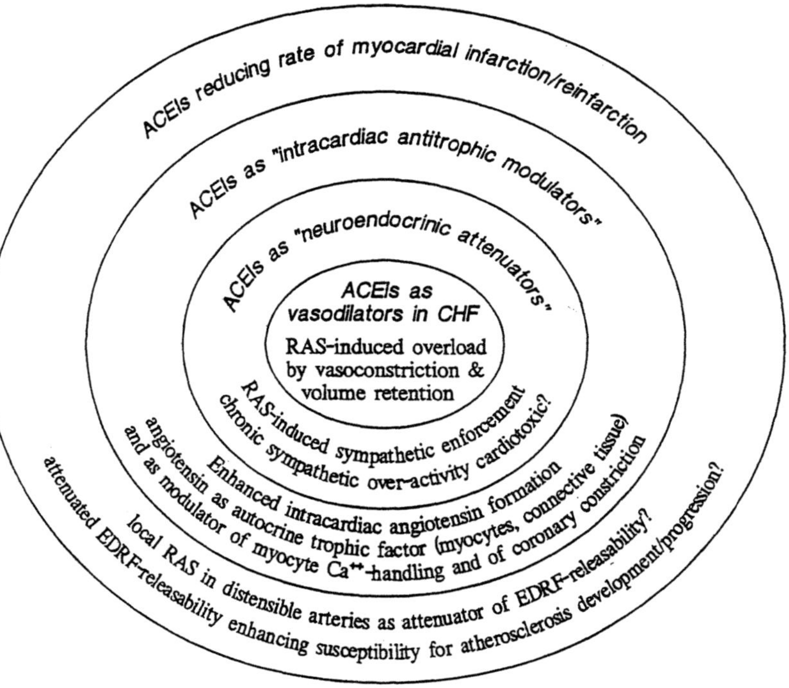

Fig. 1. The expanding preventive and therapeutic potential of angiotensin converting enzyme inhibitors (ACEIs) in congestive heart failure (CHF) indicates our growing awareness of the complexity of the pathophysiologic role of the renin-angiotensin system (RAS) in congestive heart failure. To our original view of ACEIs as vasodilators and of the RAS as a pressor system (central part of the circles), new aspects are emerging from clinical studies with the application of ACEIs in patients with CHF.

Very soon, however, it became clear that ACE-inhibition had a therapeutic potential in congestive heart failure which could not be mimicked by the combination of other systemic vasodilators and diuretics (35, 52, 53). Therefore, additional non-vasodilator actions of angiotensin were regarded, especially the enhancement of the sympathoadrenal system. A typical question out of that period was: "What is the direct cardiotoxic action of chronic neuroendocrine overactivation in congestive heart failure?," and the attenuation of this sympathetic overactivation was seen as the important addition of ACE-inhibition to its pure dilator action (69, 20).

A further expansion in the complexity of the system's pathophysiologic role in failure appeared when experimental and clinical observations indicated that angiotensin might be formed locally in the heart, that this local formation is probably enhanced in overloaded hearts, and that this locally formed angiotensin could act in an autocrine manner as a trophic factor, as a direct modulator of contraction and Ca^{++}-handling, and as a local coronary constrictor.

This setup of potential pathophysiologic actions of the RAS in heart failure was discussed in the attempt to explain the efficacy of chronic ACE-inhibition in the management of patients with overt, severe failure, as documented in recent clinical trials (18, 19). The logical next step, testing the impact of ACE-inhibitor treatment on prognosis early in developing heart failure, documented the preventive potential of this treatment (84, 85, 73). Furthermore, it added a new dimension to the complex role of the RAS in the pathophysiology of heart failure: The rate of myocardial reinfarction (or of first infarction in patients of the SOLVD trial without prior infarction) was reduced significantly by the long-term ACE-inhibition. This effect was not anticipated when these megatrials were designed, and the mechanism behind this reduction of recurrent infarction remains unexplained at present. It appears that reduction of blood pressure is not the critical mechanism for the reduction of myocardial infarction by the ACE-inhibitors. This reduction of infarction risk was demonstrable whether hypertension was present or not, whether angina or documented ischemic heart disease were present or not, and concurrent treatment with other drugs did not interfere with this ACE-inhibitor-specific effect. As stated recently: "... it is quite possible that these very large trials may have uncovered an important, previously unrecognized therapeutic action of these drugs" (17). An obvious speculation concentrates on an involvement of ACE in the pathogenesis or aggravation of arteriosclerosis, and some clinical and experimental observations can be mentioned in support of such speculation (see below). It has to be stressed: definitive proof for such an important antiatherosclerotic potential of ACE-inhibition in humans is not yet available and must await subgroup-analysis of the heart failure megatrials as well as the outcome of further ongoing clinical trials, designed specifically to address this question (such as PART: Prevention of Atherosclerosis with Ramipril Treatment; QIET: Quinapril Ischemic Event Trial). Nevertheless, an exciting and unexpected extension to the many facets of the renin-angiotensin-system and its role in heart failure is appearing (Fig. 1).

Recent reviews have discussed the pathophysiological role of the RAS in heart failure with emphasis on the classical "inner core" (Fig. 1) of the system's actions (for example, see (42)). In this text, I will consider the less well characterized, only recently identified "outher shells" (Fig. 1) of that complex field.

Intracardiac angiotensin formation

The general relevance of the so-called extrarenal "tissue renin-angiotensin systems" is illustrated by the fact that the major part of circulating angiotensins I and II is not originating in the circulating blood, but results from spill-over into the blood after local synthesis in extrarenal (and renal) tissue (12, 13, 2, 3). This conclusion was derived from the kinetic analyses of the formation and degradation of circulating angiotensins in animals and humans. It was supported by demonstrating the expression of messenger RNA and the protein synthesis of all elements of the RAS in extrarenal tissues (see also the contribution of Dzau in this volume). The messenger RNAs for angiotensinogen, prorenin, and ACE have been detected in cardiac tissue of rats (7), and, recently, the expression of ACE was also measured after standard-calibrated amplification by a RNA polymerase chain reaction in human ventricular myocardium (87).

The evidence that angiotensins can be formed locally in the heart is of great importance for understanding potential cardiac actions of the RAS. Circulating blood levels of angiotensin-II, even in severe heart failure, do not reach concentrations necessary for acute actions on myocyte contraction and Ca^{++}-handling, presynaptic modulation of transmitter release from sympathetic nerve endings or coronary constriction. Similarly, trophic actions of angiotensin-II in cell culture systems are only demonstrable at concentrations for the above blood levels in vivo. However, if local formation at the site of intracardiac action is demonstrable, all these angiotensin actions are possible in the heart in a paracrine manner.

While there is little doubt with regard to the possibility of intracardiac angiotensin formation, its exact quantification is difficult. Furthermore, possible contributions from nephrogenic renin to this local intracardiac formation are unclear. While prorenin synthesis might occur in many tissues (as concluded from mRNA detection), the cleavage of prorenin to active renin has not yet been documented in tissues outside the kidneys. In extracts from cardiac tissue, renin activity is demonstrable, and functional data in isolated, perfused hearts indicate intracardiac renin activity (see below). However, it is not clear to what extent this cardiac renin activity results from uptake and binding of circulating renal renin, local cleavage of cardiac prorenin to active renin or from cleavage-independent activation of prorenin due to alteration of its configuration during binding. For the moment, the cardiac RAS cannot be regarded as entirely independent from the circulating, "nephrocentric" RAS, which does not invalidate the arguments for intracardiac angiotensin formation.

Besides the classical pathway for angiotensin-II formation via renin and ACE, other pathways are possible in many tissues (for review see (24)), including a "chymostatin-sensitive angiotensin generating enzyme". In human myocardial tissue, such an enzyme was identified, purified and characterized as a neutral serine protease (91). The gene for this human cardiac enzyme with high specificity for the conversion of angiotensin-I to angiotensin-II (45) has been cloned and sequenced (92). Its genomic structure indicates homology to the chymase enzyme family and it is considered as a mast-cell-specific enzyme (43). This "human heart chymase" (hHC) represents roughly 90% of the angiotensin-II-forming capacity detectable in tissue extracts from human myocardium. This capacity is insensitive to ACE-inhibition and does not degrade bradykinin. However, these data from tissue extracts do not indicate that hHC is the major pathway for cardiac angiotensin formation in vivo. In-situ hybridization and immuno-cytochemistry indicates that hHC is formed and stored in granules of the mast-cells. Once released after mast-cell activation, it is bound to interstitial proteins of connective tissue and appears to retain some of its activity. Thus, the intercellular connective tissue of the human heart seems to act as a secondary pool for this enzyme after mast-cell challenge. Preparation of cardiac tissue extracts must include activity of a mast-cell specific enzyme. However, the contribution of this mast-cell derived hHC to intracardiac angiotensin-II formation under physiological conditions in vivo without mast-cell activation is entirely unknown.

Most studies on the functional role of intracardiac angiotensin formation and its sensitivity to ACE-inhibition have been performed in the rat. However, an angiotensin-II-forming enzyme analogous to hHC appears not to exist in the heart of rats. Thus, the relevance of the ACE-inhibitor sensitive pathway of intracardiac angiotensin-II formation must not be identical between man and rat. This species difference requires caution in extrapolating from experimental data to the clinical situation.

Enhanced angiotensin formation in growing or failing myocardium?

Augmentations in the expression of mRNA for angiotensinogen and for ACE in ventricular tissue have been described in various models of cardiac overload and failure (8, 78, 30, 54). The cardiac expression of angiotensinogen mRNA is roughly two decades lower than the respective expression in the liver (25), but it results in the synthesis of the mature, renin-accessible propeptide: in isolated perfused hearts, angiotensin-I release can be enhanced by adding active renin to the perfusate (53). Enhanced myocardial angiotensinogen mRNA is found in several rat models of cardiac overload: left ventricular hyperthrophy induced by hypertension (8), hypertrophied left ventricular rest-myocardium in rats surviving myocardial infarction (54), and failing, dilated left ventricular myocardium without hypertrophy in the tachypacing-induced congestive heart failure (30). In the infarction model, the overexpression of angiotensinogen mRNA was transient and appeared to be associated with enhanced systolic wall stress (54). In the tachypacing model, ectopic distribution of the pacing-evoked action potential might have resulted in localized presystolic stretch of not yet activated myocytes by early contracting myocytes, and this heterogeneous stretching has been discussed as a potential activator of angiotensinogen overexpression (40). However, the regulation of enhanced angiotensinogen expression in cardiac overload is largely unknown.

Overload-induced increases in cardiac ACE expression (78) and in ACE activity have been documented by several groups: elevated ACE activity (measured as hydrolysis of an ACE-specific substrate) was observed in myocardial tissue extracts of hypertrophied left ventricles in rats with hypertension due to suprarenal coarctation of the abdominal aorta (8, 75), of noninfarcted rest-myocardium of normotensive rats with chronic infarctions (38), of hypertrophied rat ventricles after isoproterenol treatment (66) and in hypertrophied right ventricles of rats with pulmonary artery banding (unpublished from our laboratory). Enhanced ventricular ACE concentration has also been measured by a radioligand binding assay in rats with chronic experimental heart failure (29). In isolated perfused hearts with overload-induced hypertrophy, enhanced conversion of perfusate angiotensin-I to angiotensin-II (78) and enhanced hydrolysis of an ACE-specific substrate in the perfusate (unpublished from our laboratory) has been documented.

The critical question is whether these observations on enhanced cardiac ACE in rats can be extended to the situation in the overloaded human myocardium (see above). Therefore, we developed a standard-quantified RNA polymerase chain reaction for measuring cardiac ACE-mRNA abundancy, which is extremely low in human ventricular tissue (87). By this technique, we observed a twofold higher level of left ventricular ACE-mRNA per total RNA in patients with end-stage heart failure, compared to the ventricular levels of potential heart donors, whose hearts were not used for transplantation. The elevated ACE-expression was similar in transplant recipients with dilated cardiomyopathy or with coronary artery disease (87). This result indicates that the observations on overload-induced enhancement of ACE expression in rats can be extended to humans, regardless of the species differences in mast-cell specific heart chymase (see above).

The mechanism triggering the augmentation of cardiac ACE expression is not clear. By comparing the various rat models with enhanced myocardial tissue ACE activity, one might speculate that enhanced diastolic and/or systolic wall stress yields the trigger for that alteration in expression (for discussion see (39)). The augmentation of ventricular tissue ACE after the induction of hemodynamic overload is a rather delayed response and therefore might be secondary to the formation of unidentified trophic signals within the overloaded, growing myocardium. It is not known exactly to what extent different cell types within the ventricular tissue contribute to the enhanced cardiac ACE-expression, but the weight of functional analyses indicates that the coronary endothelium is the major source of cardiac ACE, both in normal and overloaded hearts (60, 27, 40). The enhanced expression of ACE-mRNA in patients with endstage heart failure (87) is compatible with the hypothesis of an upregulation of expression by elevated wall stress. However, the scatter of expression within donor hearts and within failing hearts was very large as compared to the differences in mean values between these two groups (87). Since this scatter cannot be due to methodological imprecision, other factors must contribute substantially to the regulation of ACE expression in the human hearts.

While experiments in rats documented an enhanced number of mast cells in overloaded ventricles, it is not clear whether the hHC is augmented in human cardiac hypertrophy, either within the mast-cell granules or in its released, interstitially bound form. The releasability of an angiotensin-II-forming enzyme by inflammatory cells (mast-cells) in human hearts and preliminary reports on angiotensin-II formation by activated leukocytes indicate that angiotensin might contribute to the large group of trophic stimuli activated during processes of tissue damage and repair. Certainly, the rapid induction of enhanced hemodynamic overload in experimental models or in clinical myocardial infarction includes homologies to the inflammatory pattern of damage and repair reactions. Elevations in local myocardial renin activity in failing hearts could reflect contamination from enhanced circulating renin activity and cannot yet indicate alterations in local renin formation and/or activation.

In summary: there is little doubt about an enhanced intracardiac angiotensin-II formation in cardiac overload, but the exact quantification of this enhancement is still imprecise and requires speculative assumptions.

Functional consequences of the activated cardiac renin-angiotensin system in overload hypertrophy

The existence of such functional effects of an activated cardiac RAS is concluded indirectly from monitoring acute cardiac effects of intracoronary infusion of ACE-inhibitors at dosages without systemic effects in patients (32, 34) and from analyzing the effects of ACE-inhibitors in the perfusate of isolated perfused, hypertrophied rat hearts (58).

In patients with left ventricular hypertrophy due to aortic stenosis, the intracoronary infusion of enalaprilat caused reduced enddiastolic pressure, improved diastolic distensibility and somewhat lowered peak systolic pressure in the left ventricles, but showed no effects on the systemic circulating RAS or on right heart loading (34). A similar intracoronary infusion in patients with dilated cardiomyopathy improved left-ventricular diastolic function, moderately reduced left ventricular contractility and lowered coronary vascular resistance without causing systemic hemodynamic effects (32). These observations are consistent with the hypothesis that an enhanced, ACE-mediated angiotensin formation in failing human hearts impairs diastolic left ventricular function, marginally contributes to the maintenance of systolic function, and reduces myocardial perfusion by coronary constriction.

Qualitatively similar conclusions can be obtained from experiments with isolated perfused, hypertrophied rat hearts: ACE-sensitive conversion of perfusate angiotensin-I to angiotensin-II is enhanced in the these hypertrophied hearts (78), and ACE-inhibition in the perfusate improves diastolic relaxation (78) or attenuates the deterioration of diastolic function caused by low-flow ischemia (26); both effects could not be explained by improvements of coronary perfusion. Furthermore, angiotensin-II in the perfusate caused a significantly stronger impairment of diastolic function in hypertrophied hearts compared to control hearts, and this effect was not explained by stronger coronary constriction and was blocked by AT_1 receptor antagonists (56).

The most straight forward explanation for these clinical and experimental observations is the assumption of an enhanced intracardiac angiotensin-II formation in hypertrophied failing human hearts in vivo and in hypertrophied isolated rats hearts in vitro, sufficient for directly affecting contractile performance of myocytes (58). Acute cardiac actions of angiotensin-II encompass coronary vasoconstriction and presynaptic enhancement of sympathetic neurotransmission (94, 71) and a direct, positive inotropic action (highly variable between species) without acceleration diastolic relaxation (28, 53, 7). Several mechanisms are discussed as a basis for these myocyte effects of angiotensin-II: receptor-mediated activation of phosphlipase C with formation of inositol trisphosphate promoting Ca^{++}-release from the sarcoplasmic reticulum; activation of diacyl glycerol and the protein kinase C system promoting enhanced Ca^{++}-influx via L-type channels and enhanced myofilament Ca^{++}-sensitivity due to intracellular alkalosis (41). The enhanced cytosolic Ca^{++}-load under angiotensin-II action could impair diastolic relaxation in hearts with fragile Ca^{++}-homeostasis due to lowered expression of the sarcoplasmic Ca^{++}-ATPase (see below), especially in cases with hypoperfusion-induced impairment of sarcoplasmic reticulum Ca^{++}-ATPase.

It should be stressed that in all these clinical and experimental examples, the ACE-inhibitor could have affected diastolic function, not only by suppressing intracardiac angiotensin-II formation, but also by releasing an unknown mediator due to reduced degradation of another peptide (e.g., bradykinin). However, intracoronary application of AT_1-receptor antagonists in similar settings in vivo and in vitro is now possible and should demonstrate (in my expectation) that the acute intracardiac effects of ACE-inhibitors on diastolic function are mediated to a larger part by suppression angiotensin-II formation. This remains to be shown.

Trophic effects of an activated cardiac renin-angiotensin system

The interest in such a trophic role results from in vitro studies on angiotensin effects in cultured cardiomyocytes and from in vivo studies in rats with the chronic application of ACE-inhibitors or angiotensin-II. Because of the species differences in the pathways of angiotensin-II formation between human and rat (see above), results on regression or prevention of overload hypertrophy by ACE-inhibitors in rats must not necessarily be applicable to humans.

However, the available clinical evidence indicates that treatment by ACE-inhibitors is effective, indeed, in regressing human cardiac hypertrophy. In a recent meta-analysis of 104 studies on the regression of left ventricular hypertrophy as assessed by echocardiography, various forms of antihypertensive treatment were compared (21). According to this meta-analysis, ACE-inhibitors are significantly more effective in reversing left ventricular mass than β-blockers or Ca^{++}-antagonists, and this difference was independent from the duration of treatment and from the obtained decline in blood pressure (21). This overview yields solid proof for a direct antitrophic action of ACE-inhibition on human cardiac hypertrophy, parallel to the observations in rats.

Several studies documented regression or prevention of left ventricular hypertrophy by a direct action of ACE-inhibitors in spontaneously hypertensive rats (by comparison with the effect of sympatholythics or vasodilators (81, 72), in the renin-independent model of hypertension due to suprarenal aortic coarctation (by low, non-hypotensive doses of ACE-inhibition (8, 5) and in a high-renin model of renal hypertension (also by low, non-hypotensive dosage of ACE-inhibition (55). An increase in left ventricular mass was observed with chronic infusions of angiotensin-II in rats in subpressor doses (7). In the rat model of coarctation hypertension, treatment by non-hypotensive doses of two AT_1-receptor antagonists partially normalized the left ventricular hypertrophy (Holtz et al. submitted). In addition to these in vivo studies, recent observations in vitro documented a direct trophic action of angiotensin-II in cultured embryonic cardiocytes of chickens (1, 6) and in cardiocytes from neonatal and adult rats (7).

Together with the documented enhancement of intracardiac angiotensin-II formation (see above), these data are regarded as indicating a direct, pressure-independent antitrophic action of ACE-inhibition by reducing the intracardiac formation of the cardiotrophic factor angiotensin-II.

However, this conclusion is probably an over-simplification! In two rat models of hypertension-induced hypertrophy, the antitrophic effect of non-hypotensive ACE-inhibition on the heart was attenuated or abolished by chronic co-administration of a bradykinin-2 receptor antagonist (5, 55). This co-treatment by the bradykinin-receptor antagonist was without any effect on blood pressure and indicated that the ACE-inhibition could have acted antitrophically by reducing the availability of bradykinin (5). As explained in the last chapter of this text, some indirect arguments indicate that bradykinin can upregulate the EDRF-releasability from endothelial cells, probably by inducing enhanced expression of endothelial nitric oxide synthase. EDRF from the coronary microcirculation can affect contractile performance of the heart (31, 82). In many cells systems, nitric oxide exerts an antiproliferative or antitrophic action (62). It is well conceivable that coronary ACE modulates trophic reactions of the myocardium, not only by angiotensin-II formation, but also via up- or downregulation of the endothelial nitric oxide synthase.

Since the enhanced ACE activity in the hypertrophied myocardium is an integral part of the activated cardiac renin-angiotensin system, any cardiotrophic modulation by ACE via nitric oxide formation would still be a trophic action of the cardiac RAS, but an action independent from angiotensin. Probably, the activated cardiac RAS modulates the myocardial hypertrophy by an angiotensin-dependent and an angiotensin-independent pathway.

Hypertrophy-induced myocyte dedifferentiation and instabilization of Ca^{++}-homeostasis

The cardiac hypertrophy in response to hemodynamic overload is regarded as an adaptive response, reducing the overload-induced enhancement of myocardial wall stress by enhancing wall thickness, specifically by adding new contractile units to the overloaded heart. This addition occurs by myocyte hypertrophy and is associated with substantial phenotype changes of the growing myocytes due to an altered program of gene expression (for recent reviews see (79, 44, 64, 14)). This program results in a more fetal- or neonatal-like phenotype of the myocytes and it can be considered as a preparation of the cells for proliferation, which normally does not or only seldom occurs in cardiocytes of adult mammals. The overload-induced cardiac enlargement has been described as an "arrest in hypertrophy prior to proliferation" (83). The term "dedifferentiation" has been used for this altered myocyte phenotype resulting from the growth-induced, altered program of gene expression (39).

The clinical interest in the concept of myocyte dedifferentiation during overload hypertrophy results from the fact that it offers attractive explanations for the diastolic dysfunction of hypertrophied myocardium and for the enhanced cardiovascular risks associated with overload-induced enlargement of cardiocytes (39). Other changes in hypertrophied myocardium with relevance for diastolic dysfunction and for enhanced cardiovascular risk are alterations in the coronary system and enhanced interstitial fibrosis. They have been discussed in recent reviews (15, 86, 93) and will not be considered here.

The critical features of dedifferentiated myocardium have been summarized as a "fragile Ca^{++}-homeostasis" (88). The phenotype changes of dedifferentiated myocytes contributing to this instable CA^{++}-homeostasis are summarized in Table 1 together with the potential consequences of these alterations. As can be seen from this table, these consequences include an enhanced susceptibility for arrhythmias of various types, a myocyte-derived diastolic dysfunction independent from altered interstitial connective tissue, and a myocyte-derived lability of systolic function during enhanced frequencies of contraction, independent from the problem of tachycardia-induced hypoperfusion. Furthermore, the table demonstrates that the features of an instable myocyte Ca^{++}-homeostasis are found in human cardiac failure.

Experimental evidence in rats indicates that the enhanced cardiac ACE contributes directly to these phenotype changes, and that treatment by ACE-inhibition can induce a reversal of these critical phenotype alterations (40). Again, the critical question remains: can we conclude from the experience in rats that these phenotype changes in humans are reversible, too, under appropriate ACE-inhibitor treatment? This remains to be demonstrated. However, we have good reason for optimism: a recent study demonstrated reversibility of myocyte phenotype changes in man under therapeutic correction of hypothyreoidism (48) in exactly the same manner, as it had been demonstrated previously in rats (23). In rats, the reduction of hypertension-induced hypertrophy by non-hypotensive ACE-inhibitor treatment (which normalizes the elevated myocardial ACE activity) is associated with a renormalization of the depressed expression of the sarcoplasmic reticulum Ca^{++}-ATPase, the hallmark of the instable Ca^{++}-homeostasis (40).

Table 1. Labile myocyte Ca^{++}-homeostasis in overload cardiomyopathy

Alterations in phenotype	*Potential consequences of alteration*
Depressed expression of sarcoplasmic Ca^{++}-ATPase and of phospholamban (47, 65, 22, 59, 76, 77, 89)	Reduced rate of endsystolic, sarcoplasmic Ca^{++}-reaccumulation, resulting in reduced relaxation of myofibrils; aggravation of this relaxation disturbance during enhanced frequency of contraction or postextrasystolic potentiation (70); incomplete refilling of the sarcoplasmic reticulum and enhanced transsarcolemmal Ca^{++}-export (see below) cause reduced systolic sarcoplasmic Ca^{++}-release, resulting in a depressed myocardial force-frequency relation (37, 63)
Prolonged plateau-phase of action potential due to enhanced availability of channels for the transient outward current (A-channels, 90), but no reduction in density or activation of voltage-operated L-type Ca^{++}-channels	No reduction of transsarcolemmal Ca^{++}-influx during activation by action potential
Enhanced expression of sarcolemmal Na^{+}/Ca^{++}-exchanger (77)	Enhanced contribution of Na^{+}/Ca^{++}-exchanger to the elimination of cytosolic Ca^{++}-load; since the exchanger operates rheogenic (influx of 3 Na^{+} per 1 Ca^{++} exported, 74), transsarcolemmal export by this exchanger results in a depolarizing inward current Downregulated sarcoplasmic Ca^{++}-ATPase and maintained Ca^{++}-influx enhance the susceptibility for diastolic, sarcoplasmic Ca^{++}-induced Ca^{++}-release (49), causing delayed afterdepolarizations (by activating the enhanced rheogenic exchanger and Ca^{++}-activated K^{+}-channels, 33) and diastolic aftercontractions. *Consequence:* Susceptibility for non-reentrant arrhythmias and diastolic dysfunction
Delayed intermyocyte conduction of activation (probably due to altered isoform expression of gap-junction proteins and due to enhanced interstitial fibrosis)	Reduced stabilization of membrane polarization against localized depolarizing stimuli due to attenuated coupling of polarized cells (67); however, still sufficient coupling for conduction of suprathreshold depolarization *Consequence:* Susceptibility for non-reentrant and reentrant arrhythmias Aggravation of heterogenities of conduction, if hypertrophy-induced susceptibility for Ca^{++}-overload and ischemia-induced cytosolic acidification are combined (46) *Consequence:* Susceptibility for reentrant arrhythmias

Modified and extended from ref. 39

Vascular renin-angiotensin system as modulator of susceptibility for atherosclerosis?

As mentioned in the introduction, the results of the megatrials on ACE-inhibition in mild, developing heart failure brought this or similar speculative questions to the notion of the medical community. These questions are still vague. Nevertheless, they triggered the design and the start of clinical trials testing the anti-atherosclerotic potential of chronic ACE-inhibition (see introduction). Furthermore, these observations on the reduction of recurrent myocardial infarction in the heart failure trials coincided with other recent clinical and experimental observations, dealing with the question formulated in the headline. They will be listed here briefly and will be incorporated into a preliminary and very speculative proposal for a unifying hypothesis (Fig. 2).

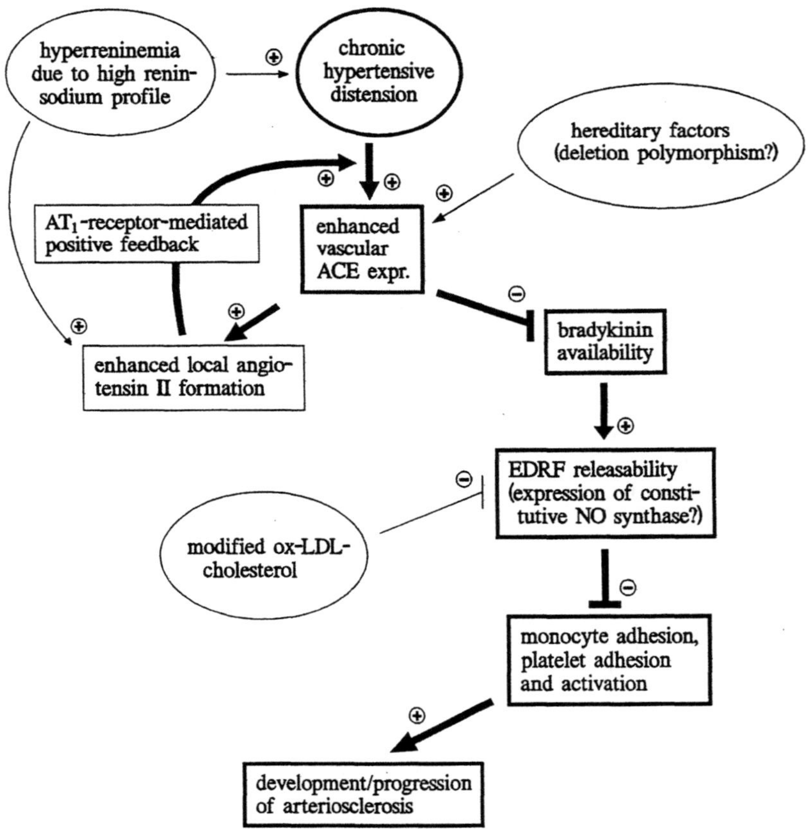

Fig. 2. Hypothetic scheme incorporating the vascular renin-angiotensin system as a modulator of the susceptibility for atherosclerosis in large, distensible arteries. Abbreviations: EDRF: endothelium-derived relaxing factor; NO: nitric oxide; ox-LDL: oxidatively modified low density lipoprotein; ACE: angiotensin converting enzyme; AT: angiotensin-II. Central elements of this hypothesis are: 1) the inhibitory effect of EDRF on monocyte adhesion, on expression of monocyte chemoattractant protein, and on platelet adhesion and activation; 2) the reduced EDRF-releasability in states with enhanced vascular ACE; 3) the distension-associated overexpression of vascular ACE in large, distensible arteries.

In analyzing the genetic factors contributing to the large interindividual variation in plasma levels of ACE activity in humans, the group of Soubrier and Alhenc-Gelas identified a deletion polymorphism in the noncoding region of the human ACE gene, which contributed to hereditary elevations of plasma ACE. This deletion polymorphism proved to be a potent risk factor for myocardial infarction (11). It is not yet clear to what extent this deletion polymorphism had contributed to the large scatter of cardiac ACE expression observed in our study in heart donors and transplant recipients (87). For the hypothesis outlined in Fig. 2, the question from this study is whether the identified deletion polymorphism determines elevated ACE expression in elastic conductance arteries.

Another recent clinical study with 8.3 years of follow-up of 1717 subjects with mild to moderate hypertension identified a significant association of the renin-sodium profile with the risk of myocardial infarction (4). The classification of patients according to their relation of plasma renin activity to urinary sodium excretion per day was introduced two decades ago by Laragh and coworkers in an effort to identify subgroups of hypertensives with different mechanism of blood pressure regulation (51). Later, it became clear that nephron heterogeneity due to focal arteriolar narrowings is the renal basis for different renin-sodium profiles in patients with essential hypertension (80, 50). The follow-up study indicated that hypertensives with kidney affections resulting in high renin release relative to the sodium balance have 3.2-fold higher risk of myocardial infarction compared to the hypertensives with normal or low renin-sodium profiles (4) after adjustment of other risk factors including blood pressure, history of cardiavascular treatment or use of beta-blockers. The question derived from this study with regard to the hypothesis in Fig. 2 is: can inappropriate, repeated elevation of circulating renin contribute to enhanced local angiotensin formation and upregulation of ACE expression in distended elastic conductance arteries after vascular binding of the circulating renin?

Vascular ACE activity is upregulated in many rat models of genetic or experimental hypertension. A detailed analysis in the model of suprarenal aortic coarctation indicated that this elevated ACE expression is reactive to the elevation in arterial pressure and is not the cause for the hypertension: the elevation is only observed in elastic arteries proximal to the coarctation, regardless of the site of coarctation (36). It occurs only in large distensible arteries and not in peripheral microcirculations exposed to the hypertension (unpublished from our laboratory). However, it occurs also in the coronary system of the left ventricles exposed to the enhanced afterload (5, 75). A reduced endothelium-dependent, EDRF- (or nitric oxide-) mediated dilation in large arteries has been observed in human hypertension as well as in many models of experimental hypertension. Since this reduction is not paralleled by a reduced dilatory responsiveness to nitric-oxide releasing nitrovasodilators, a reduced releasability of EDRF or nitric oxide is assumed as one mechanism of this dilatory dysfunction. In the coarctation model it was shown that this endothelial dysfunction is strictly restricted to the segments with enhanced ACE activity, which are exposed to the distending hypertension (36). Chronic, non-hypotensive treatment with low-dose ACE-inhibition reduced the local ACE-activity in the distended arteries and largely normalized the depressed EDRF releasability to stimuli such as acetylcholine or histamine, which are not subject to ACE-mediated degradation (36). This observation indicates that high vascular ACE downregulates and treatment-induced lowering of vascular ACE upregulates local EDRF-releasability, independently from the pressure effects of the treatment. An enhanced efficacy of ACE-inhibition in restoring depressed EDRF-releasability in large arteries, superior to the restoration by other antihypertensives, has been shown by many studies (for early examples, see (61, 10)). In the coarctation model, the recovery of EDRF-releasability induced by non-hypotensive treatment with ACE-inhibition is abolished by coadministration of bradykinin-2 receptor antagonist (36). These experimental observations are compatible with two hypotheses incorporated in the scheme outlined in Fig. 2: First, vascular ACE activity is upregulated by hypertension-induced chronic distension of large, elastic arteries, and secondly, enhanced vascular ACE activity downregulates local EDRF-releasability by reducing bradykinin availability.

The somewhat vague term "EDRF-releasability" used in this context probably reflects up- or downregulation of the endothelial nitric oxide synthase, forming NO, the active principle of EDRF. This enzyme is present in endothelial cells (and therefore has been regarded as "constitutively expressed" in endothelial cells) and requires an elevation in cytosolic Ca^{++} for its calmodulin-dependent activation. In cultured endothelial cells, the expression of this endothelial NO-synthase is upregulated (Harrison, personal communication) by the chronic application of shear stress (which is a physiologic activator of the endothelial NO formation and release). Similarly, chronic exercise training in dogs upregulates expression of NO-synthase in aortic endothelium probably by the same mechanism (Hintze, personal communication). Thus, it appears that chronic activation of the endothelial NO synthase upregulates the expression of this enzyme, thereby enhancing EDRF-releasability by any synthase-activating stimulus. The enhanced local availability of bradykinin under ACE-inhibition could act as such an unspecific, "activation-dependent" inductor for the expression of endothelial NO synthase. Conversely, distension-induced enhancement of local ACE activity could diminish bradykinin availability and thus decrease the expression of NO synthase. This hypothesis is incorporated into the speculative proposal summarized in Fig. 2.

Much to our surprise, we observed a normalization of the enhanced vascular ACE activity and a recovery of the depressed EDRF releasability in hypertension-exposed aortic segments of rats with coarctation hypertension under chronic, nonhypotensive treatment with angiotensin receptor antagonists of the AT_1-receptor (Goetz, Kuch, Holtz, submitted). This observation indicates that the distension-induced upregulation of vascular ACE expression must include an AT_1-receptor mediated positive feedback, depending on local angiotensin-II formation. By this feedback, the intermittent hyperreninemia in hypertensives with the high renin profile could contribute to the progression of atherosclerotic disease, and by interrupting this presumed feedback, chronic AT_1-receptor blockade can restore the depressed endothelial EDRF releasability in distended arteries. These hypothetic steps are included in Fig. 2.

An attenuated releasability of EDRF has been repeatedly associated with the risk of arteriosclerosis. In this context it is of relevance that nitric oxide has an inhibitory effect on monocyte chemotaxis and adhesion to cultured endothelial cells (9), reactions which are regarded as crucial for induction of atherosclerosis in vivo. The mechanism of the NO-induced inhibition of monocyte chemotaxis and adhesion has been analyzed recently (77a): suppression of NO formation in cultured endothelial cells by L-arginine derivatives enhanced the expression of the MCP_1 (monocyte chemotactic peptide$_1$) and of the adhesion molecule fibronectin, while addition of exogenous NO from nitrovasodilators lowered these expressions. Similarly, minimally oxidatively modified LDL, which is known to interfere with EDRF releasability, enhanced these expressions. It appears that these experiments illustrate important elements in the antiatherosclerotic potential of an intact EDRF-releasability. Together with the well known inhibitory actions on NO adhesion and activation of platelets, they may explain the last step in the speculative scheme of Fig. 2.

The overall relevance of the proposed sequences summarized schematically in Fig. 2 should be testable by chronic application of ACE-inhibition in experimental models of atherogenesis. This has been done recently in the Watanabe heritable hyperlipidemic rabbit (16). In this model, chronic therapy with captopril over 9 months reduced the aortic atherosclerosis, measured as aortic cholesterol content and aortic surface involvement by lesions (16). While this observation is compatible with the speculations summarized in Fig. 2, it is not clear whether and to what extent the captopril-induced hypotension had contributed to the observed effect.

Presently, the scheme in Fig. 2 represents only a summary of testable hypotheses, incorporating several recent observations with potential relevance to the "previously unrecognized therapeutic action of ACE-inhibitors," which may have been uncovered by the large heart failure prevention trials (17). As is documented by the surprising reduction in recurrent myocardial infarction by ACE-inhibition in these trials, the role of the renin-angotensin system in the pathophysiology of heart failure still includes unexpected and unexplained mechanisms.

References

1. Aceto JF, Baker KM (1990) [Sar^1]angiotensin II receptor-mediated stimulation of protein synthesis in chick heart cells. Am J Physiol 258:H806—H813
2. Admiraal PJJ, Derkx FHM, Danser AHJ, Pieterman H, Schalekamp MADH (1990) Metabolism and production of angiotensin I in different vascular beds in subjects with hypertension. Hypertension 15:44—55
3. Admiraal PJJ, Derkx FHM, Danser AHJ, Pieterman H, Schalekamp MADH (1990) Intrarenal de novo production of angiotensin I in subjects with renal artery stenosis. Hypertension 16:555—563
4. Alderman MH, Madhavan S, Ooi WL, Cohen H, Sealey JE, Laragh JH (1991) Association of the renin-sodium profile with the risk of myocardial infarction in patients with hxpertension. N Engl J Med 324:1098—1104
5. Allgeier J, Goetz RM, Studer R, Reinecke H, Holtz J (1992) Involvement of bradykinin in the cardioreparation be chronic quinapril in rats with hypertensive left ventricular hypertrophy (Abstr). Circulation 86:I—329
6. Baker KM, Aceto JF (1990) Angiotensin II stimulation of protein synthesis and cell growth in chick heart cells. Am J Physiol 259:H610—H618
7. Baker KM, Booz GW, Dostal DE (1992) Cardiac actions of angiotensin II: Role of an intracardiac renin-angiotensin system. Annu Rev Physiol 54:227—241
8. Baker KM, Chernin MI, Wixson SK, Aceto JF (1990) Renin-angiotensin system involvement in pressure-overload cardiac hypertrophy in rats. Am J Physiol 259:324—332
9. Bath PM, Hassall DG, Gladwin AM, Palmer RM, Martin JF (1991) Nitric oxide and prostacyclin: divergence of inhibitory effects on myocyte chemotaxis and adhesion to endothelium in vitro. Arterioscl Thromb 11:254—260
10. Becker RHA, Wiemer G, Linz W (1991) Preservation of endothelial function by ramipril in rabbits on a long-term atherogenic diet. J Cardiovasc Pharmacol 18 (suppl 2): 110—115

11. Cambien F, Poirier O, Lecerf L, Evans A, Cambon JP, Arveiler D, Lut G, Bard JM, Bara L, Ricard F, Piret L, Amouyel P, Ahlenc-Gelas F, Soubrier F (1992) Deletion polymorphism in the gene for angiotensin converting enzyme is a potent risk factor for myocardial infarction. Nature 359:641—644
12. Campbell DJ (1985) The site of angiotensin production. J Hypertension 3:199—207
13. Campbell DJ (1987) Circulating and tissue angiotensin system. J Clin Invest 79:1—6
14. Chien KR, Knowlton KU, Zhu H, Chien S (1991) Regulation of cardiac gene expression during myocardial growth and hypertrophy. Molecular studies of an adaptive physiologic response (Review), FASEB J 5:3037—3046
15. Chilian WM, Marcus ML (1987) Coronary vascular adaptations to myocardial hypertrophy Ann Rev Physiol 49:477—487
16. Chobanian AV, Haudenschild CC, Nickerson C, Drago R (1990) Antiatherogenic effect of captopril in the Watanabe heritable hyperlipidemic rabbit. Hypertension 15:327—331
17. Cohn JN (1992) The prevention of heart failure: a new agenda. N Engl J Med 327:725—727
18. Cohn JN, Johnson G, Ziesche S, Cobb F, Francis G, Tristani F, Smith R, Duncman WB, Loeb H, Wong WZ, Bhat G, Goldman S, Fletcher RD, Doherty J, Hughes CV, Carson P, Cintron G, Shabetai R, Haakenson C (1991) A comparison of enalapril with hydralazine-isosorbide dinitrate in the treatment of chronic congestive heart failure. N Engl J Med 325:293—302
19. Consensus trial study group (1987) Effects of enalpril on mortality in severe congestive heart failure: results of the Cooperative North Scandinavian Enalapril Survival Study (Consensus). N Engl J Med 316:1429—1435
20. Crozier IG, Theo R, Kay R, Nicholls G (1989) Sympathetic nervous system during converting enzyme inhibition. Am J Med 87 (suppl 6b):29s—32s
21. Cruickshank JM, Lewis J, Moore V, Dodd C (1992) Reversibility of left ventricular hypertrophy by differing types of antihypertensive therapy. J Human Hypert 6:85—90
22. De La Bastie D, Levitski D, Rappaport L, Mecardier JJ, Marotte F, Wisnewsky C, Brovkovich V, Schwartz K, Lompré AM (1990) Function of the sarcoplasmic reticulum and expression of its Ca^{2+}-ATPase gene in pressure overload-induced cardiac hypertrophy in the rat. Circ Res 66:554—564
23. Dillman WH, Rohrer D, Popovich B, Barrieux A (1987) Altered thyreoid function and the heart. Horm Metab Res (suppl) 17:26—29
24. Dzau VJ (1989) Multiple pathways of angiotensin production in the blood vessel wall: evidence, possibilities and hypotheses. J Hypertension 7:933—936
25. Dzau VJ, Ellison KE, Brody T, Ingelfinger J, Pratt R (1987) A comparative study of the distribution of renin and antiogensinogen messenger ribonucleic acids in rat and mouse tissues. Endocrinology 120:2334—2338
26. Eberli FR, Apstein CS, Ngoy S, Lorell BH (1992) Exacerbation of left ventricular ischemic diastolic dysfunction by pressure-overload hypertrophy. Modification by specific inhibition of cardiac angiotensin converting enzyme. Circ Res 70:931—943
27. Ehlers MRW, Riordan JF (1989) Angiotensin converting enzyme: new perspectives concerning its biological role. Biochemistry 28:5311—5318
28. El Amrani AIK (1991) Dual effect of angiotensin II and load on intrinsic myocardial contractility. Heart Failure 7:97—103
29. Fabris B, Jackson B, Kohzuki M, Perich R, Johnston CI (1990) Increased cardiac angiotensin-converting enzyme in rats with chronic heart failure. Circ Res 59:475—482
30. Finckh M, Hellmann W, Ganten D, Furtwängler A, Allgeier J, Boltz M, Holtz J (1991) Enhanced cardiac angiotensinogen gene expression and angiotensin converting enzyme activity in tachypacing-induced heart failure in rats. Basic Res Cardiol 86:303—316
31. Fort S, Shah AM, Lewis MJ (1992) Endothelium-derived relaxing factor (EDRF) can modulate cardiac contraction in the intact heart (Abstr). Eur Heart J 13:324s
32. Foult JM, Tavolaro O, Antony I, Nitenberg A (1988) Direct myocardial and coronary effects of enalaprilat in patients with dilated cardiomyopathy: assessment by a bilateral intracoronary infusion technique. Circulation 77:337—344

33. Fozzard HA (1992) Afterdepolarizations and triggered activity. In: Holtz J, Drexler H (eds) Cardiac adaption in heart failure: risks due to myocardial phenotype changes. Steinkopff, Darmstadt pp 105—113
34. Friedrich SP, Lorell BH, Douglas PS, Gordon S, Grossman W, Benedict C, Hess OM, Krayenbuehl HP, Eberli F, Rousseau MF, Pouleur H (1992) Intracardiac ACE-inhibition improves diastolic distensibility in patients with left ventricular hypertrophy due to aortic stenosis (Abstr). Circulation 86:I—119
35. Furberg CD, Yusuf S (1985) Effect of vasodilators on survival in chronic congestive heart failure. Am J Cardiol 55:1110—1111
36. Goetz RM, Krivokuca M, Holtz J (1992) Local activity of angiotensin converting enzyme and local endothelium-dependent dilatory reactivity in coarctation hypertension (Abstr). Circulation 86:I—558
37. Hasenfuss G, Mulieri LA, Leavitt BJ, Allen PD, Haeberle JR, Alpert NR (1992) Alteration of contractile function and excitation-contraction coupling in dilated cardiomyopathy. 70:1225—1232
38. Hirsch AT, Talsness CE, Schunkert H, Paul M, Dzau VJ (1991) Tissue-specific activation of cardiac angiotensin converting enzyme in experimental heart failure. Circ Res 69:475—482
39. Holtz J (1992) Bedeutung der Myokard-Hypertrophie bei Herzinsuffizienz. Z Kardiol 81 (suppl 4):41—48
40. Holtz J, Studer R, Reinecke H, Just H, Drexler H (1992) Modulation of myocardial sarcoplasmic reticulum Ca^{++}-ATPase in cardiac hypertrophy by angiotensin converting enzyme? In: Holtz J, Drexler H, Just H (eds) Cardiac adaptation in heart failure: risks due to myocardial phenotype changes, Steinkopff, Darmstadt pp 191—204
41. Ikenouchi H, Bridge JHB, Lorell BH, Zhao L, Barry WH (1992) Effects of angiotensin II on $[Ca^{2+}]_i$, motion, Ca^{2+}-current, and pH_i in adult rabbit ventricular myocytes (Abstr). Circulation 86:I—218
42. Ikram H (1989) Haemodynamic effects of ACE-inhibition in heart failure. ACE Report 63:1—7
43. Jenne DE, Tschopp J (1991) Angiotensin II-forming heart chymase is a mast-cell specific enzyme. Biochem J 276:567—568
44. Katz AM (1990) Cardiomyopathy of overload: a major determinant of prognosis in congestive heart failure. N Engl J Med 322:100—110
45. Kinoshita A, Uratah H, Bumpus FM, Husain A (1991) Multiple determinants for the high substrate specificity of an angiotensin II-forming chymase from the human heart. J Biol Chem 266:19192—19197
46. Kleber AG (1992) The potential role of Ca^{2+} for electrical cell uncoupling and conduction block in myocardial tissue. In: Holtz J, Drexler H (eds) Cardiac adaption in heart failure: risks due to myocardial phenotype changes. Steinkopff, Darmstadt pp 131—143
47. Komuro I, Kurabayashi M, Shibazaki Y, Takaku F, Yazaki Y (1989) Molecular cloning and characterization of the Ca^{2+} + Mg^{2+}-dependent adenosine triphosphatase from rat cardiac sarcoplasmic reticulum. J Clin Invest 83:1102—1108
48. Ladenson PW, Sherman SI, Baughman KL, Ray PE, Feldman AM (1992) Reversible alterations in myocardial gene expression in a young man with dilated cardiomyopathy and hypothyroidism. Proc Natl Acad Sci 89:5251—5255
49. Lakatta EG (1989) Chaotic behaviour of myocardial cells: possible implications regarding the pathophysiology of heart failure. Perspect Biol Med 32:421—433
50. Laragh JH (1989) Nephron heterogeneity: clue to the pathogenesis of essential hypertension and effectiveness of angiotensin-converting enzyme inhibitor treatment. Am J Med 87 (suppl 6B)2s—14s
51. Laragh JH, Baer L, Brunner HR, Bühler FR, Sealey JE, Vaugham ED (1972) Renin, angiotensin and aldosteron system in pathogenesis and management of hypertensive vascular disease. Am J Med 52:633—652
52. Lee WH, Packer M (1986) Prognostic importance of serum sodium concentration and its modification by converting enzyme inhibition in patients with severe chronic heart failure. Circulation 73:257—267

53. Lindpainter K, Ganten D (1991) The cardiac renin-angiotensin system. An appraisal of present experimental and clinical evidence. Circ Res 68:905—921
54. Lindpainter K, Lu W, Niedermaier N, Schieffer B, Just H, Ganten D, Drexler H (1993) Selective activation of cardiac angiotensinogen gene expression in post-infarction ventricular remodeling in the rat. J Moll Cell Cardiol (in press)
55. Linz W, Schölkens BA (1991) Bradykinin receptor antagonist abolishes the antihypertrophic effect of ramipril. In: The role of bradykinin in the cardiovascular action of ramipril, Eds: Bönner G, Schölkens BA, Scicli AG; Media medica, Wiessbaden; pp 85—89
56. Lopez JJ, Tang SS, Diamant D, Ingelfinger JR, Weinberg EO, Schunkert H, Lorell BH (1992) Distribution and function of angiotensin AT_1 and AT_2 receptor subtypes in hypertrophied rat hearts (Abstr). Circulation 86:I—838
57. Lorell BH, Wexler LF, Momomura S, Weinberg EO, Apstein CS (1986) The influence of pressure overload left ventricular hypertrophy on diastolic properties during hypoxia in isovolumically contracting rat hearts. Circ Res 58:653—663
58. Lorell BH (1993) Diastolic dysfunction in pressure-overload hypertrophy and its modification by angiotensin II: current concepts. In: Holtz J, Drexler H, Just H (eds) Cardiac adaptation in heart failure: risks due to myocardial phenotype changes, Steinkopff, Darmstadt pp 163—172
59. Mercadier JJ, Lompré AM, Duc P, Boheler KR, Fraysse JB, Wisnewsky C, Allen P, Komajda M, Schwartz K (1990) Altered sarcoplasmic reticulum Ca^{2+}-ATPase gene expression in the human ventricle during end stage heart failure. J Clin Invest 85:305—309
60. Meulemans AL, Andries LJ, Brutsaert DL (1990) Does endocardial endothelium mediate positive inotropic responses to angiotensin I and angiotensin II? Circ Res 66:1591—1601
61. Miller VM (1990) Does antihypertensive therapy improve the function of the vascular endothelium? Hypertension 16:541—543
62. Moncada S (1993) The L-arginine: nitric oxide pathway. J Cardiovasc Pharmacol (suppl 3): 1—9
63. Mulieri LA, Hasenfuss G, Leavitt B, Allen P, Alpert NR (1992) Altered myocardial force-frequency relation in human heart failure. Circulation 85:1743—1750
64. Nadal-Ginard B, Mahdavi V (1990) Molecular basis of cardiac performance. J Clin Invest 84:1693—1700
65. Nagai R, Zarain-Herzberg A, Brandl CJ, Fuji J, Tada M, MacLennan DH, Alpert NR, Periasamy M (1989) Regulation of myocardial Ca^{2+}-ATPase and phospholamban mRNA expression in response to pressure overload and thyroid hormone. Proc Natl Acad Sci USA 86:2966—2970
66. Nagano M, Higaki J, Nakamura F, Higashimori K, Nagano N, Mikami H, Ogihara T (1992) Role of cardiac angiotension II in isoproterenol-induced left ventricular hypertrophy. Hypertension 19:708—712
67. Nordin C (1989) Abnormal Ca^{2+} handling and the generation of ventricular arrhythmias in congestive heart failure. Heart Failure 5:143—154
68. Packer M (1987) Comment. N Engl J Med 316:1471—1472
69. Packer M, Lee WH, Kessler PD, Gotlieb SS, Bernstein JL, Kukin ML (1987) Role of neurohormonal mechanisms in determining survival in patients with severe chronic heart failure. Circulation 75 (suppl IV):80—92
70. Paulus WJ, Sys SU, Nellens P, Heyndrickx, Andries E (1988) Failure of inactivation of hypertrophied myocardium: a cause of impaired left ventricular filling in hypertrophic cardiomyopathy and aortic stenosis. In: Grossman W, Lorell BH (eds) Diastolic relaxation of the heart, Nijhoff, Boston, pp 291—304
71. Perondi R, Saine A, Tio RA, Pomidossi G, Gregorini L, Alessio P, Morganti A, Zanchetti A, Mancia G (1992) ACE-inhibition attenuates sympathetic coronary vasoconstriction in patients with coronary artery disease. Circulation 85:2004—2013
72. Pfeffer JM, Pfeffer MA, Mirsky I, Braunwald E (1982) Regression of left ventricular hypertrophy and prevention of left ventricular dysfunction by captopril in the spontaneously hypertensive rat. Proc Natl Acad Sci 79:3310—3314

73. Pfeffer MA, Braunwald E, Moyé LA, Basta L, Brown EJ, Cuddy TE, Davis BR, Geltman EM, Goldman S, Flaker GC, Klein M, Lamas GA, Packer M, Rouleau J, Rouleau JL, Rutherford J, Wertheimer JH, Hawkins CM (1992) Effect of captopril on mortality and morbidity in patients with left ventricular dysfunction after myocardial infarction: Results of the Survival and Ventricular Enlargement Trial. N Engl J Med 327:669—677
74. Philipson KD (1992) Cardiac sodium-calcium exchange research. Trends Cardiovasc Med 2:12—14
75. Reinecke H, Studer R, Goetz RM, Drexler H, Just H, Holtz J (1992) Die Genexpression der SR-Ca^{++}-ATPase und des Connexin-43 bei kompensierter linksventrikulärer Hypertrophie (LVH) ist nur vorübergehend vermindert. Z Kardiol 81 (suppl 1):120
76. Reinecke H, Bilger J, Hollmann A, Holtz J, Just H, Müller B, Philipson KD, Studer R, Drexler H (1992) Veränderung der Genexpression von SR-Ca^{2+}-ATPase und Na^+/Ca^{2+}-Exchanger im Restmyokard nach Infarkt bei der Ratte. Z Kardiol 81 (suppl 1):113
77. Reinecke H, Studer R, Philipson KD, Bilger J, Eschenhagen T, Böhm M, Just H, Holtz J, Drexler H (1992) Myocardial gene expression of Na^+/Ca^{++}-exchanger and sarcoplasmic reticulum Ca^{++}-ATPase in human heart failure (Abstr). Circulation 86:I—860
77a. Schray-Utz B, Zeiher A, Busse R (1993) The expression of monocyte chemo-attractant protein (MCP-1) mRNA in human endothelial cells is modulated by nitric oxide (Abstr). FASEB J (in press)
78. Schunkert H, Dzau VJ, Tang SS, Hirsch AT, Apstein CS, Lorell BH (1990) Increased rat cardiac angiotensin converting enzyme activity and mRNA expression in pressure overload left ventricular hypertrophy. J Clin Invest 86:1913—1920
79. Schwartz K, Mercadier JJ, Swynghedauw B, Lompré AM (1988) Modifications of gene expression in cardiac hypertrophy. Heart Failure 4:154—163
80. Sealey JE, Blumenfeld JD, Bell GM, Pecker MS, Sommers SC, Laragh JH (1988) On the renal basis for essential hypertension: nephron heterogeneity with discordant renin secretion and sodium excretion causing a hypertensive vasoconstriction-volume relationship. J Hypert 6:763—777
81. Sen S, Tarazi RC, Khairallah PA, Bumpus FM (1974) Cardiac hypertrophy in spontaneously hypertensive rats. Circ Res 35:775—781
82. Shah AM, Evans HG, Lewis MJ (1992) The characteristic effect of emdothelium-derived relaxing factor (EDRF) on myocardial contraction is mimicked by interleukin-1β (Abstr). Circulation 86:I—82
83. Simpson PC (1990) Regulation of hypertrophy and gene transcription in cultured heart muscle cells. In: Roberts R, Schneider MD (1990) Molecular biology of the cardiovascular system. Alan R Liss Inc 125—133
84. SOLVD Investigators (1991) Effect of enalapril on survival in patients with reduced left ventricular ejection fractions and congestive heart failure. N Engl J Med 325:293—302
85. SOLVD Investigators (1992) Effect of enalapril on mortality and the development of heart failure in asymptomatic patients with reduced left ventricular ejection fractions. N Engl J Med 327:685—691
86. Strauer BE (1987) Structural and functional adaption of the chronically overloaded heart in arterial hypertension. Am Heart J 114:948—957
87. Studer R, Müller B, Reinecke H, Just H, Holtz J, Drexler H (1992) Quantified RNA-polymerase chain reaction demonstrates augmented gene expression of angiotensin converting enzyme in ventricles of patients with heart failure (Abstr). Circulation 86:I—119
88. Swynghedauw B (1990) Heart failure: a disease of adaptation. Heart Failure 6: 57—62
89. Takahashi T, Allen PD, Izumo S (1992) Expression of A-, B-, and C-type natriuretic peptide genes in failing and developing human ventricles: correlation with expression of the Ca^{++}-ATPase gene. Circ Res 71:9—17

90. Ten Eick RE, Whalley DW, Rasmussen HH (1992) Connections: heart disease, cellular electrphysiology, and ion channels. FASEB J 6:2568—2580
91. Urata H, Kinoshita A, Misono KS, Bumpus FM, Husain A (1990) Identification of a highly specific chymase as the major angiotensin II-forming enzyme in the human heart. J Biol Chem 265:22348—22357
92. Urata H, Kinoshita A, Perez DM, Misono KS, Bumpus FM, Graham RM, Husain A (1991) Cloning of the gene and cDNA for human heart chymase. J Biol Chem 266:17173—17179
93. Weber KT, Brilla CG (1992) Factors associated with reactive and reparative fibrosis of the myocardium. In: Hasenfuss G, Holubarsch C, Just H, Alpert NR (eds) Cellular and molecular alterations in the failing human heart, Steinkopff, Darmstadt, pp. 291—301
94. Xiang JZ, Linz W, Becker H, Ganten D, Lang RE, Schölkens B, Unger T (1985) Effects of converting enzyme inhibitors: ramipril and enalapril on peptide action and sympathetic neurotransmission in the isolated heart. Eur J Pharmacol 113:215—223

Author's address:
Prof. Dr. med. J. Holtz
Martin-Luther-Universität
Institut für Pathophysiologie
Magdeburger Allee 6
O-4020 Halle/Saale

Angiotensin-converting enzyme inhibitors in the treatment of clinical heart failure

H. Pouleur

Department of Physiology and Pharmacology and Division of Cardiology, University of Louvain, School of Medicine, Brussels, Belgium

Summary: During the last decade, angiotensin-converting enzyme inhibitors (ACE-I) have become cornerstones in the treatment of clinical congestive heart failure. There is convincing evidence that they improve survival and that, in this respect, they are superior to ordinary vasodilators. ACE-I administration also improves New York Heart Association functional class and the left-ventricular function, but their long-term effects on exercise tolerance and quality of life appear modest. During prolonged administration to patients with ischemic left-ventricular dysfunction, ACE-I also significantly reduce the incidence of new ischemic events (myocardial infarction, unstable angina).

Key words: Enalapril; captopril; left-ventricular function; heart failure; survival

During the last decade, captopril and enalapril, rapidly followed by several other angiotensin-converting enzyme inhibitors (ACE-I) have become corne stones in the treatment of patients with congestive heart failure. However, if the clinical benefit of these agents has been established beyond any doubt by a large number of long-term and well designed clinical studies, the fact remains that heart failure still is a 100% lethal disease. In this perspective, it may be useful to critically review what ACE-I can and cannot do in heart failure, what can predict a favorable response and what appears to be, in 1992, the optimal use of these compounds.

For that purpose, we will focus first on the main goals of the therapy, which are to improve the symptoms of the patients and to prolong their life. We will then examine the effects of ACE-I on objective parameters like exercise duration and ventricular function, which may explain some, but probably not all, the clinical benefits observed. Finally, we will examine several hypotheses that may explain the failure of ACE-I in various clinical circumstances, including also the problem of adverse events.

Effects of ACE-I on subjective symptoms and quality of life

One of the major goals of the therapy in heart failure is obviously to relieve the symptoms of dyspnea and fatigue present during daily activities and sometimes even at rest. In the large, multicenter, placebo-controlled SOLVD (Studies of Left Ventricular Dysfunction) Trial (19, 20), this issue was addressed by examining the effects of enalapril or placebo, added to conventional therapy, on the frequency of periods of shortness of breath. The evaluation was done by the patient in a self-administered quality-of-life questionnaire. As shown in Table 1, enalapril administration significantly reduced the frequency of the episodes of dyspnea. The benefit was already present at 6 weeks and was well maintained throughout the trial. Similarly, the functional class of the New York Heart Association (NYHA), a parameter graded by the physician, also showed a significant improvement during the first 2 years of treatment, tapering-off after 3 years (Table 1). Several other trials have also shown that NYHA class improved over time with captopril, lisinopril or enalapril (2, 3, 4, 5, 10, 14, 15, 17) when compared to placebo treatment.

Thus, there is good evidence that ACE-I improve some subjective symptoms that can be "quantified" (albeit imperfectly) by the patient or the physician. The same, unfortunately, cannot be said for the "quality" of life of the patients. Although the elaborate, 28-page quality-of-life questionnaire used in SOLVD easily discriminated at baseline between the patients with heart failure and those with asymptomatic LV dysfunction or the age and sex-matched normal controls, it failed to detect a significant improvement in quality of life beyond 6 weeks.

Most other studies were also unable to demonstrate a positive effect of ACE-I on this variable. Several hypotheses may explain this discrepancy between subjective improvement in shortness of breath and functional class and the lack of prolonged benefit on quality-of-life evaluation. First, "quality" is, by definition, different from "quantity" and does not lend itself to be measured. Second, the longer the study, the more the data become biased against ACE-I, as a number of patients with severe heart failure have died in the placebo group but remain in the enalapril group. For ethical reasons also, it is difficult to administer the questionnaire in end-stage heart failure patients. Whatever the explanation, it seems clear, not only from the data derived from various instruments used to evaluate quality of life, but also from the clinical judgement, that ACE-I cannot produce a dramatic and sustained improvement in the quality of life in heart failure patients.

Effects of ACE-I on exercise tolerance

An exhaustive review of the published and non-published data on the effects of ACE-I on exercise capacity has been made by Held and Swedberg (7). From the 10 to 15 trials reviewed, less than a third reported a significant improvement in the active treatment group compared with the placebo group. Held and Swedberg concluded that the "generally held impression of a strong effect (of ACE-I on exercise capacity) is perhaps not true" (7). This conclusion is extremely important, not only because an improvement in excercise capacity is frequently regarded as a major end-point by regulatory authorities, but also because there appears to be a discrepancy between the modest effect of ACE-I on exercise capacity and the highly consistent impact of this therapy on survival (see below).

Effects of ACE-I on survival and hospitalizations for congestive heart failure

Three large trials with enalapril (6, 18, 19) and one with captopril (SAVE, Survival and Ventricular Enlargement) have shown significant improvement in survival when

Table 1. Cardiovascular symptomatology. Frequency of periods of shortness of breath (quality-of-life questionnaire, SOLVD treatment trial).

	Placebo		Enalapril		
	N	(%)	N	(%)	p-value
Pretreatment					
Distribution					>0.25
Every day	271	(22.4)	262	(21.7)	
Several days a week	258	(21.3)	272	(22.5)	
About once a week	143	(11.8)	128	(10.6)	
2 or 3 times a month	157	(7.4)	105	(8.7)	
About once a month	90	(7.4)	105	(8.7)	
Not at all	292	(24.1)	293	(24.2)	
6 weeks following randomization					
Distribution					0.001**
Every day	189	(17.8)	142	(13.1)	
Several days a week	204	(19.2)	167	(15.3)	
About once a week	109	(10.3)	149	(13.7)	
2 or 3 times a month	123	(11.6)	132	(12.1)	
About once a month	103	(9.7)	114	(10.5)	
Not at all	334	(31.5)	384	(35.3)	
12 months following randomization					
Distribution					0.021*
Every day	157	(18.3)	143	(16.1)	
Several days a week	152	(17.7)	139	(15.7)	
About once a week	95	(11.1)	95	(10.7)	
2 or 3 times a month	109	(12.7)	103	(11.6)	
About once a month	87	(10.1)	101	(11.4)	
Not at all	258	(30.1)	307	(34.6)	
Final visit					
Distribution					0.027*
Every day	232	(20.6)	194	(17.0)	
Several days a week	177	(15.7)	181	(15.8)	
About once a week	118	(10.5)	128	(11.2)	
2 or 3 times a month	143	(12.7)	133	(11.6)	
About once a month	123	(10.9)	128	(11.2)	
Not at all	334	(29.6)	380	(33.2)	

*, ** Indicate significantly less shortness of breath in the enalapril group than in the placebo group, with $p \leqslant 0.05$ and $p \leqslant 0.01$, respectively.

compared to placebo or vasodilators (6). This benefit of the order of 16% was sustained up to 4 years and was present in all classes of heart failure and in all etiologies. Moreover, it was accompanied by a significant reduction in hospitalization for congestive heart failure. These data therefore justify the early use of ACE-I in all forms of heart failure. Interestingly, all trials used a relatively high target dose of ACE-I (enalapril 10 mg/b.i.d., captopril 50 mg/t.i.d.). There is limited evidence that higher doses of enalapril or captopril provide a better clinical result and a better control of the neuro-humoral activation than lower doses (11, 23). Whether or not this better control of neuro-hormones results in a greater benefit on survival remains to be demonstrated; a large trial (ATLAS) comparing the effects of a low (2.5 to 5) and a high (32.5 to 35) dose of lisinopril on survival is now ready to start and should help in answering this question.

In this respect, an important observation was made by the CONSENSUS investigators. In this study, the benefit of enalapril on survival appeared to be largely confined to a subgroup with large (above median) activation of all neuro-hormones studied (16). In the subgroup with less neuro-humoral activation, the mortality was lower, and comparable with placebo and enalapril. In the SOLVD Prevention trial, in which patients with modest neuro-humoral activation were enrolled, no effect of enalapril on mortality could be detected for at least 18—24 months (21). Thus, both in class I—II and in class IV patients, the level of neuro-humoral activation might perhaps be one of the predictors of a positive response to ACE-I. Today, however, it is too early to suggest that measurements of neuro-humoral activation have a role in clinical decision making.

It is also noteworthy that strong arteriodilators like hydralazine or flosequinan improve exercise capacity consistently better than ACE-I, but that their effects on survival are significantly less favorable (6).

Effects on left-ventricular function

In most studies showing an improved survival with ACE-I, the benefit appeared related to a reduction in death from progressive pump failure rather than from sudden, supposedly arrhythmic death (18, 20). In a substudy of the SOLVD, iterative evaluations of right- and left-ventricular performance were performed, using radionuclide angiography and left-heart catherization (9). The data indicate that with conventional therapy, left-ventricular dysfunction continued to progress, as evidenced by progressive increases in end-diastolic and end-systolic volumes and by a fall in ejection fraction. In contrast with enalapril therapy, further left-ventricular dilatation was prevented and a partial reversal was generally observed, resulting in an improved ejection fraction. It is tempting therefore to link the improved survival observed with ACE-I to an effect on left-ventricular function.

Interestingly, improvements in ejection fraction of greater magnitude than with enalapril have been reported with the association hydralazine-isosorbide (6); nevertheless, despite more pronounced effects on pump performance, this association had less favorable effects on survival. We believe, however, that the mechanisms underlying the chronic changes in ventricular function are substantially different between hydralazine and enalapril. Hydralazine acts primarily as an afterload reducing agent. Enalapril, on the other hand, produced only minor changes in systolic pressure, but there was evidence of a qualitative change in ventricular wall properties (13).

An unexpected finding made in SOLVD and later confirmed in SAVE has been the highly significant reduction in unstable angina pectoris and new myocardial infarction in the actively treated group. Although several mechanisms related to ACE-inhibition may underly this property (blood pressure lowering, effect on

EDRF ...), it is possible that the prevention of left-ventricular dilatation could also play a role. Indeed, ventricular dilatation undoubtedly increases the shear stress on epicardial vessels and this might result in plaque rupture.

Limitations of ACE-I in the treatment of congestive heart failure

The problems of reduced glomerular filtration rate and hyperkaliemia are well understood and the steps to avoid or minimize these potential complications are now universally recommended: reduction in diuretic dosage, correction of hypovolemia, progressive titration of the ACE-I and regular control of renal function and ionogram, particularly when therapy is initiated. Angioneurotic edema is a rare but serious complication and patients should be warned of this possibility so that adequate treatment can be provided at the first clinical signs. A dry cough has been observed with all ACE-I in approximately 10—15% of the patients, sometimes requiring withdrawal of therapy.

Despite all their beneficial effects, ACE-I in heart failure are not a cure and patients may "escape" after a variable period of time. Plasma angiotensin II levels and aldosterone levels increase again and heart failure symptoms worsen. The reasons for the loss of the full clinical benefit is not entirely clear. Tissue-converting enzymes insensitive to ACE-I, like the human heart chymase may be part of the problem (8, 22). New studies with angiotensin II antagonists should help in elucidating these mechanisms. It is also clear that the neurohumoral activation in heart failure is complex and that stimulation of other factors such as endothelin and norepinephrine may play a role in the disease progression. Finally, the aging process itself contributes to impair ventricular function.

Mechanisms of action of the angiotensin-converting enzyme inhibitors in heart failure

Considering the complexity of the action of angiotensin II on the cardiovascular system and the multiple sites of action of most ACE-I, in addition to the inhibition of the systemic conversion of angiotensin I in angiotensin II, it is not surprising that the mechanisms underlying the beneficial effects of these agents in patients with left-ventricular dysfunction have not yet been fully elucidated. There are at least four major possible targets: the heart, the kidney, the peripheral circulation, and the central nervous system.

At the cardiac level, angiotensin II is a well known growth factor, acting not only on the myocyte, but also on the fibroblast. Together with aldosterone, angiotensin II may modify in a complex way the type and the amount of collagen present in the collagen matrix; it may also stimulate myocyte hypertrophy (12, 24). Thus, ACE-inhibitors may reduce hypertrophy, not only in hypertension, but probably also in heart failure patients. In addition, recent experimental data indicate an improvement in the turn-over rate and type of collagen synthetized in heart failure animals treated with captopril (1). Clinical data indicate that enalapril not only stops the progression of left-ventricular dilatation, but probably also partially reverses left-ventricular remodeling (9, 13). Accordingly, part of the benefit of ACE-inhibitors on prognosis in heart failure and, more particularly, the reduction in pump failure deaths, could be related to the reduction of the angiotensin II effects on cardiac fibroblasts and myocytes.

Angiotensin II is also a powerful vasoconstrictor, but many studies suggest that the vasodilation observed after ACE-inhibition also largely depends on other factors, such as an increased half-life of bradykinin, an increased production of prostaglandin or of EDRF. A direct reduction in the vasoconstrictor stimuli, modulated through the reduction of the stimulation of the orthosympathetic system by angiotensin II is also likely to participate in the afterload reduction. Now that specific antagonists are becoming available for angiotensin II, bradykinin, aldosterone, and other potential culprits like endothelin, it is hoped that some light will soon be shed on these fascinating properties of ACE-I.

In conclusion, ACE-I are a major step forward in the treatment of heart failure, and probably also in the prevention of the development of congestive heart failure when administered early after acute myocardial infarction or in other forms of asymptomatic left-ventricular dysfunction.

Acknowledgement. The author thanks Ms. Isabelle Mottard for her careful secretarial assistance.

References

1. Araki T, Shimizu M, Sugihara N, Takeda R (1992) Effect of angiotensin converting enzyme inhibitor on myocardial collagen metabolism in cardiomyopathic hamsters. J Moll Cell Cardiol 24:S56
2. Bussman WD, Störger H, Hadler N (1987) Long-term treatment of severe chronic heart failure with captopril: a double-blind, randomized, placebo-controlled, long-term study. J Cardiovasc Pharmacol 9:S50—S60
3. Captopril Multicenter Research Group (1983) A placebo-controlled trial of captopril in refractory chronic congestive heart failure. J Am Coll Cardiol 2:755—763
4. Chalmers JP, West MJ, Cyran J (1987) Placebo-controlled study of lisinopril in congestive heart failure: a multicenter study. J Cardiovasc Pharmacol 9:S89—S97
5. Cleland JG F, Dargie HJ, Ball SG (1985) Effects of enalapril in heart failure: a double-blind study of effects in exercise performance, renal function, hormones, and metabolic state. Br Heart J 54:305—312
6. Cohn JN, Johnson G, Ziesche S, Cobb F, Francis G, Tristani F et al. (1991) A comparison of enalapril with hydralazine-isosorbide dinitrate in the treatment of chronic congestive heart failure. N Engl J Med 325:303—310
7. Held P, Swedberg K (1992) ACE-inhibitors in the treatment of heart failure. In: Barnett D, Francis G, Pouleur H (eds) Heart failure: newer therapeutics. Marcel Dekker, Inc. (in press)
8. Hirakata H, Fouad-Tarazi FM, Bumpus FM, Khosla M, Healy B, Husain A et al. (1990) Angiotensins and the failing heart. Enhanced positive inotropic responce to angiotensin I in cardiomyopathic hamster heart in the presence of captopril. Circ Res 66:891—899
9. Konstam MA, Rousseau MF, Kronenberg MW, Udelson JE, Melin J, Stewart D et al. (1992) Effects of the angiotensin converting enzyme inhibitor enalapril, on the long-term progression of left ventricular dysfunction in patients with heart failure. Circulation 86:431—438

10. McGrath BP, Arnolda L, Matthews PG (1985) Controlled trial of enalapril in congestive cardiac failure. Br Heart J 54:405—414
11. Pacher R, Globits S, Bergler-Klein J, Kratochwill C, Stefenelli T, Baumgartner W et al. (1992) Clinical and neurohumoral response of patients with severe congestive heart failure treated with two different captopril dosages. J Am Coll Cardiol 19:317
12. Pfeffer MA, Braunwald E (1990) Ventricular remodeling after myocardial infarction Experimental observations and clinical implications. Circulation 81:1161—1172
13. Pouleur H, Konstam MA, van Eyll C, Melin J, Gallagher P, Yusuf S, Rousseau MF, for the SOLVD Investigators (1992) Long-term effects of enalapril on left ventricular diastolic properties: evidence for "reversed remodeling". Circulation 86:I—120
14. Remes J, Nikander P, Rehnberg S (1986) Enalapril in chronic heart failure, a double-blind placebo-controlled study. Ann Clin Res 18:124—128
15. Sharpe DN, Murphy J, Coxon R, Hannan SF (1984) Enalapril in patients with chronic heart failure: a placebo-controlled, randomized, double-blind study. Circulation 70:271—278
16. Swedberg K, Eneroth P, Kjekshus J, Wilhelmsen and CONSENUS Trial Study Group (1990) Hormones regulating cardiovascular function in patients with severe congestive heart failure and their relation to mortality. Circulation 82:1730—1736
17. The captopril-digoxin multicenter research group (1988) Comparative effects of therapy with captopril and digoxin in patients with mild to moderate heart failure. JAMA 259: 539—544
18. The CONSENSUS Trial Study Group (1987) Effects of enalapril on mortality in severe congestive heart failure Results of the Cooperative North Scandinavian Enalapril Survival Study (CONSENSUS). N Engl J Med 316:1429—1435
19. The SOLVD Investigators (1990) Studies of left ventricular dysfunction (SOLVD) — Rationale, design and methods: two trials that evaluate the effect of enalapril in patients with reduced ejection fraction. Am J Cardiol 66:315—322
20. The SOLVD Investigators (1991) Effect of enalapril on survival in patients with reduced left ventricular ejection fraction and congestive heart failure. N Engl J Med 325:293—302
21. The SOLVD Investigator (1992) Effects of enalapril on mortality and the development of heart failure in asymptomatic patients with reduced left ventricular ejection fraction. N Engl J Med 327:685—691
22. Urata H, Healy B, Stewart RW, Bumpus FM, Husain A (1990) Angiotensin II-forming pathways in normal and failing human hearts. Circ Res 66:883—890
23. Vagelos R, Yee G, Boyle M, Moore C, Prikaszky L, Willson K et al. (1992) Failure of low but not high dose chronic enalapril therapy to suppress serum angiotensin converting enzyme (ACE) activity in heart failure. J Am Coll Cardiol 19:145
24. Weber KT, Brilla CG (1991) Pathological hypertrophy and cardiac interstitium. Circulation 83(6):1849—1865

Author's address:
Hubert Pouleur, M.D.
University of Louvain
av Hippocrate 55/5560
B-1200 Brussels, Belgium

Summary and perspective
A. Basic aspects

H. Grobecker

Institut für Pharmakologie der Universität Regensburg

During this symposium on "Angiotensin and the Heart", an appraisal of the present experimental and clinical evidence for the existence and function of the cardiac renin-angiotensin system has been made. It is now accepted that the renin-angiotensin system originally detected as a classical humoral system, which secretes active molecules from a gland reaching their receptors of a target organ via the blood, may also reside in many tissues, especially in organs involved in cardiovascular regulation like the heart and vessels (Tigerstedt and Bergman, 1897; Dzau, 1990).

The presentations during the last two days gave evidence for the physiological and pathophysiological role of the local cardiac renin-angiotensin system in development and maintenance of high blood pressure and congestive heart failure.

The impressive beneficial effects of converting enzyme inhibitors in hypertension and heart failure and the remarkable *cardioprotective action* of the ACE-inhibitors in pharmacological and clinical-pharmacological experiments has lead to a breakthrough in these lethal cardiovascular diseases.

Not only the angiotensin converting enzyme has been identified in the heart (Yamada, 1991), but also all other components of the enzyme cascade of the renin-

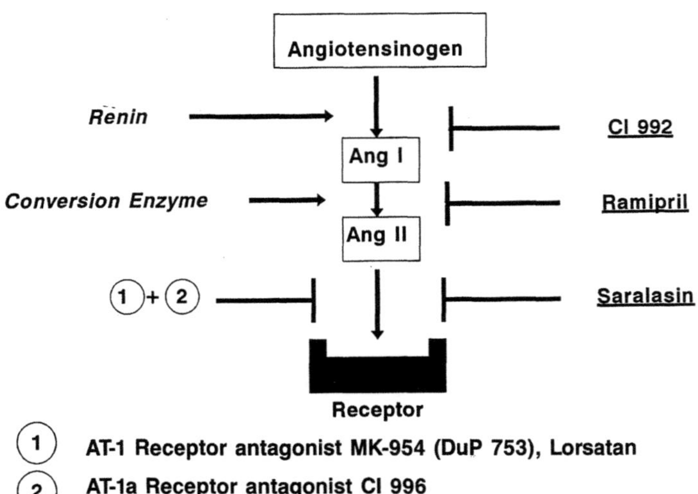

Fig. 1. Inhibition of Renin-Angiotensin-System on different levels of the cascade

angiotensin system are present in the myocardium. The local renin-angiotensin system in the heart exhibits paracrine and autocrine functions (Dzau, 1988).

In recent experiments in different tissues, e. g., in rat testis a different molecular structure of the converting enzyme has been detected which exhibits only one active site in contrast to two active sites of the enzyme in the heart for the substrate Angiotensin I (Johnston, 1992).

Also, the receptors for Angiotensin II have recently been divided into subpopulations like AT_1 and AT_{1a} receptors which can be blocked by specific antagonists (Fig. 1).

One of the tools to elucidate the role of angiotensin II receptors in cardiovascular regulation, especially in hypertension, is the nonpeptide DuP 753 which exhibits selective and competitive blockade at AT_1 receptors after oral application in both animals and man (Wong et al., 1990; Christen et al., 1991).

In SHR the AT_1 receptor antagonist reduced blood pressure dose-depently, but had no bradykinin potentiating effect (Fig. 2).

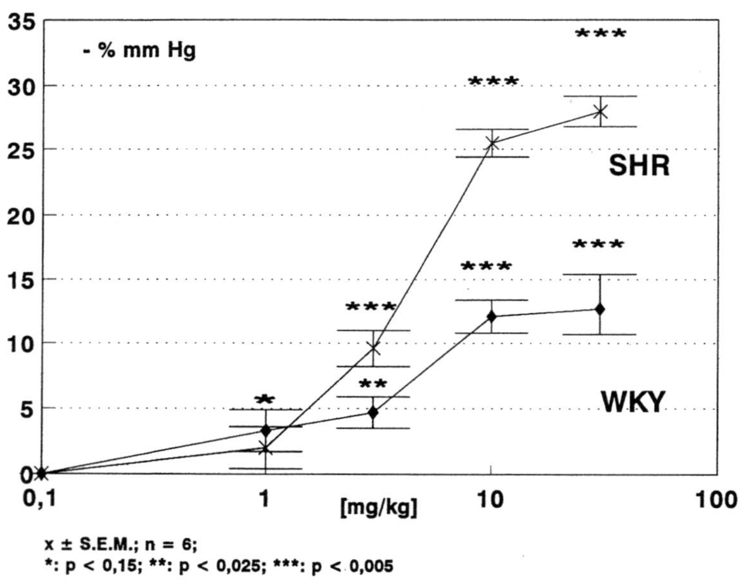

Fig. 2. Dose-response curves established with AT-1 receptor antagonist MK-954 (DuP 753) in SHR and WKY; 12 weeks of age

However, after administration of angiotensin converting enzyme inhibitors like ramipril or quinapril, the reduction of blood pressure in SHR could be partially prevented by the bradykinin antagonist Hoe 140. The bradykinin potentiating effects of ramipril or quinapril contributed up to 40% of the total blood-pressure-lowering effect of the drugs, as calculated from experiments using both receptor antagonists DuP 753 and Hoe 140 (Fig.3).

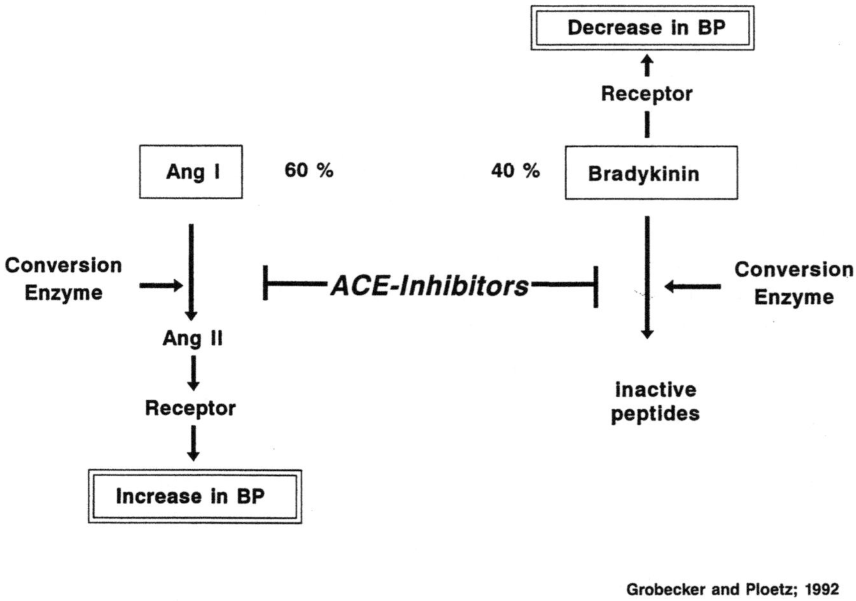

Fig. 3. RAS and Kinin-System

Moreover, HOE 140 in contrast to DuP 753 was able to partially prevent the improved glucose disposition after application of quinapril in diabetic rats after administration of streptozoticin or in genetic diabetic rats (Table 1).

Table 1

Substance		**d-SHR** (n = 6) effect on blood glucose	**d-WKY** (n = 6) effect on blood glucose
Quinapril	20 mg/kg	—25 +/—2.0%	—33 +/—3.5%
Quinapril HOE 140	20 mg/kg 1 mg/kg	—6.9 +/—1.3%	—10.4 +/—4.4%
MK-954	10 mg/kg	—12.3 +/—2.0%	—13.4 +/—1.8%

Since under these conditions the insulin receptor seems to be intact (Häring, 1991) an action of accumulated bradykinin due to inhibiton of kininase II (conversion enzyme) on the transduction system of the insulin receptor seems to be likely.

Highlights of the presentations of Drs. 1) Dzau, 2) Lüscher, 3) Heusch, 4) Nadal-Ginard, 5) Vatner, 6) Weber, 7) Przyklenk, 8) Bolli and 9) Holtz were:

ad 1: In the first contribution the role of short-term action of the circulating renin-angiotensin system (RAS) versus the long term actions of RAS on cardiovascular system was carefully analyzed (cf. also Dzau, 1990, Dzau and

Gibbons, 1991). Angiotensin II as end-product of the renin-converting-enzyme-cascade is a potent growth factor in vascular smooth muscle leading either to hypertrophy or hyperplasia. In hypertension not only vacular hypertrophy is modulated by the endogenous RAS, but also the development of left-ventricular hypertrophy. Moreover, cardiac RAS plays a crucial role in the pathophysiology of heart failure leading from compensatory mechanism to a circulus vitiosus. Investigating the mechanism of action of inhibitors of converting enzyme, e.g., pharmacodynamic effects resulting form actions on tissue RAS and interesting pharmacokinetic parameters has brought insight into the pathophysiology of cardiovascular diseases like atherosclerosis, congestive heart failure and high blood pressure.

ad 2: The interactions of the renin-angiotensin-system and endothelium — derived vasoactive substances as regulators of vascular tone have been discussed. Bradykinin was recognized as potent activator of the L-arginine nitricoxide system (endothelium derived relaxing factor). Therefore, the vasodilator actions of ACE-inhibitors as acute effects via the bradykinin — NO — mechanism of action is important for the decrease of high blood pressure, both in animals and man. On the other hand the vasoconstrictor action of angiotensin II activates vasopressor systems with transmitters like endothelin, noradrenaline or serotinin. Chronic administration of ACE-inhibitors seem to sensitize the endothelical cells in hypertensive states for agonists, like NO or the endotheline derived hyperpolarizing factor, thus keeping the blood vessel wall in a continuous state of vasodilation. Taking the acute and chronic effects of ACE-inhibitors together, these mechanism of actions may account for an important *vascular protective effect* of the drugs.

ad 3: Experiments in anesthetized dogs infusing angiotensin II in coronary arteries caused constrictions and reduction of coronary blood flow lasting for a few minutes. In consequence, deterioration of regional myocardial wall function occurred, possibly leading to ischemic reactions of the myocardium. The potential anti-ischemic mechanisms by which ACE-inhibitors may attenuate myocardial ischemia are: 1) Improvement of the driving pressure gradient for coronary blood flow. 2) Reduction of myocardial oxygen consumption. 3) Decrease of coronary vasomotor tone.
However, the authors could not demonstrate acute effects of ACE-inhibitors on coronary blood flow. This does not exclude a benificial effect of ACE-inhibitors after chronic administration on the ischemic myocardium.

ad 4: In this communication the genes encoding contractile proteins of the myocardium have been characterized. The authors could demonstrate that work overload hypertrophy induced the re-expression of several fetal isoforms in the post-natal myocardium. In human atria which normally expresses α-MHC, a switch to β-MHC (myosin heavy chain) is apparent in response to increased pressure. Therefore, in the hypertrophic myocardium the MHC phenotype is simular to that in fetal states, with high levels of β-MHC. Cells which receive growth stimuli react with induction of protooncogenes, such as c-fos and c-myc leading to a cascade of events to reach cell division.
Also, the mRNA for the major stress protein HSP 70 is increased within 30 min after increasing aortic pressure. These factors play a causative role in

the hypertrophic response of the heart. There is evidence that work overload may induce gene expression through mechanism similar or shared by the growth factor receptors for basic fibroblast growth factor (bFGF) or transforming growth factor β (TGFβ). The fetal isoforms of MHC have been shown to be bioenergetically more efficient than that of the adult heart cells. Furthermore, the authors gave evidence that thyroid receptors are transcriptional regulators of cardiac MHC gene expression.

Finally, the authors presented evidence for the hypothesis that direct injection of genes in the myocardium of large mammals is a useful model to study gene expression under experimentally controlled physiological conditions. The model of gene transfer by injection of plasmid DNA in vivo, e.g., in transgenic animals, offers a potential route for gene therapy in human disease.

ad 5: The authors demonstrated that in dogs with LV hypertrophy an impaired subendocardial coronary reserve which is caused not only by the hypertrophy but also by hemodynamic changes, e.g., the LV subendocardial wall stress, which increased markedly upon exercise. Subendocardial hypoperfusion and depression in subendocardial wall thickening observed during more severe exercise in dogs with LV hypertrophy was prevented by treatment with β-adrenergic receptor blockade (propranolol).

ad 6: In this report the replacement and reactive fibrous tissue responses of rat myocardium in response to effector hormones of the renin-angiotensin-aldosterone system has been described. Increased plasma angiotension II concentrations are associated with acute cardiac myocyte necrosis and chronic elevations in plasma aldosterone concentrations relative to sodium intake caused perivascular and intestitial fibrosis of coronary arteries. Elevated plasma aldosterone concentrations leading to mineralocorticoid excess also caused cardiac myocyte necrosis and scarring. ACE-inhibitors applied chronically lead to a regression in reactive myocardial fibrosis. Thus ACE-inhibitors can protect the myocardium against pathologic structural remodeling created by the reactive and replacement — reparative — fibrosis.

ad 7: The communication carefully reviews the question whether ACE-inhibitors have "cardioprotective" actions, i.e., attenuation of myocardial injury, dysfunction and necrosis. In animal models of permanent coronary artery occlusion captopril, enalapril and ramipril have been reported to acutely limit myocardial injury necrosis. The cardioprotective actions of ACE-inhibitors are complex, but they certainly influence the kinin-systems of the heart, e. g., bradykinin and, or prostaglandin metabolism. ACE-inhibitors are beneficial in states of "stunned" myocardium in the early hours following relief of ischemia. With enalapril both positive and negative results in stunned hearts have been reported.

However, in cardiomyopathic hamsters, quinapril significantly prolonged survival time (cardioprotective action). In conclusion, despite many efforts, the cardioprotective action of ACE-inhibitors *in acute myocardial ischemia* and infarction is not established.

ad 8: The presentation also deals with the effects of ACE-inhibitors on myocardial ischemia and reperfusion injury. The mechanism discussed are summarized in the Fig. 1 of the paper Zughaub et al. The conclusions reached are simular to those discussed in the paper by Przyklenk and Kloner (see ad 7). Nevertheless, ACE-inhibitors are already a cornerstone in therapeutic interventions in cardiac diseases, such as congestive heart failure.

ad 9: This paper deals with basic aspects of the pathophysiological mechanism in the development of congestive heart failure. From the convincing benefits after therapeutic use of conversion enzyme inhibitors in congestive heart failure it soon became evident that the cardiac RAS plays a crucial role in the development of heart failure. The full cardiac RAS has been characterized by messenger RNAs for angiotensinogen, prorenin and conversion enzyme both in rat heart and human ventricular myocardium (RNA polymerase chain reaction). However, interactions between circulating RAS and cardiac RAS cannot be ruled out today. It seems to be clear that enhanced intracardiac angiotensin II formation during cardiac overload takes place, but no quantitative data are available. The activated cardiac RAS possibly modulates the myocardial hypertrophy by an angiotensin-independent pathway.
In addition, hypertrophy myocyte dedifferention and instabilization of Ca^{++}-homeostasis ("fragile Ca^{++}-homeostasis") has been discussed (cf. Table 1 of the paper, p. 192). These changes contribute considerably to diastolic and systolic dysfunction, as well as to impairment of Ca^{++}-transport in sacroplasmatic reticulum by depressed expression of the SR-Ca^{++}-ATPase in human cardiac failure. In this context cardiac converting enzyme contributes directly to phenotype changes of myocytes. Finally, the vascular renin-angiotensin-system as modulator of susceptibility for atherosclerosis has been considered. Hereditary elevations of plasma converting enzyme is considered to be a risk factor for myocardial infarction. Also, patients with high blood pressure and high kidney renin release relative to sodium balance have an increased risk for myocardial infarction compared to patients with normal or low renin-sodium profils. The author and his group investigated the question of if repeated elevations of circulating renin contribute to increased local angiotensin formation and, consequently, to upregulation of ACE expression in elastic conductance arteries after vascular binding of circulating renin. A hypothesis for a modulating function of the renin-angiotensin system in promotion of atherosclerosis in these arteries has been presented. Central elements of this hypothesis are: 1) the inhibitory effect of EDRF on monocyte adhesion, on expression of monocyte chemoattractant protein, and on platelet adhesion and activation; 2) the reduced EDRF-release in states with enhanced vascular ACE; 3) the distension-associated overexpression of vascular ACE in large, distensible arteries.

The results reviewed and discussed during the symposium "Angiotensin and the Heart" provides conclusive evidence that the cardiac tissue renin-angiotensin system is integrated in the function of myocardium under physiological and pathophysiological conditions. Furthermore, the symposium was effective in promoting the interaction between basic research and clinical practice in order to improve our therapeutic interventions in lethal diseases like congestive heart failure and high blood pressure.

References

1. Christen Y, Waeber B, Nussberger J, Porchet M, Borland RM, Lee RJ, Maggon K, Shum L, Timmermans PBMWM, Brunner HR (1991) Oral administration of DuP 753, a specific angiotensin II receptor anatgonist, to normal male volunteers; inhibition of pressor response to exogenous angiotensin I and II. Circulation 83:1333—1342
2. Dzau VJ (1990) Mechanism of action of angiotensin — converting inhibitors in hypertension and heart failure. Role of plasma versus tissue ACE. Drugs 39, suppl 2
3. Dzau VJ, Gibbons GH (1991) The role of the endothelium in vascular remodeling. In: Cardiovascular Significance of Endothelium-Derived Vasoactive Factors. Rubanyi GM (ed) New York: Futura Publishing, pp. 281—291
4. Dzau VJ (1988) The tissue renin-angiotensin-system: implications for angiotensin converting enzyme inhibition. Curr. Opinion Cardiol. 3, suppl 1, 97—102
5. Grobecker H, Ploetz H (1992) Effect of ACE-inhibitor quinapril on blood pressure and glucose disposition in diabetic spontaneously hypertensive rats (SHR). J of Hypertension 10, suppl 4, S100
6. Johnston CJ (1992) Tissue ACE-inhibition — Clinical Implications: in Focus on ACE-Inhibition: Implications for cardiovascular Structure and Function: Reaven Health Care Communications; Division of Raven Press Ltd.; New York
7. Tigerstedt R, Bergman PG (1897) Niere und Kreislauf. Skand. Arch. Physiol. 8, 223
8. Wong PC, Price WA, Chiu AT, Carini DJ, Duncia JV, Johnson AL, Wexler RR, Timmermans PBMWM (1990) Nonpeptide angiotensin II receptor antagonists: studies with EXP 9270 and DuP 753. Hypertension 15:823—834
9. Yamada H, Fabris B, Allen AM, Jackson B, Johnston CI, Mendelsohn FAO (1991) Localisation of angiotensin converting enzyme in the rat heart. Circ Res 68:141—149

Author's address:
Prof. Dr. med. H. Grobecker
Institut für Pharmakologie
der Universität Regensburg
Universitätsstr. 31
8400 Regensburg

Summary and perspective
B. Clinical aspects

B. E. Strauer

Abteilung für Kardiologie, Pneumologie,
Med. Klinik und Poliklinik B der Heinrich-Heine-Universität Düsseldorf

Perspectives in clinical research: Angiotensin, ACE inhibition, Tissue ACE

1) Arterial hypertension, the increase in systolic wall stress and left ventricular hypertrophy (LVH) per se may be associated with increased concentrations of tissue ACE. The final trigger mechanisms are unknown. Hypothesis: the initiating factor represents the increase in systolic wall stress. Therefore, comparative studies are needed in hypertensive hypertrophy without and with increased systolic wall stress to determine regional tissue ACE concentrations. Different patient groups are necessary:

   — hypertensive hypertrophy with normal wall stress (= appropriate hypertrophy)
   — hypertensive hypertrophy with low wall stress (= irregular, inappropriate hypertrophy)
   — hypertensive hypertrophy with high wall stress (= inappropriate, dilated hypertrophy).

   One of the main problems in these studies is the availability of analytic methods to analyze and quantitatively to determine tissue ACE from human myocardial biopsy specimens.

2) Normotensive hypertrophy, as in hypertrophic cardiomyopathy, may or may not have altered tissue ACE levels. Angiotension and ACE concentrations may modulate LVH by trophic influence. Conservative therapy in hypertrophic cardiomyopathy is considerably limited. Thus, the use of ACE inhibitors in hypertrophic cardiomyopathy could be of invaluable clinical-therapeutical significance, provided that tissue ACE concentrations are increased in these diseases and that by the therapeutical ACE inhibition both, reduction of ACE levels and regression of LVH occur. Again, myocardial biopsy studies are required to determine:

   — degree of LVH (myocyte hypertrophy)
   — interstitial fibrosis (plus collagen content)
   — tissue ACE and angiotensin concentrations.

3) The reasons for the transition from (clinically compensated) concentric (or irregular) LVH to (clinically decompensated) eccentric LVH are unknown. Trophic factors, e.g., an increase in the tissue activities of the renin-angiotensin system and in ACE levels may play a role. Coronary microangiopathy, abnormal protein synthesis, modulation of the ADP/ATP-carrier, immunological (self-perpetuating) mechanisms and many others may be important. If the ACE system and related hormonal activities are of trophic influence, then ACE inhibition could be beneficial in these diseases. Again, tissue analyses of angiotensin and/or of the

ACE by human myocardial biopsies studies are necessary in the three crucial functional states of the human left ventricle: in the normal heart, in LVH, and in the dilated and failing heart.

4) The importance of coronary microangiopathy for both coronary hemodynamics and for left ventricular function has recently been developed and investigated by the Düsseldorf group. Depressed coronary reserve, media and adventitia hypertrophy (resistance vessel), myocyte hypertrophy, and increased amount of "small scars" and an increased collagen content have been demonstrated for hypertensive hypertrophy. Moreover, the reversibility of these abnormal changes by long-term ACE-inhibition has been shown. Thus, the existence of small vessel involvement in hypertensive LVH, their influence on myocardial structure and ventricular function (diastolic, systolic) and its functional reversal by ACE inhibition is proven. Two of the final pathophysiological and clinical points are open! Can ACE inhibition also reverse media hypertrophy and the myocyte as well as the changes in interstitial fibrosis and collagen augmentation? And can ACE inhibition therefore contribute to the prevention of late cardiac failure in hypertensive hypertrophy? Again, myocardial biopsy studies are required in hypertensive patients to resolve these problems of marked therapeutical relevance, here with the aim of quantitative determinations of the structural myocardial and coronary vascular changes in the progression and regression of hypertensive heart disease.

5) The problem of re-stenosis following coronary angioplasty (PTCA) is of considerable clinical importance. Many attempts in the recent past have been made, and many therapeutical observations have been reported in both experimental models and in clinical studies. Low molecular heparine, Ca-channel blocking agents, nitrates, spasmolytic agents (cicletanine, magnesium etc.), glucocorticoids, cytostatics and others have been tried. Mercator I was designed to prove the effectiveness of ACE inhibition on the re-stenosis rate after PTCA. This study failed. However, negative results are also important and sometimes encouraging. Thus, Mercator follow-up studies are in preparation using different dosages and application forms. Nevertheless, the beneficial use and influence of ACE inhibition in the invasive management of acute myocardial infarction (AMI) by PTCA has not yet been evaluated. If the EDRF-hypothesis is valid, then the additive use of ACE-inhibition in AMI in conjunction with invasive measures could be effective.

6) Myocardial imaging by Tl-scintigraphy, by SPECT-techniques and by PET has demonstrated inhomogenous myocardial perfusion ("speckled type") in myocardial hypertrophy due to hypertension and to other forms of LV hypertrophy. Except for myocardial hypertrophy, the involvement of small coronary resistance vessels may modify the perfusion of the hypertrophied myocardium. ACE inhibition could be appropriate to improve myocardial perfusion by its EDRF enhancement, by the regression of LVH and of interstitial fibrosis, and by the regression of media hypertrophy and of adventitia fibrosis, thus improving the overall and the local oxygen availability to the myocardium. Comparative studies in patient groups with normotensive (hypertrophic cardiomyopathy, dilated, cardiomyopathy, aortic stenosis, and aortic incompetence) as well as with hypertensive hypertrophy are needed to determine the possible influence of ACE inhibition on regional myocardial perfusion.

7) Hypertrophic heart disease (normotensive, hypertensive) represents a significant risk factor for both malignant rhythm disturbances and sudden cardiac death. This arrhythmogenicprone feature of hypertrophic heart disease may be referred to an increased arrhythmogenic potential of the hypertrophied myocardial muscle cell as well as to primary non-myocyte structured changes (interstitial fibrosis, scars, coronary microangiopathy). ACE inhibition could contribute to the reversal of the inherent structural changes. Thus, rhythmological studies by the analysis of late potentials, of heart rate variability, of ST-monitoring and, if clinically indicated, by programmed ventricular (right) stimulation are desirable.

8) The natural history of coronary artery disease as well as the progression of coronary artherosclerosis are dependent on multiple risk factors of the cardiovascular system. Pharmacotherapeutical interventions have to be specifically considered with regard to their possible (and desired) influence on i) the coronary arteries and the plaque formation or plaque regression respectively, ii) the progression of left ventricular dysfunction and its improvement by inotropic or unloading measures. Many studies and trials (Consensus, Save, etc.) have shown beneficial effects of ACE inhibition on the outcome of coronary patients after AMI. Here, however, strict differentiation is necessary to separate possible and desired effects on the process of coronary artherosclerosis (which is completely unknown) from the unloading (= passive) effects on the left ventricle (which may be beneficial in coronary heart disease.). In my opinion, a normally or almost sufficiently contracting left ventricle with coronary artery disease will not profit from ACE inhibition, whereas the same coronary condition in a dilated and compromised heart may attain better ventricular function. Therefore, future trials concerning this problem should focus more precisely (concomitant to coronary artery disease) on the problem of left ventricular function.

9) Except for systolic left ventricular function (or dysfunction) diastolic dysfunction develops parallel to myocardial hypertrophy due to arterial hypertension (hypertensive heart disease). This is not neccassarily relevant for the same amount of LVH in aortic stenosis, in aortic incompetence or in other forms of LVH (congenital and aquired heart disease). Therefore, the diastolic properties of the hypertrophied left ventricular myocardium depend not only on myocyte hypertrophy, but also on non-myocyte factors. Interstitial fibrosis, as has been demonstrated by the Missouri and the Düsseldorf groups may play a crucial role. Hypertensive hypertrophy — in contrast to non-hypertensive hypertrophy (as, for example, in aortic stenosis) is associated with marked interstitial fibrosis and myocardial collagen content. ACE inhibition may profoundly reverse the fibrotic structure of the left ventricle in hypertensive heart disease. An improvement of diastolic dysfunction can therefore be expected. Future studies should focus more precisely on the diastolic properties of the left ventricle in LVH in order to differentiate systolic from diastolic dysfunction in hypertrophic heart disease.

10) Beta receptor blocking agents have been proven a safe therapy after myocardial infarction. Mortality may be reduced by 10—20% 1 year following the acute event. ACE inhibitors may possibly contribute to decreased mortality in the long-term therapy after AMI. The question should be raised of whether both drugs are potent enough to more significantly reduce AMI late mortality than either of the monotherapy interventions. Is there a more profound benefit from ACE inhibitors

than from a beta-receptor-blocking agent? This problem has to be considered in future studies of survival after AMI.

11) Granulocytes may be aggressive for the cardiovascular vessel system, especially when there are eosinophilic components. The anti-granulocytic influence of ACE inhibition has been discussed. If relevant, positive clinical-therapeutical interactions may be present in clinical heart disease associated with myocarditis, vasculitis or both.

12) One last point, possibly relevant for future, long-term trials, refers to the discussed antiatherosclerotic effects of ACE inhibitors. Clinical sonographic and angiographic observations (peripheral arteries, coronary arteries) could help to contribute to the outcome of this question. Atherectomy specimens with adequate analyses of endothelial cells, of smooth musculature and of collagen content, as well as vascular responsiveness tests (e.g., with acetylcholine) and blood flow reserve determinations are important.

Author's address:
Med. Klinik und Poliklinik B
der Heinrich-Heine-Universität
Abt. für Kardiologie, Pneumologie
Moorenstr. 5
4000 Düsseldorf 1

Subject Index

α-, β-myosin heavy chain 65
α-adrenoceptors 25
ACE-inhibitors 25, 43
acute myocardial infarction 43
aldosterone 107
angiotensin 25
angiotensin II 1, 107
angiotensin-converting enzyme 1
angiotensin-converting enzyme inhibitors 155
arterial hypertension 43

β-adrenergic receptor blockade 81
bradykinin 15

captopril 155, 203
cardiac angiotensin formation 183
cardiac development and hypertrophy 65
cardiocyte Ca^{++}-homeostais 183
cardiocyte dedifferentiation 183
collagen 107
congestive heart failure 43
coronary artery disease 43
coronary artery occlusion 139
coronary artery reperfusion 139
coronary circulation 81
coronary microcirculation 97
coronary reserve 25
coronary vasomotor tone 25
creatine kinase 139

enalapril 155, 203
endothelial function 183
endothelin 15

gene regulation 65
gene transfer 65
growth factors 1

heart failure 203
hypertensive hypertrophy 97

in vitro and in vivo gene regulation 65
inhibitors 1

L-arginine 15
left ventricular dysfunction 125
left ventricular function 203
left ventricular hypertrophy 107

mineralocorticoids 107
myocardial and coronary reparation 97
myocardial contractile function 139
myocardial hypertrophy 81, 183
myocardial infarction 1, 125
myocardial infarct size 139
myocardial ischemia 25, 81

nitric oxide 15

postischemic myocardial dysfunction 155
prostaglandins 15

regional wall thickening 81
remodeling 125
reperfusion arrhythmias 155
reperfusion injury 155
repression of hypertrophy 97

sarcoplasmic reticulum Ca^{++}-ATPase 183
survival 203

thyroid hormones 65
transcription factors 65
transmural blood flow 81
transmural function 81

vascular hypertrophy 1

zofenopril 155

Batch number: 10577969

Printed by Printforce, the Netherlands